€MT
manual

Michael K. Copass, M.D.

Professor, Department of Medicine
School of Medicine, University of Washington
Director, Emergency Trauma Center
Harborview Medical Center
Director, Seattle Fire Department Medic One
Seattle, Washington

Louis Gonzales, B.S., Paramedic

King County Medic One
Emergency Medical Services Division, Seattle-King County
Department of Public Health, Seattle, Washington
Early Defibrillation Program Coordinator
Emergency Medical Services Division, Seattle-King County
Department of Public Health, Seattle, Washington

Mickey S. Eisenberg, M.D., Ph.D.

Professor, Department of Medicine
School of Medicine, University of Washington
Director, Emergency Medicine Service
University of Washington Medical Center
Co-Director, Center for Evaluation of Emergency Medical Services
Emergency Medical Services Division, Seattle-King County
Department of Public Health, Seattle, Washington

Roy G. Soper, Paramedic

Medical Services Officer
King County Medic One
Emergency Medical Services Division, Seattle-King County
Department of Public Health, Seattle, Washington

THIRD EDITION

EMT
manual

W. B. SAUNDERS COMPANY
A Division of Harcourt Brace & Company
Philadelphia, London, Toronto, Montreal, Sydney, Tokyo

W. B. SAUNDERS COMPANY
A Division of Harcourt Brace & Company

The Curtis Center
Independence Square West
Philadelphia, Pennsylvania 19106

Library of Congress Cataloging-in-Publication Data

EMT manual / Michael K. Copass . . . [et al.]. — 3rd ed.
    p.   cm.
    Rev. ed. of: EMT manual / Michael K. Copass, Roy G. Soper, Mickey
S. Eisenberg. 2nd ed. 1991.
    Includes index.
    ISBN 0–7216–6965–4
    1. Emergency medicine—Handbooks, manuals, etc.   I. Copass,
Michael K.
    [DNLM: 1. Emergencies handbooks.   2. Emergency Medical
Technicians handbooks. WB 39 E555 1998]
    RC86.8.C66   1998
    616.02′5–dc21
    DNLM/DLC   97-47600

EMT MANUAL   ISBN 0–7216–6965–4

Printed in the United States of America.

Last digit is the print number: 9   8   7   6   5   4   3   2   1

On a personal note, I wish to thank my wife, Marianne, and my children for their patience and support during the creation of this third edition.

Louis Gonzales

Preface

Emergency medical technicians (EMTs) face one of the most challenging jobs in the world of medical care. They must care for patients in living rooms, in shopping centers, and on streets, and they must perform their medical evaluations without benefit of laboratory tests or radiographs. On the basis of less than adequate information in less than ideal and safe physical surroundings, they must make critical decisions and initiate treatment. The purpose of this book is to assist EMTs in their difficult task.

This third edition of the *EMT Manual* has been updated to be consistent with the current National Standard EMT-Basic curriculum. The information contained in this book should be considered enrichment material for the core EMT-Basic curriculum. This information can be used by the EMT seeking to gain additional knowledge and to review patient assessment skills. This book should also be utilized as a convenient source of useful emergency medical information. It is meant to be carried in the pocket (or with other references in an emergency vehicle). It can also be referred to when some question arises about the recognition or management of a patient's condition. This will probably not occur during active emergency patient care; rather, this book will be most useful after an emergency call as a review, or it may be used while responding to a call (assuming all eyes are not needed to monitor traffic flow). When early patient information indicates the possibility of an assessment challenge, the EMT may wish to refer to this manual. These challenges often occur in patients who present with problems or complaints that are not frequently seen. If this manual is useful in these settings, then it has accomplished its purpose.

The EMT instructor/educator may also find this book useful as an adjunct to course textbooks, or as an aid for continuing education classes. The design of this manual is such that the student will find here all the essential information about EMT emergency medical care. However, this book cannot serve as a replacement for a textbook. We have intentionally not included physiology or detailed anatomy. Our goal was to keep the material concise, specific, and immediately relevant. In essence, this is a reference manual for the practicing EMT as well as the EMT educator.

Some recommendations for therapy in this book may not agree with local protocol. The authors would like to stress that the EMT should always follow local guidelines, protocols, and medical control directives.

We hope this book helps in the task of providing good emergency care.

Acknowledgments

We thank the EMTs, firefighters, and paramedics of Seattle and King County for their continued professionalism and commitment to excellent patient care. As experienced professionals, they have taught us much. We in turn have tried to pass this knowledge on to new EMT students as well as experienced professional EMTs. We also are thankful to the many physician, paramedic, and EMT educators who satisfy a quest for knowledge in EMT students.

We are especially grateful to Leonard Cobb, M.D., for his tremendous contributions to emergency medical services. His vision and diligence have had a positive impact on EMS providers throughout the world.

We also wish to thank the King County Emergency Medical Services Division for sharing their valuable prehospital experiences, and Physio Control Corporation for their assistance in the development of Appendix I.

Artwork was provided by Dinah Stone, who worked closely with us to get the illustrations "just right." We are also appreciative of the continual editorial support offered by Selma Kaszczuk and Rachael Kelly.

Contents

Section IV
Procedures and Medical Equipment

SECTION I

PATIENT CARE: SKILLS AND PRINCIPLES

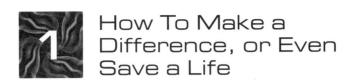

How To Make a Difference, or Even Save a Life

■ AN EMT's PROFESSIONAL ATTITUDE

The attitude you, as an EMT, bring to your performance directly affects your patient's care.

- EMTs must have a strong desire to help people. EMTs do this by providing the best care and comfort possible.
- Concern for a patient's needs must be the EMT's first and foremost priority. All personal feelings and prejudices must be set aside. Focus on the patient's well-being.
- An EMT must act professionally at all times. Disagreements with coworkers should be settled after the patient is treated. Legal problems can be prevented through careful delivery of service within the scope of your training and medical direction.
- An effective EMT is a team player. Take full advantage of all available assistance, using coworkers, family members, and bystanders as part of your team.
- An EMT works safely and avoids unnecessary risks. Injury to yourself, coworkers, or bystanders only adds to the overall problem and requires additional resources.
- An EMT must be prepared. Regular checks and maintenance of equipment are essential. The EMT must take to the patient's side any equipment that may be needed to immediately manage the acutely ill patient (airways, suction unit, ventilation devices, patient assessment tools, defibrillator, and personal protective equipment).

These superior EMT attitudes are demonstrated in the following ways:

Contact.   Maintain eye-level contact. Make physical contact with the patient quickly. Palpating the radial pulse is helpful for early assessment of the patient and also provides a nonthreatening impression that treatment has begun.

Confidence.   Conduct the interrogation and physical exam systematically. This indicates to the patient that a specific purpose is in mind. It builds patient confidence in your EMT abilities and knowledge.

Curiosity.   Learn as much about the patient's problem as you can. Look around the scene for further clues about what has occurred. You are the eyes and ears of the rest of the EMS team, who will not have as accurate a view of the situation. Ask, don't assume: "Why did you call?" "Why do you take this medicine?" "Where do you hurt?"

Compassion. Be soothing and empathetic. Warn the patient before doing anything that will cause pain or anxiety, particularly before exposing skin. Protect the patient's modesty from curious onlookers. Talk to all patients, even those who are unconscious, as if they can hear you.

Common Sense. Be flexible. Be able to make rapid adjustments in assessment and management based upon minute-to-minute changes in the patient's status and the setting. Take several sets of vital signs to monitor changes in the patient's condition.

■ Applying Your Knowledge: Recognizing the Acutely Ill Patient

The most important EMT skill is the ability to distinguish an acutely ill patient from one who is not (rapid patient assessment). In some instances, the difference will be obvious. Other cases are more difficult. Experience and intuition (clinical judgment) will help you make this distinction.

Take a quick but careful look at the patient, and form a **general impression**.

- Does the **environment pose a risk** to the patient or the EMS team?
- What is the patient's **appearance**? (Awake, alert? Eye contact? Motor function? Color?)
- How hard is the patient **working to breathe**? (Airway open? Ventilations effective?)
- What are the **pulse and skin** like? (Radial pulse present? Skin temperature, color and texture? Capillary refill time?)

The number one question on your mind as you approach the patient is:

"How sick (or injured) is this person?"

Tables 1–1 and 1–2 present two guides to recognizing acutely ill patients. Table 1–1 utilizes the EMT's general observations to identify the acutely ill patient, while Table 1–2 uses the EMT's initial assessment. People who meet these acute illness criteria often need rapid transport to a hospital, advanced life support, or consultation with a base station physician.

■ An EMT's Skills and Scope of Practice: The Team Concept

An EMT does not practice emergency treatment in a vacuum. You act as a member of an emergency medical services (EMS) system.

Table 1-1 General Observations of the Acutely Ill Patient

Posture	Slumped or leaning forward
	Leaning to one side
	Tripod position
Level of consciousness	Unresponsive
	Responds only to painful stimuli
	Responds to verbal stimuli
	Disoriented
Symmetry	Face or mouth sagging
	Eyelid drooping
	Arm(s) and/or leg(s) hanging limp
Speech	Slurred
	Garbled
	Absent
	Rapid
	Short phrases
Eyes	Lackluster
	Roving
	Deviated to one side
Skin color	Pale or chalk white
	Ashen gray
	Cyanotic (blue)
	Red (flushed, cherry color)
	Yellow (jaundiced)
Skin texture	Moist or wet
	Dry (loss of turgor)
	Hot
	Cold
Pupils	Dilated
	Constricted
	Unequal
	Unreactive
Motor function	Stiff neck
	Cannot move
	Can only move one side of body
Initial vital signs	
Respirations	Rapid (>30/min)
	Slow (<12/min)
	Absent
	Labored
	Noisy
	Irregular with periods of apnea
Pulse	Rapid (>120/min)
	Slow (<55/min)
	Absent
	Thready
	Irregular
Blood pressure	<90 mm Hg systolic
	>180 mm Hg systolic
	>120 mm Hg diastolic
	Postural hypotension

Table 1-2	**Recognizing the Acutely Ill Patient by Initial Assessment**

Acute illness is present in the patient

- With a poor general appearance
- Unresponsive or with an altered mental status (disoriented and/or unable to follow commands)
- Unable to maintain an open airway and/or spontaneous breathing without assistance
- Not breathing
- With difficult or ineffective breathing
- With an absent carotid pulse
- With cardiac arrest not responding to therapy
- Who is in the postresuscitation period
- With seizure activity that does not stop
- With evidence of shock (hypoperfusion)
- Who has had a near-drowning event
- With significant trauma, including burns and electrical injuries
- With blood loss in large volumes
- With an extremely high or low body temperature
- Experiencing a severe allergic reaction
- Experiencing chest pain of possible cardiac origin
- With severe pain originating from any part of the body
- Who is pregnant with impending delivery (especially if complications are suspected)
- Who has ingested poisons, including an overdose of medicines or recreational drugs

EMTs are not usually the first contact with the EMS system during an emergency. Someone had to recognize a problem and call the EMS system. Often an emergency medical dispatcher (EMD) has taken the call for help and may be assisting bystanders with prearrival instructions, or extracting vital information. EMTs usually will receive a short report from the EMD providing information about the emergency in progress.

A team of two EMTs per patient provides optimal care with a minimum of confusion. Additional resources may be called upon, if necessary. One of the two EMTs in the team is in charge to provide leadership and avoid confusion. An understanding of who will assume the position of the EMT in charge must be established before the team arrives at the scene. The EMT in charge is also responsible for overall patient management at the scene. He/she is responsible for the patient write-up; he/she must *never* leave the task of writing the report to an EMT not involved in the actual interrogation and

Table 1–3   EMT Team Concept: Division of Patient Care Responsibilities

EMT in Charge of Patient	EMT Partner	Additional EMTs/Responders
Assess ABCDs	Obtain vital signs (every 5–10 minutes): blood pressure, pulse, respiratory rate	Assist with CPR team
Assess level of consciousness		Assist with management of ABCDs
Conduct patient assessment		Assist with treatment as directed
Perform physical examination		Runner for equipment
Determine course of treatment	Administer oxygen	Assist with other patient(s) as directed
Complete reports (written and verbal)	Assist with treatment as directed	
Determine method of transportation	Attach ECG monitor (if available)	
Function as medical group supervisor (multiple patient incidents)	Interrogate family/witnesses	
	Obtain patient's medicine list	
	Triage (multiple patient incidents)	

physical examination of the patient. Table 1–3 outlines the division of responsibilities among the initial EMS responders.

Management includes establishment of a resource pool (often referred to as staging), traffic control, extrication, additional equipment, support of EMTs, and incoming transportation. These duties are to be assumed until a more senior responsible person arrives at the scene. In situations involving several patients, the EMT in charge of the patients should now be responsible for all medical issues (often referred to as the medical group supervisor). The EMT in charge is the last person to assume responsibility for treating a particular patient when sufficient resources are available. It is essential that the EMT in charge maintain close communication with the senior officer at the scene (usually referred to as the incident commander, or IC). The second EMT is now responsible for patient triage (usually referred to as the triage officer). Chapter 2 provides additional details on multiple patient incidents.

■ Role of Other EMS Team Members

The following summaries describe the roles played by other members of the EMS team.

EMDs-Dispatchers

- Obtain critical information about a call for help
- Decide on the response level and required resources
- Provide prearrival instructions to bystanders or the patient
- Provide EMTs with a short report about the situation, including:
  - Age and sex
  - Chief complaint
  - EMS response level and other agencies responding
  - Injuries and/or symptoms described by the caller
  - Significant medical history (if relevant)
- Act as a communication link by relaying information or contacting other resources

Bystanders

- May offer assistance if they have not already done so prior to the arrival of the EMS team
- May be used to perform simple prearrival care such as cardiopulmonary resuscitation (CPR) and bleeding control
- Can provide information about the events prior to the emergency and prior to the arrival of the EMS team
- May have personal knowledge of the patient's medical condition and history
- May be upset and actually be in need of care themselves when the emergency is over
- Should be used by the EMS team as much as possible

First Responders

- May be the first professional responder at an emergency scene
- May be police officers, firefighters, school teachers, security officers, or any other person with some training in first aid, CPR, or emergency medical care
- Sometimes have received specialized training, including basic cardiac life support and initial care of illnesses and injuries (training usually consists of about 40 hours as outlined by the U.S. Department of Transportation)
- In some locations, may also be trained to provide automated external defibrillation
- Provide reports that can give you valuable information about the emergency and the patient's condition before your arrival

Advanced Life Support Providers (Paramedics)

- May perform advanced interventions in prehospital emergency care
- Take command of patient care from the EMT after receiving a short report

- Will need the EMT to continue basic life support and other assistance as necessary
- Have a scope of practice that varies with the standards of each community and service provider, but typically includes starting intravenous lines, insertion of advanced airway protection devices, chest decompression, emergency drug administration, electrocardiogram (ECG) interpretation, obtaining a 12-lead ECG, and defibrillator operation
- Will need the EMT's report and assessment findings as soon as possible
- Make decisions regarding mode and destination of transport
- Request assistance from EMTs in carrying out these procedures

In some communities, specific advanced life support procedures may be provided by EMTs or intermediate EMTs.

Physician Medical Director (PMD)

- Establish an expected standard of practice for EMTs within an EMS system
- Provide EMTs with standing orders and/or protocols that guide the EMT's patient care practices
- May assist in training EMTs to provide care according to these standards
- Ensure the EMT knows and follows the system's standing orders and protocols
- Encourage the EMT to continue his/her education with each patient contact and training session
- Work with the EMT to provide the best out-of-hospital care the community can offer
- May be available (or appoint a designee) by telephone or radio to provide online advice for difficult decisions or advanced emergency care
- Review the performance of the EMT and the overall system as part of an ongoing quality improvement program

Quality Improvement (QI) Team

- Oversees the review of all aspects of EMS operations to assure the highest quality of care is being provided
- Focuses on ensuring that the EMS system's objectives are being met
- Attempts to identify which system objectives are not being met, reasons this may be occurring, methods to improve performance, improvement implementation plans, and methods for continued measurement and review

The QI program may address clinical and operation issues such as

- Documentation reviews
- Case reviews
- Clinical assessments and decision making
- Physician, nurse, and patient feedback
- Continuing education
- Maintenance and failure rates of supplies and equipment
- Skills maintenance
- Response times

- Directly observed patient contact, assessment, and treatment skills
- EMT injuries, exposures, and accidents

EMTs often hold informal QI sessions with their partners following an EMS response in order to identify ways of making the next call more effective.

2 Patient Assessment

An understanding of the patient's mental and physical condition requires the EMT to use the senses of sight, smell, hearing, touch, and (possibly) taste. These senses are used to accumulate a history and to understand the patient's symptoms (what the patient, family, and witnesses told you in their own words about the patient's current problem) and signs (what you find out about the patient through examination). As stated in Chapter 1, EMTs must be able to recognize the acutely ill patient. They must also be able to identify those patients who have the potential for becoming acutely ill.

Keep in mind that the patient assessment will require the EMT to ask questions and perform an examination that may make the patient feel very uncomfortable. Before beginning the patient examination, consider these hints regarding the patient interview and contact process.

1. You are a visitor to this patient's home.
   - Treat the patient's home with respect.
   - Unless there is a life-threatening emergency, avoid causing damage to or soiling the patient's home.
   - Knock before entering. This also serves as a protective measure for the EMT.

2. You are a stranger when you first meet the patient.
   - Polite introductions are always in order.
   - Use terms of respect such as Sir, Ma'am, Mr. Smith, or Miss Jones. Ask permission to address the patient by first name unless they introduce themselves by their first name.
   - Avoid terms of endearment such as "honey," "sweetie," or "sweetheart." Many people will find this disrespectful.

3. Maintain eye contact. Keep an appropriate distance to allow time for the patient to become comfortable with you (particularly with children).

4. Gain the patient's confidence by acting, speaking, and appearing professionally.
   - Use appropriate language. Vulgar or demeaning language can quickly change the patient's impression of the EMT.
   - Speak in terms the patient can understand.
   - Explain the examination and your actions as you proceed.

A systematic approach to the patient assessment and examination will assist the EMT in identifying the acutely ill patient. The EMT must consider three components of assessment: inspection, interrogation, and palpation. (*Note:* Although auscultation is considered another component of assessment, this component is limited to blood pressures and lung sounds in the EMT's assessment.)

■ Patient Examination

Inspection

Make a rapid visual inspection of the patient's surroundings (medicine bottles nearby, home oxygen or nebulizer), mechanism of injury, general posture, and physical state. Quickly identify potential hazards to the patient and to the EMS providers.

- Does the patient look and act sick (pale, diaphoretic, anxious, agitated, in pain)?
- Is the patient's mental state appropriate considering the circumstances?
- Are there any obvious abnormal signs, particularly signs of respiratory distress (gasping for breath)?

Observe the reactions of the friends and family members to the patient's condition.

Interrogation

Trauma Questions

Trauma patients sustain injury from accidents that are unexpected, and these patients can be approached in a straightforward manner. It is particularly appropriate to inquire directly about areas of pain or discomfort with a trauma patient. Quickly introduce yourself and explain what you are about to do.

1. Do you have any difficulty breathing? Are you comfortable with the way you are breathing?
2. Do you hurt anywhere? (Have the patient point to the affected area.)
3. What happened? Include questions about patient protection (seat belts, helmets), weapons involved (gun caliber, knife size and shape), height of fall, or voltage/current of electrical device.
4. Do you have any current medical problems? Are you being treated by a doctor for anything?
5. Are you taking any medications? Any taken today?
6. Are you allergic to any medications?

Medical Questions

Patients should be made to describe their complaints in their own words without much prompting or leading questions. Begin with open-ended questions (e.g., "What is the problem?"). Then add closed or specific questions (e.g., "Exactly where is this pain in your chest?").

1. What is the problem? (Interrupt only to keep the patient discussing the current problem. However, the EMT must keep the patient focused on those problems that may require immediate or urgent treatment.)

2. When did it begin?
3. What were you doing when it began? How did it begin?
4. Did this ever happen to you before? If so, what was done to alleviate this problem?
5. Does anything make it better or worse?
6. Do you take medications for this problem? Have you taken any today?
7. Do you have any other current medical problems? Are you being treated by a doctor for anything?
8. Do you take any other medications?

If the complaint is about pain, have the patient point to the affected area and describe the nature of the pain (i.e., sharp, dull, cramping, pressure, steady, intermittent).

Palpation

■ Determine general skin conditions (temperature, moisture); Check capillary refilling by compressing fingernail.

■ Use gentle but firm pressure, starting at areas distant from reported pain and moving slowly toward the painful area. Note pain response to palpation.

■ In the trauma patient, touch every accessible bone and every joint.

■ Use your stethoscope as an additional device for palpating to confirm questionable areas of tenderness. The patient's reaction to the pressure of the stethoscope should be the same as to the pressure of your hand.

■ INITIAL PATIENT ASSESSMENT

The primary, basic function of all persons involved in emergency medical care is the rapid assessment, management, and reassessment of a patient's ABCDs: airway, breathing, circulation, and disability/defibrillation.

The EMT has the added responsibility to perform a rapid assessment of the scene to determine (1) environmental dangers, (2) the number of patients to be treated, (3) the mechanism of injury, (4) additional resources required, and (5) the problems of immediate extrication or patient access. In serious illness or trauma, aggressive management of major ABCD problems is vital. This places particular importance on the rapid extrication of the trapped or entangled patient by people trained to perform such activities. The patient will die if these primary functions are neglected or managed carelessly.

A = Airway

■ *Is it open?* Check for the movement of air: look to see if the chest rises; listen for airflow; feel the chest wall for movement and crepitus; check for a stoma.

■ *Is the patient positioned properly?* Use the head tilt and chin lift method to open the airway. Use the jaw thrust or chin lift methods for face or suspected neck trauma (maintaining in-line cervical stabilization). Ensure that the child's occiput is not causing airway closure due to neck flexion.

■ *Are respirations noisy, gurgling, or labored?* Visually check for partial obstruction, fluids, frothy sputum, excess salivation (drooling).

■ *Is the airway obstructed?* Look for inspiratory retractions at supraclavicular and intercostal spaces, and diaphragmatic movement only without airflow. If a complete obstruction is suspected, immediately begin procedures for the removal of foreign body obstructions.

B = Breathing

■ *Is the patient breathing?* If not, ventilate using the mouth-to-mask method until a bag-valve mask (or other manual ventilating device) is available. Add oxygen supply to the bag-valve mask as soon as possible. Also, assist ventilations if the patient states he/she has difficulty breathing or appears to be too exhausted to continue his/her spontaneous respiratory drive. Does the patient have a lingering cough and/or other signs of possible tuberculosis? If so, immediately consider implementing appropriate protective measures.

■ *What is the depth of respirations?* Inspect chest movement. Are respirations very shallow? Are the respirations deep but very slow? Are the respirations agonal? Begin assisting the patient's ventilations as necessary with a bag-valve mask (or other manual ventilating device) using 100% oxygen supply.

■ *Are there gasping respirations?* Palpate, observe, and listen for a flail chest or sucking chest wound. Place an occlusive dressing over the sucking chest wound. Immediately treat with high-flow oxygen or assist ventilations with a bag-valve mask (or other manual ventilating device) using 100% oxygen supply.

■ *What is the respiratory rate?* Rates less than 12/min should be assisted using a bag-valve mask (or other manual ventilating device) connected to a 100% oxygen supply. Rates greater than 30/min may indicate respiratory distress. Immediately treat with high-flow oxygen.

■ *Are there unusual respiratory patterns?* Observe the respiratory pattern. Cerebral insults and certain metabolic abnormalities may produce specific patterns that should be documented.

C = Circulation

■ *Is there a palpable pulse?* Check carotid pulses; if there are none and the patient is unconscious, begin CPR. Use the femoral pulse to assess circulation during CPR.

■ *Is the pulse rate less than 55/min or greater than 120/min?* Check for signs of inadequate perfusion. If one is available and you are trained to operate it, attach an ECG monitor in order to record the ECG rhythm. Provide the recording to the advanced life support responders or the receiving hospital.

■ *Is the pulse irregular?* Compare apical and radial pulses for discrepancy, then check irregularities with an ECG monitor, if one is available (and you are trained to use it). Document discrepancies.

■ *Is there visible external hemorrhage?* Control external bleeding. Keep the patient calm and supine (or semireclined) if at all possible. In the acutely ill patient, focus first on severe external hemorrhage. Control minor bleeding when time and resources allow.

■ *Is there suspected internal bleeding?* Begin treatment for shock. Reassess the patient frequently. Consider rapid transport to an appropriate hospital or to a meeting point with advanced life support personnel.

D = Disability (or Defibrillation in Cardiac Arrest)

Level of Consciousness

In addition to the assessment of the ABCs, it is necessary to make an initial assessment of the patient's level of consciousness. A quick assessment can be performed by determining the Glasgow Coma Scale score (see Appendix F). Other measures of neurologic status include state of mind, responsiveness, and pupillary condition.

STATE OF MIND

■ Is the patient oriented? Does the patient know who he/she is, where he/she is, the approximate time of day, and the circumstances of the event.

■ To what degree is the patient oriented?

RESPONSIVENESS

■ *Alert:* completely awake, acting appropriately, and aware of surroundings
■ *Lethargic:* sleepy, but aware of surroundings
■ *Stuporous:* will awaken to verbal stimuli, prefers to remain asleep
■ *Obtunded:* will awaken to painful stimuli only
■ *Comatose:* nothing will awaken patient, does not respond to painful or verbal stimuli, has no gag reflex

Note: Medical terms such as "stuporous" or "obtunded" can be imprecise, meaning different things to different people, even within the medical community. An alternative approach that characterizes levels of consciousness on the basis of response is often referred to using the mnemonic "AVPU":

■ *Alert:* completely awake, acting appropriately, and aware of surroundings
■ Responsive to *verbal* stimuli: awakens only when spoken to
■ Responsive to *painful* stimuli: awakens only when ears are pinched or other pain stimulus is applied
■ *Unresponsive:* does not awaken to any stimulus

PUPILLARY CONDITION

What is the pupillary response to bright light? Do the pupils constrict? Are the pupils constricted or dilated initially? Check for a deviated gaze. Are the eyes deviated to one side? Check pupillary size. Are the pupils equal in size?

Chronic Illness

If the patient is conscious, inquire about chronic illnesses, current medications, and allergies. If the patient is unconscious, check for a medical alert wallet card, bracelet, or necklace. Knowing the patient's medication names may provide clues to his/her medical conditions.

Defibrillation in Cardiac Arrest

In the sudden cardiac arrest patient, the EMT should think of *defibrillation* immediately after assessing the ABCs and initiating CPR. The patient who experiences sudden death has at least a 50% probability of having ventricular fibrillation as his/her initial terminating rhythm. Because of this, an EMT equipped with and trained to use a defibrillator should immediately attach the device to the patient to determine if a defibrillatory shock should be administered to the patient. The combination of early CPR and defibrillation provides the patient with the best chance of survival. Cardiac arrest patients who are not in ventricular fibrillation will require continued CPR and advanced life support. Follow local protocols for defibrillator use.

■ FOCUSED HISTORY AND PHYSICAL EXAMINATION

The history provides a general description of the patient's medical status. The head-to-toe exam is called the physical examination and provides additional and specific information about the patient's condition. Such information is best obtained by focusing the history taking and physical exam based on the patient's complaint or the mechanism of injury. As this is being done, ask the patient about the chief complaint and associated symptoms. Problems identified in the physical exam are generally not treated immediately, with the exception of life-threatening problems (ABCDs). Repeat the assessment of ABCDs during the physical exam and treatment phase to make sure that the patient's condition is not worsening. Evaluation of pulse rate, respiratory rate, and blood pressure should be repeated at 10-minute intervals.

The focused physical exam is divided into medical and trauma sections. This helps refine the approach to the special problems in each category. The focused exam is often modified to center on the patient's chief complaint or specific injuries. The equipment required includes a stethoscope, blood pressure cuff, and penlight.

History-Taking Tools

In obtaining the patient's history, the EMT may find it useful to utilize mnemonic reminders. Two mnemonics often used when obtaining focused histories are "SAMPLE" and "OPQRST." "SAMPLE" should be used for all patients because the information obtained is valuable to both trauma and medical patients. "OPQRST" is particularly useful in the communicative patient with a pain complaint.

SAMPLE

Signs and symptoms
Allergies
Medications
Past medical history
Last oral intake
Events leading up to this incident

OPQRST

Onset
Provocation
Quality
Radiation
Severity
Time

Examination of the Medical Patient

The focused physical examination in patients with medical problems depends upon a careful interrogation and elicitation of past history (SAMPLE). This directs the examiner to specific problem areas. Begin with a quick, initial set of vital signs (pulse rate, respiratory rate, blood pressure). Then proceed with a physical examination that focuses only on those body systems that may be associated with the patient's complaints or your initial rapid assessment findings.

Head, Eyes, Ears, Nose, Throat/Neck (HEENT)

- *Look* for skin discoloration, moisture, drooling, blood, nasal flaring, pursed lips, anxious facial expressions, frothy or bloody sputum, bloody emesis, facial sagging, drooping eyelid(s), deviated gaze, unequal pupils, eyelids held closed by patient, color of conjunctiva, distention of neck veins, retractions of accessory muscles at base of neck, presence of stoma, deviated trachea.
- *Listen* for stridorous speech, whispered speech, snoring, gurgling, coughing, grunting, wheezing.
- *Feel* for tenderness, subcutaneous air, stiffened neck, bulging fontanel (infants), skin temperature
- *Smell* for ketones, vomit, alcohol, fecal-like odor, ordinary household chemicals, home medicinal remedies (particularly those that are common to specific cultures).

Chest

- *Look* for respiratory rates and patterns: rapid (tachypnea), slow (bradypnea), shallow, irregular, painful (splinted), periodic patterns (Cheyne-Stokes, Kussmaul). Look for chest wall movement: intercostal retractions, barrel chest, and obvious malformations. Look for scars and skin discoloration, including rashes.
- *Listen* for absence of lung sounds, presence of rales or wheezes in either lung field, stridor at upper airway.

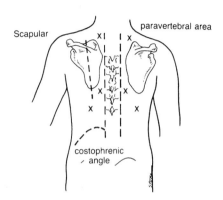

Figure 2-1

Surface anatomy of the back. The Xs indicate six places where lung sounds are auscultated on the back.

- Patients who can sit: use stethoscope to listen to posterior thorax at apex, midscapula, and base, starting at the base and moving toward the head to compare both sides (Fig. 2–1). Have the patient breathe deeply with mouth open while stethoscope is being used.
- For patients who are unable to sit, listen to anterior part of chest at second intercostal space lateral to sternum and at midaxillary line near armpit.

Abdomen

- *Look* for changes in general contour, distention, presence of pulsatile mass lateral to midline. Note scars, rashes, and their locations.
- *Feel* for tenderness, muscle resistance, masses.
  - With the patient lying down, start at the point furthest from area stated to be painful by patient. Patient may flinch or tense the muscles because of ticklishness or the examiner's cold hands. Confirm all reactions with patient verbally.
  - Begin with gentle palpation: move fingers of one hand over the entire abdominal area, noting areas of tenderness, increased muscle resistance (spasm), or solid masses.
  - Continue with deep palpation: with second hand pressing on top of the fingers of the first hand, slowly compress to a depth of 4 to 5 cm. Palpate the complete abdomen, noting tenderness or solid masses.
  - If there is a pulsating mass along the midline between the epigastrium and umbilicus, identify and mark the extent of the pulsatile mass. Check femoral pulses bilaterally for equal strength.

Extremities

- *Look* for skin discoloration, moisture, texture, obvious deformities, symmetry, inflammation, edema of ankle and lower leg (note and mark extent), scars, skin rashes, needle marks, cyanosis of nail beds, or yellowing of fingertips and nail beds.

■ *Feel* for bilateral radial and/or pedal pulses, skin turgor of hands and arms, pitting edema (ankles, lower legs), equal bilateral grip strength, foot extension strength, equal movement, and range of motion. Touch for sensation and skin temperature.

Examination of the Trauma Patient

The severely injured trauma patient must have a head-to-toe (neck/head-to-toe) systematic physical examination. Knowing the mechanism of injury is important in understanding the potential extent of injury to the trauma patient. The EMT in charge, or his/her partner, must assess the accident scene for possible mechanisms of injury. When the extent of injury appears minor, the physical examination may be modified to focus on body areas that appear injured or are causing symptoms. Remove or rearrange enough clothing to examine all parts of the body in order to avoid missing hidden injuries.

HEENT

Neck (Anterior and Posterior)

■ *Look* for wounds, distended neck veins, stoma, deviated trachea, and suprasternal retractions.
■ *Feel* for bony deformities, tenderness, muscle spasm, and subcutaneous air.

The neck must remain stable during the exam, maintaining anatomically normal alignment. Direct the application of a cervical collar as soon as possible (if there is suspected cervical spine injury).

Scalp

■ *Look* for areas of hemorrhage, hematoma, depressions, punctures.
■ *Feel* for deformity, blood.

The neck must remain stable during the exam, maintaining anatomically normal alignment. Note pain or tenderness in response to palpation.

Ears

■ *Look* at outer ear and inside canal. Look for hemorrhage, drainage of clear or pink fluid, discoloration behind ear (mastoid area).

Eyes

■ *Look* for constriction/dilation of pupils, unequal pupil size, deviated gaze, contact lenses, foreign objects, conjunctival discoloration, ecchymosis around eyes (raccoon eyes), or other gross injuries. With penlight, check pupillary response to light and ability to follow an object through the full range of motion.
■ *Feel* for resistance by patient to opening eyelids, if behavioral disorder is suspected.

NOSE

- *Look* for hemorrhage, deformity, drainage of clear or pink fluid, nasal flaring.

FACE

- *Look* for wounds, discoloration.
- *Feel* for deformity of cheekbones, instability of upper and lower jaw.

MOUTH

- *Look* for wounds, hemorrhage, blood drainage from nasopharynx, discoloration (cyanosis, ecchymosis around lips), foreign objects, loose or missing teeth, dentures.
- *Listen* for stridor, gurgling, partial obstruction.

Chest and Lumbar Spine

- *Look* for supraclavicular or intercostal retractions, wounds, discoloration, paradoxical respiratory movement (flail, diaphragmatic breathing), deformity, penetrating injuries.
- *Listen* for sucking wounds, altered or asymmetrical breath sounds (diminished or absent), wheezes or rales (anterior at second intercostal space and at midaxillary line near armpit), muffled or distant heart sounds (at apex, under left nipple).
- *Feel* for deformity, symmetrical chest wall movement, tenderness, crepitus, and muscle spasm. Compress midsternum gently, then firmly. If the patient is supine, palpate the spine and back for deformities or wounds.

Abdomen

- *Look* for wounds, discoloration, distention, guarding, bruising, or evisceration.
- *Feel* for tenderness, muscle spasm (voluntary and involuntary), and rigidity. Palpate all four quadrants gently, then deeply.

Pelvis

- *Look* for wounds, discoloration, deformity.
- *Feel* for deformity, tenderness, stability. Gently, then firmly, compress iliac crests toward midline, then downward. Palpate femoral pulses bilaterally for equality.

Buttocks/Genitalia

- *Look* for wounds, discoloration, deformity.
- *Feel* for tenderness.

Extremities

GENERAL

- *Look* for wounds, deformity (swelling, angulation), discoloration (especially check skin color distal to an injury). Look for ability to move spontaneously and on command, symmetry, and abnormal movement or posturing.

■ *Feel* for tenderness, deformity, skin temperature. Before and after splinting, check
  –*Sensation:* response to gentle touch (with patient looking away), then to painful stimuli
  –*Movement:* pain on movement, ability to move spontaneously and against resistance
  –*Pulses:* distal circulation

LEGS

  ■ *Look* for ability to wiggle toes. Note any rotation or shortening of one leg.
  ■ *Feel* for ability of foot to push against resistance.

ARMS

  ■ *Look* for ability to wiggle fingers.
  ■ *Feel* for strength and equality of grasp.

Reassess ABCDs and Vital Signs

Reassess ABCDs

Treat ABCD problems immediately.

  ■ If necessary, ventilate with oxygen and begin CPR.
  ■ Apply supplemental oxygen and maintain cervical spine stabilization.
  ■ Treat sucking chest wounds with an occlusive dressing.
  ■ Control severe bleeding.
  ■ Package patient, using spinal immobilization device if necessary, and prepare for rapid transport to an appropriate hospital.

Reassess Vital Signs

If time permits, reassess vital signs or reassess during transport.

  ■ *Respiratory rate:* Increase supplemental oxygen delivery or assist ventilations with bag-valve mask if rate or depth decrease significantly or patient's general appearance has deteriorated.
  ■ *Pulse rate:* Treat for shock if significant volume loss is suspected, particularly when the pulse rate is fast.
  ■ *Blood pressure:* Determine in both arms. Elevate the patient's head (raise head of bed or backboard slightly) if blood pressure is high.
  ■ *Skin temperature, color, and moistness:* Maintain body heat, particularly in cold environments, to prevent additional losses. Avoid rapid cooling of very warm patients to avoid shivering (with the exception of heat stroke patients).
  ■ *State of consciousness:* Reassess the level of consciousness and calculate the Glasgow Coma Scale score (Appendix F).
  ■ Calculate the Revised Trauma Score, if indicated (see Appendix F).

History

Obtain a SAMPLE history, if possible, before or during transport.

■ REPORTING METHODS

Just as important as the ability to perform rapid and concise assessment and treatment is the ability to report these findings and treatment in an organized manner to persons giving the next level of medical care. The most practical and professional method is a written form, which is sent with the patient (e.g., fire department releasing the patient to an ambulance for transport) or left with the patient at the hospital by the treating EMT, if the patient is transported (Figs. 2–2, 2–3, 2–4, and 2–5). Written professionally, this report will be important for the physician. Hospitals make this report part of the patient's permanent medical record. It is a legal record and provides documentation of the out-of-hospital findings and the care given. The EMT in charge of the patient must write this report; it cannot be left to another EMT, who may have only a partial idea of the details concerning the patient's condition and treatment.

Narrative Format

The most widely accepted format—SOAP—is patterned after the method used by much of the medical profession. It is a simple format that follows the same logic used in the patient interrogation and examination.

S = Subjective

The subjective portion of the report includes the patient's chief complaint(s), associated symptoms, and the events leading up to calling EMS, as well as activity at onset, actions taken by the patient to alleviate symptoms or treat injury, and the time of onset as described by the patient, family, and witnesses. Include a brief past history, current medications, when taken, and allergies. Condense the information to a brief format, but use the patient's language. For trauma patients, include information learned from others regarding accident description, seat belts or helmet worn, airbag deployed, and other information obtained second hand from other parties.

O = Objective

The objective portion of the report contains signs the examiner sees, feels, and so on. It describes the general conditions of the patient, including age, sex, level of consciousness, emotional state, position or location, environmental conditions, general appearance, and impression of acute illness as actually seen by examiner. Include other exam findings such as ECG, vital sign changes, smell of alcohol on the breath, and improvement or deterioration following treatment. Describe abnormal findings of each of the major body areas. Include, when applicable, pertinent negatives as well (e.g., chest expansion is symmetrical, clear lung sounds in patient with complaint of shortness of breath, no swelling or deformity in an extremity suspected of being

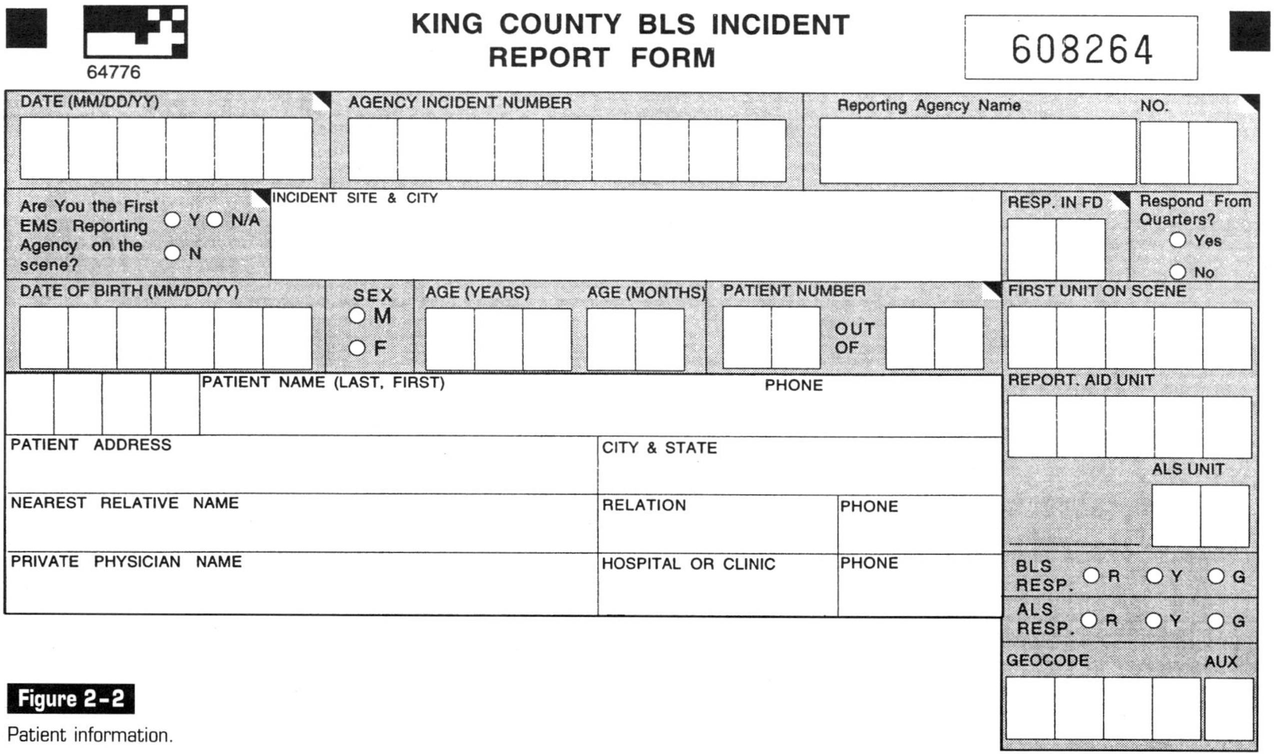

KING COUNTY BLS INCIDENT REPORT FORM

608264

64776

DATE (MM/DD/YY)	AGENCY INCIDENT NUMBER	Reporting Agency Name	NO.

Are You the First EMS Reporting Agency on the scene?   ○ Y ○ N/A ○ N

INCIDENT SITE & CITY

RESP. IN FD

Respond From Quarters? ○ Yes ○ No

FIRST UNIT ON SCENE

DATE OF BIRTH (MM/DD/YY)

SEX ○ M ○ F

AGE (YEARS)   AGE (MONTHS)   PATIENT NUMBER   OUT OF

REPORT. AID UNIT

ALS UNIT

PATIENT NAME (LAST, FIRST)   PHONE

PATIENT ADDRESS   CITY & STATE

NEAREST RELATIVE NAME   RELATION   PHONE

PRIVATE PHYSICIAN NAME   HOSPITAL OR CLINIC   PHONE

BLS RESP. ○ R ○ Y ○ G
ALS RESP. ○ R ○ Y ○ G

GEOCODE   AUX

Figure 2-2
Patient information.

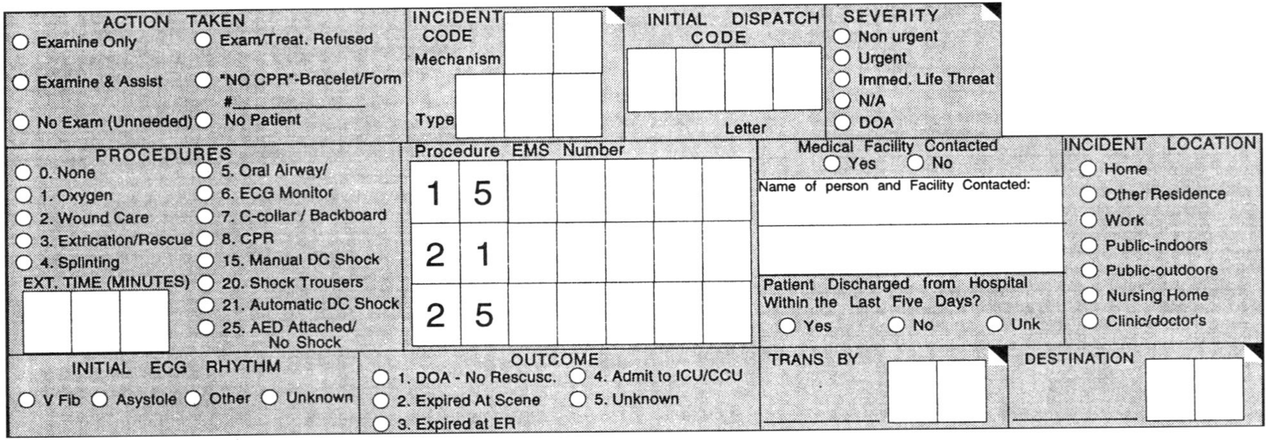

Figure 2–3

Procedures of incident data.

fractured). Note findings of the exam performed on the following areas:

- General appearance
- HEENT: head, eyes, ears, nose, throat/neck, and cervical spine
- Chest: thorax, front and back
- Abdomen; list lumbar spine and pelvis separately when applicable
- Extremities: arms/legs, hands/feet, including pulses, motor function, and sensation
- Neurologic: level of consciousness, ability to move all extremities, any sensory loss

A = Assessment

The assessment portion of the report contains the EMT's conclusions and/or impressions of the patient's condition. Using the term "rule out" (R/O) only suggests a diagnostic impression, not a firm diagnosis. It indicates what you think may be the cause of the patient's illness/injury, although you cannot be sure it definitely is or is not. More than one R/O may be listed, if applicable. Preface the conclusion with the term "possible" unless the injury is obvious.

P = Plan

The plan portion of the report describes the actual treatment, including all methods of treatment and equipment used to treat the patient, even when obvious. Note specific treatment components such as oxygen (delivery method and flow rate), patient positioning (supine, head elevated, sitting up), calming and reassurance, prolonged or rapid extrication, medical direction from medical control or advanced life support providers, or assisting the patient with home meds. A good rule of thumb is, "If it isn't written on the report, it wasn't done." Remember, this is a legal document—be accurate and truthful. The EMT may also use the report to record equipment left at the hospital with the patient, unusual circumstances surrounding the incident, and a patient's refusal of treatment. Many EMS systems have instituted specific procedures for patient refusals that utilize signed statements preprinted on the report form.

Verbal and Radio Communication

The EMT must also be able to quickly summarize the patient report and verbalize it to others. In some cases, the EMT may be required to provide the summary (short report) to higher level personnel in the EMS system (e.g., advanced life support) or to the receiving hospital when transferring the patient's care. This report may be done using radio communication or in a face-to-face manner. In either case, keep the following points in mind:

1. Identify the appropriate person to whom the report should be relayed.

CALL TIME (24 HOUR)	DISPATCHED	ARRIVED ON SCENE	PATIENT LEAVES SCENE	ARRIVES AT HOSPITAL	IN SERVICE

EMS Personnel		EMS Number		EMS Personnel		EMS Number	

FOR AGENCY USE

EQUIPMENT USED _____

SENT TO _____

FIRE REGULAR 8/96

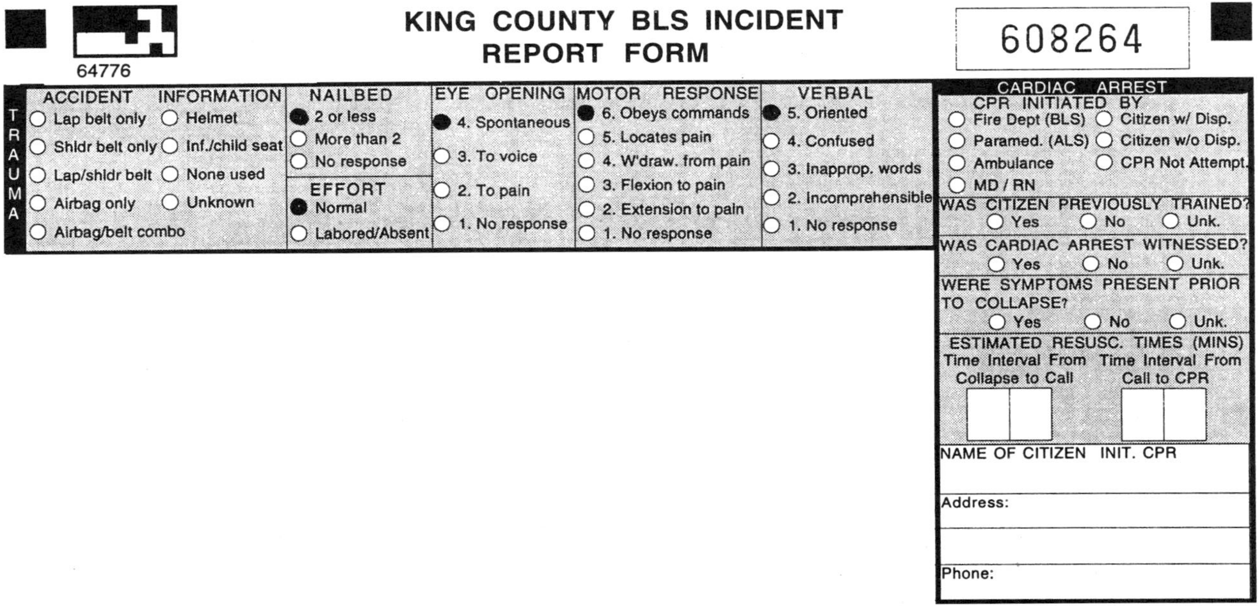

KING COUNTY BLS INCIDENT REPORT FORM

608264

64776

ACCIDENT	INFORMATION
T	○ Lap belt only ○ Helmet
R	○ Shldr belt only ○ Inf./child seat
A	○ Lap/shldr belt ○ None used
U	○ Airbag only ○ Unknown
M	○ Airbag/belt combo
A	

NAILBED
● 2 or less
○ More than 2
○ No response

EFFORT
● Normal
○ Labored/Absent

EYE OPENING
● 4. Spontaneous
○ 3. To voice
○ 2. To pain
○ 1. No response

MOTOR RESPONSE
● 6. Obeys commands
○ 5. Locates pain
○ 4. W'draw. from pain
○ 3. Flexion to pain
○ 2. Extension to pain
○ 1. No response

VERBAL
● 5. Oriented
○ 4. Confused
○ 3. Inapprop. words
○ 2. Incomprehensible
○ 1. No response

CARDIAC ARREST

CPR INITIATED BY
○ Fire Dept (BLS)   ○ Citizen w/ Disp.
○ Paramed. (ALS)   ○ Citizen w/o Disp.
○ Ambulance   ○ CPR Not Attempt.
○ MD / RN

WAS CITIZEN PREVIOUSLY TRAINED?
○ Yes   ○ No   ○ Unk.

WAS CARDIAC ARREST WITNESSED?
○ Yes   ○ No   ○ Unk.

WERE SYMPTOMS PRESENT PRIOR
TO COLLAPSE?
○ Yes   ○ No   ○ Unk.

ESTIMATED RESUSC. TIMES (MINS)
Time Interval From   Time Interval From
Collapse to Call   Call to CPR

NAME OF CITIZEN INIT. CPR

Address:

Phone:

Figure 2-4

Response, trauma registry, and cardiac arrest data.

TIME		0750	0754	0802					
F Blood Pressure		130/72	128/74	100/66					
L Pulse Rate		96	92	96					
O Respiratory Rate		24	20	20					
W Consciousness		A/O	→						
C ECG Rhythm			Sinus c̄ PVCs						
H O2			4 lpm nasal cannula →						
A									
R Nitro			0.4 mg tab						
T									
DC Shock									

Medications Taken By Patient at Home

Nitro, Cardizem, Furosemide 40mg/day,
Potassium

Allergies NKA

Narrative (Subjective, Objective, Assessment, Plan)

(S) 55 y/o ♂ C/o sudden onset of pressure in the center
of his chest. Radiates to Ⓛ arm. Pt. had some
sweating, nausea and SOB @ onset. Awakened
from sleep c̄ symptoms around 0715 hours. Rates pressure
discomfort @ "8" on "10" scale. Took Tums thinking this was

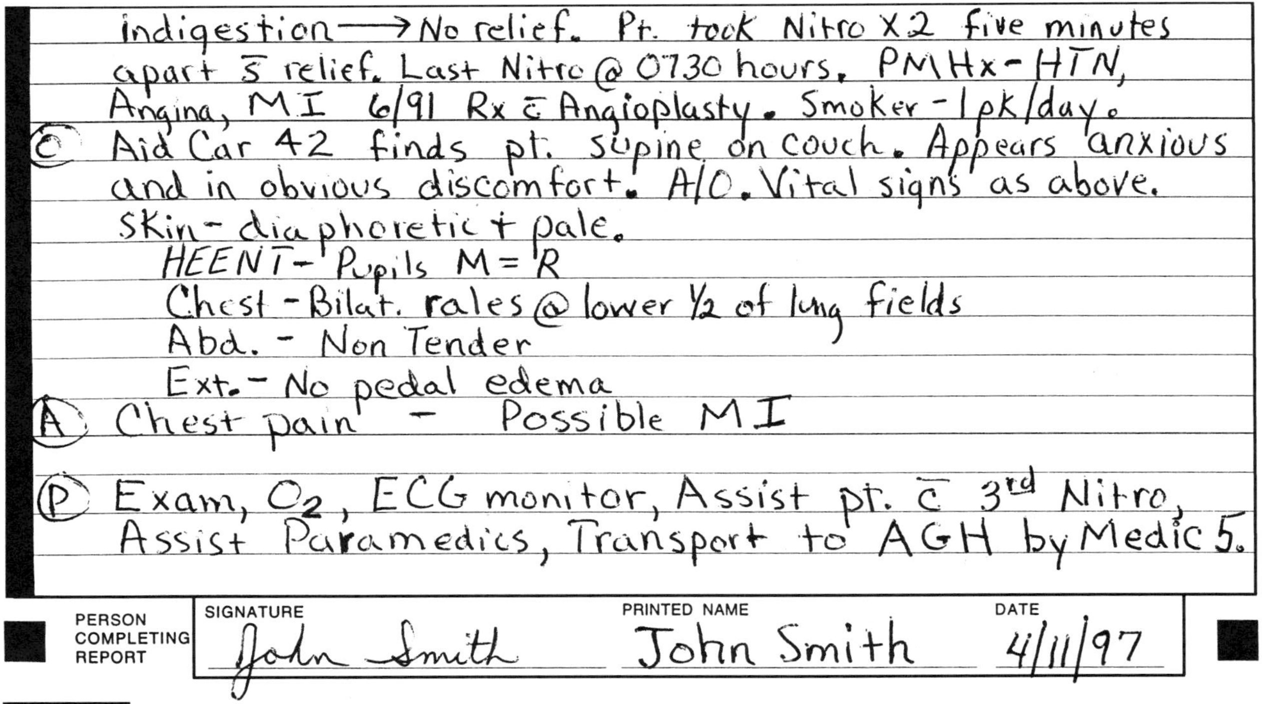

indigestion → No relief. Pt. took Nitro x2 five minutes apart c̄ relief. Last Nitro @ 0730 hours. PMHx- HTN, Angina, MI 6/91 Rx c̄ Angioplasty. Smoker- 1pk/day.

(O) Aid Car 42 finds pt. supine on couch. Appears anxious and in obvious discomfort. A/O. Vital signs as above.

Skin- diaphoretic + pale.

HEENT- Pupils M = R

Chest - Bilat. rales @ lower ½ of lung fields

Abd. - Non Tender

Ext.- No pedal edema

(A) Chest pain - Possible MI

(P) Exam, O₂, ECG monitor, Assist pt. c̄ 3rd Nitro, Assist Paramedics, Transport to AGH by Medic 5.

| PERSON COMPLETING REPORT | SIGNATURE John Smith | PRINTED NAME John Smith | DATE 4/11/97 |

Figure 2-5

Flow chart and narrative—includes vital signs, other procedures or therapies, and SOAP narrative.

2. Be brief and to the point.
3. Arrange your report in a systematic fashion similar to the patient assessment and exam:
   a. Age, sex (if by radio), and name (if face to face)
   b. Mechanism of injury and/or chief complaint — include brief review of injuries noted and/or other complaints and associated symptoms
   c. Significant findings of the patient assessment and examination
   d. Significant and pertinent past/present medical history
   e. Treatment and therapies provided and their effect, if any
   f. Patient's current status — vital signs and current complaint

4. Allow the person receiving the report a brief period to ask pertinent questions.
5. Be prepared. The ability to effectively summarize and communicate patient information requires practice, practice, and practice.

■ TRIAGE

Triage is the classification of patients according to medical need. There are three applications of this process in the early management of the trauma patient: (1) field triage; (2) interhospital triage to specialized care facilities; and(3) mass casualty triage.

Field Categorization of Trauma Patients (Field Triage)*

Trauma patients who, because of injury severity, require care at level I or level II trauma centers constitute a fraction of all patients hospitalized each year for trauma. In 1983, approximately 3.75 million patients were hospitalized for injury. In the same year, a study revealed 450 patients per million had an Injury Severity Score (ISS) of 15 or more, accounting for only 5.7% of all patients who were discharged from the hospital. Only 8.9% of the patients had scores greater than ISS 10, which incorporates just one serious body injury. Even with high overtriage rates, it is unlikely that the number of patients entering trauma centers will exceed 1000 per million per year.

It is a substantial challenge for field EMS personnel to identify that small proportion of patients who require prompt access to trauma centers. Furthermore, time is critical. Of the trauma victims who are going to die, 50 to 60% do so before reaching a hospital. Of the remaining patients who die in-hospital, about 60% do so within the first 4 hours.

---

*Resources for Optimal Care of the Injured Patient. Chicago, American College of Surgeons, 1990.

The following factors must be considered in field triage: (1) the actual or potential level of severity of the injured patient; (2) medical control; and (3) the regional resources available to treat the patient, including time and distance.

Assessment of Patient Severity

For the purpose of field triage, assessment of patient severity is based on examination of the patient for (1) abnormal physiologic signs; (2) obvious anatomic injury; (3) mechanism of injury; and (4) concurrent disease. Keep in mind that some communities also correctly classify injuries such as thermal injuries (heat and cold injuries) and diving injuries/illnesses as traumatic, requiring that these types of patients be considered for transport to a level I or level II trauma center.

A triage decision scheme based on current scientific knowledge is illustrated in Figure 2–6. It is the general intention of these triage guidelines to select patients with an ISS of greater than 15 for trauma center care. Patients with this level of ISS have at least a 10% risk of dying from a single severe or multiple serious injuries. When there is doubt, the patient is often best evaluated in a trauma center. Some notes regarding the use of these guidelines are presented here.

STEP I

Deviations from normal of the Glasgow Coma Scale score, blood pressure, and respiratory rate are associated with less than a 90% probability of survival. Used in this manner, prehospital values can be included in the admission trauma score and the quality assessment process. A variety of physiologic severity scores have been used for prehospital triage and have been found to be accurate. The scores contained in the triage guidelines, however, are believed to be the simplest to compute, and provide an accurate basis for field triage based on physiologic abnormality.

STEP II

Even in the presence of normal physiology, it is important to evaluate the likely presence of injuries that should be treated in a trauma center. A patient who has normal vital signs at the scene of an accident may still have a serious or lethal injury. Accurate diagnosis of life-threatening injury at the accident scene is unlikely. Thus, it is essential to look for indications that significant forces were applied to the body. Evidence of damage to an automobile can be a helpful guideline to the change in velocity (ΔV). A ΔV of 20 mph will produce an ISS of greater than 15 in 90% of automobile crash occupants. ΔV can be estimated if 1 inch of vehicular deformity is equated to approximate 1 mph of ΔV.

STEP III

Certain other factors that might lower the threshold at which patients should be treated in trauma centers must be considered in field triage.

TRIAGE DECISION SCHEME

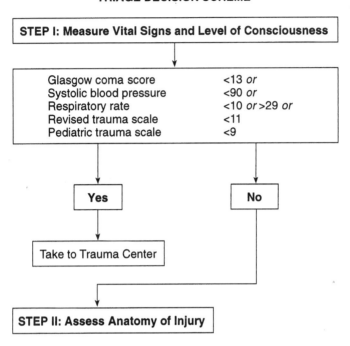

STEP I: Measure Vital Signs and Level of Consciousness

Glasgow coma score	<13 *or*
Systolic blood pressure	<90 *or*
Respiratory rate	<10 *or* >29 *or*
Revised trauma scale	<11
Pediatric trauma scale	<9

Yes **No**

Take to Trauma Center

STEP II: Assess Anatomy of Injury

• Penetrating injuries to head, neck, torso, and extremities proximal to elbow and knee
• Flail chest
• Combination trauma with burns of 10% or inhalation injuries
• Two or more proximal long bone fractures
• Pelvic fractures
• Limb paralysis
• Amputation proximal to wrist or ankle

Yes **No**

Take to Trauma Center

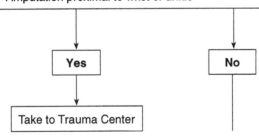

Figure 2-6

Triage decision scheme. *Illustration continued on opposite page*

STEP III: Assess Mechanism of Injury (Forces Applied to Body)

- Ejection from automobile
- Death in same passenger compartment
- Extrication time >20 minutes
- Falls >20 feet
- Rollover auto accidents
- Automobile vs. stationary solid object
- High-speed auto crash
  - Initial speed >40 mph
  - Velocity change >20 mph
  - Major auto deformity >20 inches
  - Intrusion into passenger compartment >12 inches
- Auto-pedestrian injury with significant (>5 mph) impact
- Pedestrian thrown or run over
- Motorcycle crash >20 mph or with separation of rider and bike

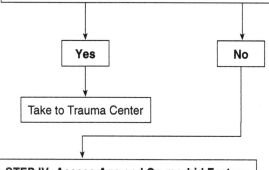

| **Yes** | | **No** |

Take to Trauma Center

STEP IV: Assess Age and Co-morbid Factors

- Age <5 or >55 years
- Known cardiac disease, respiratory disease, or use of anti-psychotic medication
- Diabetics taking insulin, cirrhosis, malignancy, obesity, or coagulopathy

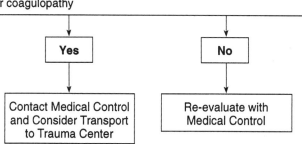

| **Yes** | **No** |

| Contact Medical Control and Consider Transport to Trauma Center | Re-evaluate with Medical Control |

WHEN IN DOUBT, TAKE TO A TRAUMA CENTER

These include the following:

- *Age:* Patients over age 55 have an increased risk of death from even moderately severe injuries. Patients younger than age 5 have certain characteristics that may merit treatment in a trauma center with special resources for children.
- *Co-morbid factors:* The presence of significant cardiac, respiratory, or metabolic diseases is an additional factor that may merit the triage of patients with moderately severe head injury to trauma centers.

Medical Control

The triage decision determines the level and intensity of initial management of the major or multiple trauma patient. The vast majority of trauma deaths occur within a few hours of injury. The triage decision is often critical to or determinant of patient survival or death. It is for this reason that the highest available level of medical expertise should be brought into the triage decision-making process. Usually this process will involve advice and guidance from physicians who provide medical control to prehospital personnel. On-line physician medical control is vitally important in emergency medical systems for the trauma patient.

Surgeons, emergency physicians, and prehospital care personnel should work together to develop prehospital triage protocols for trauma patients. In most instances of triage based on potentially severe injuries, the patient is unable to make an informed decision in selecting appropriate hospital care. The "system" is often responsible for this decision. The system must therefore make surrogate decisions. In no instance may these decisions prejudice patient outcome. Disposition decisions at the scene must hold the patient's interests and needs paramount.

Range of Resources and Time/Distance Factors

Both the level of available hospital resources and time/distance factors are also considered in making the triage decision. It must be recognized that level I through level IV trauma facilities are stratifications in a continuum of capability of commitment to trauma patient care. The system for trauma triage in an urban environment is considerably different from that in a rural environment. In the latter case, access to any level of trauma care may involve significant distance and time.

Each region must therefore structure a trauma system in a manner that ensures prompt access to appropriate care and minimizes the risk of delay in diagnosis, delay in surgical intervention, and inadequately focused care. These factors are responsible for most of the preventable deaths that occur.

URBAN TRIAGE

In most urban communities in the United States, prompt access to a level I or level II trauma center should be feasible within 30 minutes of activation of the EMS system. Many urban populations have more than reasonable access to sophisticated care because of the distribution of tertiary care hospitals that function as level I trauma centers. Other hospitals that do not offer this level of care or commitment should be bypassed in favor of access to a trauma center.

RURAL TRIAGE

In the rural environment, an injured patient may be at substantial distances from a trauma center. Such patients should initially be treated at a rural trauma hospital. In more remote rural areas, where level III facilities are not available, staff should at least be trained in advanced trauma life support. Patients with more severe injuries should then be secondarily triaged to level I or II trauma centers, should local resources prove inadequate for continued care (see Table 2–1) later in this chapter.

Just as the level II trauma center provides the highest level of care available within most communities across the country, the importance of the level III and IV trauma facilities cannot be overemphasized. Between rural and urban environments, there are geographic areas with increasing distances between hospitals and decreasing population density. Some patients may require initial triage and resuscitation at a level III or IV rural trauma hospital. This action may be preferred to primary patient transport from the scene to an urban tertiary care referral center. The EMS system should be structured to provide the patient timely access to the best available level of care indicated by the extent and nature of injuries received.

CONTINUING EDUCATION AND EVALUATION

Because of acknowledged imperfections of current field triage and the importance of this process in the delivery of trauma patient care, it is essential to involve surgeons in the continuing education of prehospital care personnel, as well as in feedback to personnel on the accuracy of their patient triage decisions. Undoubtedly, as decision rules are reviewed and the results are reported back to the prehospital care personnel, the process of triage will improve. Communities should strive to establish regional trauma data collection systems. Collected data can then be analyzed and used for quality improvement (triage and medical interventions), overall system performance, injury prevention and education, and research. Many states have passed legislation mandating the creation of such systems.

OVERTRIAGE AND UNDERTRIAGE

A system has yet to be developed that reliably and correctly selects the patients for appropriate levels of care that might be available in a given region. As a result, there will always be a certain number of patients selected for trauma center care who could very adequately be handled at a community hospital (85 to 90% of all injured patients do not need trauma center care). These patients are referred

Table 2-1   Interhospital Triage Criteria

CENTRAL NERVOUS SYSTEM

Head injury
- Penetrating injury or depressed skull fracture
- Open injury with or without cerebrospinal fluid leak
- Glasgow Coma Score (GCS) <13 or GCS deterioration
- Lateralizing signs

Spinal cord injury

CHEST

Widened mediastinum
Major chest wall injury
Cardiac injury
Patients who may require protracted ventilation

PELVIS

Unstable pelvic ring disruption
Pelvic ring disruption with shock and evidence of continuing hemorrhage
Open pelvic injury

MULTIPLE SYSTEM INJURY

Severe face injury with head injury
Chest injury with head injury
Abdominal or pelvic injury with head injury
Burns with associated injuries
Multiple fractures

EVIDENCE OF HIGH-ENERGY IMPACT

Auto crash or pedestrian injury—velocity ≥25 mph
Rearward displacement of front axle or front of car (20 inches)
Ejection of patient or rollover
Death of occupant in same car

CO-MORBID FACTORS

Age <5 years or >55 years
Known cardiorespiratory or metabolic diseases

SECONDARY DETERIORATION (LATE SEQUELAE)

Mechanical ventilation required
Sepsis
Single or multiple organ system failure (deterioration in central nervous, cardiac, pulmonary, hepatic, renal, or coagulation systems)
Major tissue necrosis

to as overtriaged. Conversely, patients who are in need of trauma center care but who fail to gain timely access to such care are referred to as undertriaged. Together, overtriaged and undertriaged patients combine to form a misclassification rate for any triage decision scheme or rule.

Overtriage and undertriage are interdependent. Considerable medical effort should be made to minimize the number of patients who are undertriaged in a trauma system, because these patients are at risk of dying. Lives may be saved or cost of care may be reduced by prompt access to the needed level of definitive care. There is also concern about the overtriage of patients; overtriage can produce overuse of trauma centers and may divert patients away from community hospitals.

Not all patients with apparent minor injuries can clearly be grouped as not needing trauma center evaluation. For example, a patient who suffers high-deceleration injuries may be found to have a widened mediastinum on x-ray film in a rural emergency department. Because of the risk of a ruptured aorta, the standard of care would dictate that such a patient be promptly evaluated in a trauma center, where an arteriogram and necessary surgical care are immediately available. A large number of patients who undergo radiographic studies for a widened superior mediastinum after trauma will not have a ruptured aorta. These patients might eventually exhibit only minimal injuries. They could represent an overtriage on trauma system statistics, yet the medical prudence of transferring such a patient for trauma center evaluation could not be argued.

Studies have shown that a 35 to 50% overtriage rate may be required to maintain an appropriate safety net for patients. It also has been estimated that, because of the small number of patients who really need to be in trauma centers, the impact of patient flow on an individual institution will be minimal should this degree of overtriage exist. Clearly, the surgical community needs to be more concerned about undertriage and the medical consequences that result from inadequate use of a trauma system.

Interhospital Triage

The criteria in Table 2–1 identify patients at a particularly high risk of dying from multiple and severe injuries. Ideally, such patients should be treated in a high-level trauma center where continued exposure of multidisciplinary teams to such patients may afford an optimum outcome. Such patients should be considered for transfer to high-level centers whenever possible.

Multiple Casualty Triage

When the EMT is faced with an incident involving a number of patients that overwhelms his/her immediately available resources, the incident is termed a multiple casualty incident (MCI). Although there are many interpretations of this term, the common theme is the lack of immediately available resources considering the patient count. Although there are many aspects and details associated with the organization of an MCI response, the following is a summation of a typical approach using the START (simple triage and rapid transport) method.

Command Structure

The EMS system must develop an MCI plan that defines a command structure and details the primary roles and responsibilities of those responding to the incident. The probability of success in an MCI response will improve significantly with:

- An effective organization and command structure
- Preplanning and practice
- Predefined roles and responsibilities
- Preplanning for adequate and appropriate equipment, supplies, and support resources

The command structure typically consists of the following personnel:

- *Incident commander* (IC)—usually the highest ranking officer at the scene. This person oversees all operations associated with the MCI.
- *Medical group supervisor* (medical group)—usually the highest ranking EMS officer at the scene or an officer designated by the IC. Initially, this role is filled by the EMT in charge of the first arriving unit. This person is responsible for all EMS-related operations of the MCI. He/she reports directly to the IC.
- *Triage team leader* (triage)—initially, this is usually the partner of the EMT in charge of the first arriving unit. This person immediately begins triage, establishes a funnel point to ensure that all patients are directed to the treatment areas, and requests necessary resources to accomplish these tasks.
- *Treatment team leader* (treatment)—this person is responsible for overseeing all patient treatment and for establishing a treatment area. He/she requests resources as needed to provide necessary treatment.
- *Transportation team leader* (transportation)—this person is responsible for overseeing and managing all aspects of patient transportation. Generally, this position is considered to be the most critical and most difficult in the MCI command structure.

The EMT in charge of the first arriving unit assumes command of the incident until relieved by a higher ranking officer.

START Triage Process

The purpose of triage is to quickly provide the best care possible for the greatest number of patients considering the available resources.

1. Patients are initially sorted into one of four categories:
   a. Red—critical and require immediate treatment
   b. Yellow—injured; however, treatment may be slightly delayed

Hint: Use the RPM mnemonic to recall the triage criteria

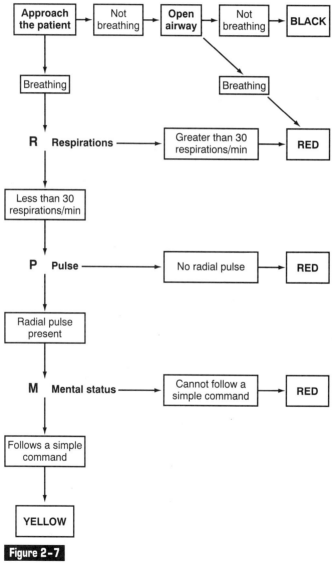

Figure 2-7

Using the START triage method.

    c. Green—minor or no injuries; often referred to as walking wounded

    d. Black—dead or mortally wounded

2. Initially, the triage team leader or designee asks that all patients who can get up and walk do so to a designated area. This area may be a bus or parking area. It should be controlled and have at least one EMT to provide simple assessments and upgrade patients if necessary.

3. The triage team leader and/or triage team members begin triaging patients. One method of noting a patient's triage category is by attaching a length of color-coded plastic tape (nonadhesive) to the patient's arm (or leg). The plastic tape color represents the triage category.

4. Triage of each patient should take no more than 30 seconds. *Hint:* One method of estimating a patient count is to tear off a small piece of the appropriate color tape for each patient triaged. After triage, the small strips can be counted, giving a relatively accurate count of the total patients in each category.

5. Once all patients are triaged, the triage team leader requests resources to move the patients to the appropriate treatment area (red or yellow).

6. Movement of patients is through a funnel point, at which time each patient has a sequential number placed on his/her forehead (or arm).

7. Once all patients are removed to the treatment area, the treatment team leader reports the total number of patients to the medical group supervisor and/or IC. The triage team resources are then reassigned to other duties.

START Triage Criteria (see Fig. 2–7)

- If the patient is not breathing, one attempt to open the airway and restore breathing is made. If the patient cannot maintain an open airway and remains apneic, the patient is coded BLACK.

- R—If the patient is breathing and respirations are greater than 30/min, the patient is coded RED.

- P—If the patient is breathing less than 30 times/min and has no radial pulse, the patient is coded RED.

- M—If the patient does have a radial pulse but cannot follow simple commands (stick out your tongue), then the patient is coded RED.

- If the patient can follow a simple command, the patient is coded YELLOW.

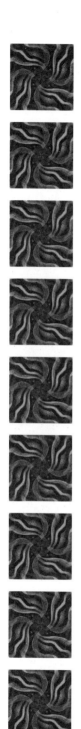

SIGNS AND SYMPTOMS

■ Organization of Section Content

This section provides an organized list of signs and symptoms in order to help guide the EMT through the steps of assessment, impression development (the most likely diagnosis), and patient management (treatment). Signs and symptoms are included here only if they either (1) may be present in more than one condition and therefore lead to the search for further signs and symptoms or (2) indicate the immediate need for some action by the EMT, such as treatment, stabilization, or rapid transport to advanced life support (ALS) services.

It is often thought that the EMT must go through the following steps in sequence:

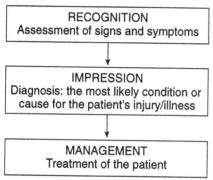

However, we believe that in many cases (particularly in the acutely ill patient) the patient is best served if the EMT progresses directly from the recognition of signs and symptoms to immediate action (management):

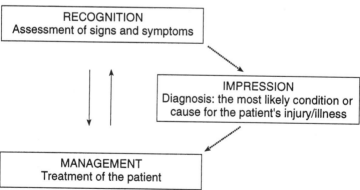

In these cases, the need for immediate action by the EMT, such as the administration of oxygen therapy, is greater than the need for a detailed or prolonged search for an exact diagnosis. Once the immediate management is provided, the EMT may continue to reassess the patient and provide additional treatment as necessary. The entries for each condition in the chapters in this section therefore have two parts: characteristics and immediate action.

Characteristics are the guide to recognition of the condition—specific indications to look for in assessing the patient. The list does not include every possible sign or symptom of a condition, only those helpful in differentiating one cause of a symptom from another. Not all patients with a particular condition will show all of the characteristics listed. In fact, many will have only one or two, but the presence of these hallmarks will suggest that the particular condition is the most likely. In this way, the EMT forms an impression. This impression of the most likely condition can direct the EMT in management of the patient.

Immediate action represents the basics only—specific indications for stabilization or rapid transport. All patient management is guided by severity of the patient's condition. The most severely injured or ill patients need the most rapid and aggressive therapy. Nevertheless, these immediate actions do not imply a halt in the thorough head-to-toe (neck/head-to-toe in trauma patients) examination of the patient. A thorough search for other conditions (medical or trauma) is essential for good patient assessment. For the most severely ill or injured patient, "rapid transport" means that much of that search will continue while en route to ALS services or an appropriate hospital.

In each chapter, the listing of the causes for a particular symptom is in rough order of the importance of immediate action. This order is modified by the frequency of occurrence of the conditions. For the most part, traumatic conditions are not included in this section. Although they have been included here where they are useful, recognition of the most likely condition is usually based upon the history of the mechanism of injury. Furthermore, even (or perhaps especially) when the impression is not obvious, all patients with significant head, chest, or abdominal trauma need rapid transport to ALS services or an appropriate hospital, not a detailed, prolonged search for an exact diagnosis.

■ NOTES ON TERMINOLOGY

Rapid Transport

The term "rapid transport" is used throughout Section II to mean rapid provision of, or transport to, ALS services. In the case of serious trauma, it includes the more specific goal of rapid transport to an appropriate hospital, preferably a level I trauma center.

In some urban and suburban communities, these services are provided in the field by paramedics in a "tiered-response" system. In these systems, the EMS communication center dispatches the closest basic life support (BLS) unit(s) and the closest ALS unit simultaneously when a life-threatening emergency is suspected. A typical characteristic of tiered-response EMS systems is that there are many more BLS units than ALS units. This commonly results in very short response times for the BLS unit and a slightly greater response time for the ALS unit. As a result, the EMT can quickly perform an assessment, provide immediately necessary treatment, and advise the responding ALS unit of the assessment findings. Often, the information obtained in the EMT's assessment will allow the arriving paramedic to expedite his/her assessment and delivery of ALS treatment. Additionally, the EMT's assessment may determine that the ALS unit is not needed, and he/she may then cancel the unit. This makes the ALS unit available for additional responses. When a life-threatening emergency was not suspected by the dispatcher but is found to be present, the EMT would then request an ALS unit to respond. In some communities, ALS unit response times are delayed or extended as a result of remote locations or limited ALS availability. In this circumstance, the EMT may arrange for an ALS unit "intercept" (or "rendezvous"). This means that the ALS unit will start traveling toward the scene or some agreed upon location. The BLS unit will simultaneously transport the patient toward the ALS unit or the agreed-upon location.

In other communities, paramedic-level ALS services are supplemented by intermediate-level EMTs. These EMTs may have additional training in specific ALS skills, such as intravenous access, advanced airway management, and the administration of specific medications. This level of EMT training is outside the scope of this book, which focuses on the EMT-Basic.

In still other communities, ALS services may not be available in the out-of-hospital setting. In this case, the EMT must recognize that rapid transport to the hospital may be the best management of the most severely ill or injured patient. The indications for "immediate action" in Section II attempt to put this need for rapid transport in the context of the patient's total needs. Naturally, the provision of airway control and ventilatory assistance, for example, must precede rapid transport. As stated earlier, for the most severely ill or injured patients, especially those with significant head, chest, or abdominal trauma, rapid transport has priority over the comprehensive patient examination. The term "rapid transport," then, is used in Section II when it is a critical part of the "immediate action."

Adrenaline Response

The term "adrenaline response" is used in Section II and throughout the book to draw attention to a common response that many acutely ill or injured patients have that makes many of the different medical conditions appear quite similar. The human body reacts to acute stress by the production of hormones, as if to prepare for what has been called "fight or flight." The preparation for "fight or flight" requires the body to increase the blood supply to vital areas and decrease it to nonessential areas. Thus, the heart rate speeds up, and blood is diverted from the skin (making it cool and pale) and from the gastrointestinal tract (causing nausea). The pupils of the eyes dilate to improve vision, and circulation is increased to the brain (causing increased awareness but also anxiety) and to the skeletal muscles. The sweat glands on the hands also are activated (possibly this helped our prehistoric ancestors hold onto their clubs).

The substance principally causing these effects is epinephrine, also known as adrenaline. Epinephrine is released when the body is trying to compensate for some acute insult. It does not matter whether the insult is a disease or an injury; the response is the same, and the signs and symptoms of that response only indicate that the body is attempting to compensate. Therefore, the observation by the EMT that a patient is exhibiting an adrenaline response is not enough for determining the underlying problem. The EMT must look further—beyond the rapid pulse; pale, cool, clammy skin; anxiety; thirst; and nausea—to the underlying cause. Instead of a separate list of all these signs and symptoms, in Section II the term "adrenaline response" is used to indicate this common compensatory action when it may be present.

The EMT must also keep in mind that some patients may not exhibit signs of an adrenaline response or may be unable to develop an adrenaline response when it normally would be expected. This may occur for a variety of reasons, the most frequent being the use of certain prescribed drugs or the presence of specific underlying diseases. Drugs such as some antihypertensives (beta blockers), antidepressants, and antiarrhythmics may prevent the patient from being able to exhibit an adrenaline response. For these reasons, the EMT must focus on the overall patient assessment, particularly the patient's general appearance, symptoms, history, and examination findings.

Respiratory Distress

■ DYSPNEA (SHORTNESS OF BREATH)

DEFINITION.   A subjective difficulty in breathing; a sensation of not getting enough air. The respiratory rate is increased and the patient may only be able to speak in short phrases.

Causes	Characteristics	Immediate Action
Congestive heart failure (CHF)/ pulmonary edema	The patient usually has a past cardiac history. Rales, frothy cough, and a nocturnal onset are characteristic signs. The patient's breathing will be positionally dependent (orthopnea).	Place the patient in an upright, sitting position. Provide high-flow oxygen. Assist ventilations if necessary. Monitor for patient exhaustion and respiratory failure.
Chronic obstructive pulmonary disease (COPD)	The patient most likely has a past history of lung disease and a recent history of yellow-green sputum. He/she may present with pursed lip breathing, dyspnea and be in a sitting position. All lung fields may be silent in severe cases.	Low-flow oxygen should be used initially. High-flow oxygen should be given only if respiratory distress does not improve. Monitor for patient exhaustion and respiratory failure. Prepare to assist ventilations if needed. Project an attitude of calmness and reassurance.
Airway obstruction (partial)	Information learned from the history of the present incident will likely lead the EMT to be suspicious of an airway obstruction. The patient may have stridor, hoarseness, dyspnea and drooling and be reluctant to swallow.	If air exchange is good, provide high-flow oxygen and transport. If air exchange is poor, assist ventilations, request ALS, and provide rapid transport. Be prepared to perform complete airway obstruction relief maneuvers.

Causes	Characteristics	Immediate Action
Croup	Croup commonly occurs between the ages of 6 months and 3 years. The patient may present with stridor and a barking cough. The presentation of symptoms may be sudden and often occurs during bedtime.	Provide cool low flow oxygen (humidified if available). Handle the patient gently. Request ALS if severe respiratory distress is present.
Epiglottitis	Signs and symptoms develop rapidly in a previously well patient. While most common in children 2–7 years of age, it can occur at any age. Symptoms include hoarseness and pain on swallowing. Signs include leaning forward with chin thrust out, drooling, stridor, use of accessory breathing muscles, and high fever.	Provide high-flow oxygen (humidified if available). Avoid any stimulation of the mouth or throat (no oral airway, no suctioning). Request ALS, and provide rapid but gentle transport.
Anaphylaxis	The patient often has a past medical history of hypersensitivity (allergic reaction) and a present history of exposure. Signs and symptoms include itching, swelling, rash, hives, hoarseness, difficulty swallowing, stridor, hypotension, and tachycardia.	Provide high-flow oxygen. If hypotensive, position flat with legs elevated. Consider military antishock trousers (MAST), preferably inflating legs only. Request ALS and provide rapid transport.
Pulmonary embolism	The onset of symptoms is sudden. There may be a history of recent inactivity (such as postsurgery), pregnancy, inflamed veins, heart valve surgery, or birth control pill use. Signs include pink sputum (hemoptysis), wheezes (audible near the pain source), and tachycardia. Progression to cardiovascular collapse and shock may occur.	Provide high-flow oxygen. Treat for shock if hypotensive. Request ALS and provide rapid transport.

Causes	Characteristics	Immediate Action
Simple pneumo-thorax (spontaneous)	Symptoms may be sudden and include sharp unilateral chest pain, a history of vigorous coughing, and decreased lung sounds unilaterally.	Provide oxygen. Avoid positive pressure ventilation if possible. Place in a position of comfort or, if lying, with affected side down (this occasionally helps).
Tension pneumothorax	Often there is a history of a simple pneumothorax or a traumatic chest injury. Signs include decreased lung sounds unilaterally, tachycardia, hypotension, and possible tracheal shift in the late stages.	Provide high-flow oxygen. Assist ventilations with bag-valve mask if necessary. Treat for shock. Request ALS and provide rapid transport.
Pneumonia	Signs and symptoms include fever, shaking, chills, chest pain on inspiration, productive cough with dark sputum, and rales or rhonchi usually involving only one lung.	Provide oxygen. If respiratory distress is present, provide high-flow oxygen. Place the patient in a position of comfort (usually a sitting position). Provide transport.

■ HYPOVENTILATION

DEFINITION.   A reduced rate and/or depth of breathing, resulting in a decreased exchange of air. Rates less than 10/min usually do not exchange enough air. The depth of ventilation is inadequate when breath sounds are audible only at the top portion of the lungs.

IMMEDIATE ACTION.   **Provide high-flow oxygen and ventilatory assistance. Provide rapid transport to ALS services.**

Causes	Characteristics	Immediate Action
Chest injury: pneumo- or hemothorax	These injuries may involve a penetrating injury with a sucking wound, or a blunt injury with multiple rib fractures. A flail chest wall segment with paradoxical chest movement may be present along with unilaterally reduced breath sounds.	Immediately seal any sucking chest wounds. Provide high-flow oxygen. Assure airway control and provide ventilatory assistance if respiratory distress continues. Position with injured side down if possible. Observe for possible progression to a tension pneumothorax.

Causes	Characteristics	Immediate Action
Cerebral injury: trauma or cerebrovascular accident (CVA)	The patient may have a traumatic head injury or may display signs of a closed head injury. Unilateral paralysis or sensory loss may be evident along with an altered level of consciousness.	Provide high-flow oxygen. Assure airway control and provide ventilatory assistance if needed.
Drugs (depressants)	There often is a past or present history of opiate or substance abuse. Pinpoint pupils and respiratory depression are the hallmark characteristics.	Provide oxygen. Increase to high-flow oxygen if respiratory distress or depression is found. Assure airway control and provide ventilatory assistance if needed. Request ALS if there is an altered mental status or inadequate ventilations.
Hypothermia	The patient typically has a history of cold exposure or, in the elderly, the exposure may be due to a cool environment with prolonged immobility (e.g., fall with trauma). The skin is cold and the mental status is altered. Drugs and/or alcohol may be involved.	Provide high-flow oxygen. Assure airway control and provide ventilatory assistance as needed. Rewarm the core before the extremities using heated oxygen and/or hot packs to the chest and neck. Request ALS and provide rapid, gentle transport.

■ Hyperventilation

Definition. An increased rate and/or depth of breathing. Rates of greater than 20/min are excessive.

Causes	Characteristics	Immediate Action
Shock	Shock may result in hypotension from hypovolemia or blood loss, cardiac pump failure, or vasodilation. Signs of adrenaline response are present, including rapid pulse, pallor, diaphoresis, and nausea.	Provide high-flow oxygen. Control any major bleeding. Maintain body heat. Consider antishock trousers (MAST) for multisystem trauma of the pelvis or lower extremities, neurogenic shock, or anaphylactic shock. Request ALS and provide rapid transport.

Causes	Characteristics	Immediate Action
COPD	The patient most likely has a past history of lung disease and a recent history of yellow-green sputum. He/she may present with pursed lip breathing, dyspnea and be in a sitting position. All lung fields may be silent in severe cases.	Low-flow oxygen should be used initially. High-flow oxygen should be given only if respiratory distress does not improve. Monitor for patient exhaustion and respiratory failure. Prepare to assist ventilations if needed. Project an attitude of calmness and reassurance.
CHF/pulmonary edema	The patient usually has a past cardiac history. Rales, frothy cough, and a nocturnal onset are characteristic signs. The patient's breathing will be positionally dependent (orthopnea).	Place the patient in an upright, sitting position. Provide high-flow oxygen. Assist ventilations if necessary. Monitor for patient exhaustion and respiratory failure.
Airway obstruction (partial)	Information learned from the history of the present incident will likely lead the EMT to be suspicious of an airway obstruction. The patient may have stridor, hoarseness, dyspnea and drooling and be reluctant to swallow.	If air exchange is good, provide high-flow oxygen and transport. If air exchange is poor, assist ventilations, request ALS, and provide rapid transport. Be prepared to perform complete airway obstruction relief maneuvers.
Pain	Usually caused by an injury or illness.	Treat the underlying cause of the pain. Project an attitude of calmness and reassurance.
Anxiety	Peripheral numbness and tingling are sometimes present. Lung sounds are normal. The patient may have a high systolic pressure with a normal diastolic pressure.	Project an attitude of calmness and reassurance. Low-flow oxygen may assist in alleviating the anxiety. If the symptoms persist, a paper bag or non-rebreather mask may be used (*use with caution*).
Drugs (stimulants)	There is likely to be a past or present history of stimulant or substance abuse. Stimulants may also be found in cola drinks, coffee, and tea. The signs and symptoms include agitation and tachycardia.	Provide low-flow oxygen. Project an attitude of calmness and reassurance. Call the local poison control center for assistance if needed.

■ DIAPHRAGMATIC BREATHING

DEFINITION.   Breathing efforts performed by the contraction of the diaphragm alone, without the assistance of the intercostal muscles. The upper abdomen often bulges with inspiration. There is minimal chest wall movement.

Causes	Characteristics	Immediate Action
Airway obstruction (complete)	Information learned from the history of the present incident will likely lead the EMT to be suspicious of an airway obstruction. There may be intercostal and supraclavicular retractions without air exchange. The patient is unable to speak.	Reposition the airway and provide abdominal thrusts for the child and adult (see Chapter 8). Reposition the airway, and provide back blows and chest thrusts for the infant (see Chapter 8).
Spinal cord injury	There is information from the history causing suspicion of a spinal cord injury above C6.	Immediately stabilize the cervical spine manually. Provide high-flow oxygen. Assist ventilations if needed. Place the patient supine and secure to a backboard.

■ ABNORMAL LUNG SOUNDS

Stridor

DEFINITION.   A shrill, high-pitched sound heard on inhalation, originating in the narrowing of the upper airway.

Causes	Characteristics	Immediate Action
Anaphylaxis	The patient often has a past medical history of hypersensitivity (allergic reaction) and a present history of exposure. Signs and symptoms include itching, swelling, rash, hives, hoarseness, difficulty swallowing, stridor, hypotension, dyspnea, and tachycardia.	Provide high-flow oxygen. If hypotensive, position flat with legs elevated. Consider antishock trousers (MAST), preferably inflating legs only. Request ALS and provide rapid transport.

Causes	Characteristics	Immediate Action
Croup	Croup commonly occurs between the ages of 6 months and 3 years. The patient may present with stridor, dyspnea, and a barking cough. The presentation of symptoms may be sudden and often occurs during bedtime.	Provide cool low flow oxygen (humidified if available). Handle the patient gently. Request ALS if severe respiratory distress is present.
Epiglottitis	Signs and symptoms develop rapidly in a previously well patient. While most common in children 2–7 years of age, it can occur at any age. Symptoms include hoarseness and pain on swallowing. Signs include leaning forward with chin thrust out, drooling, stridor, dyspnea, use of accessory breathing muscles, and high fever.	Provide high-flow oxygen (humidified if available). Avoid any stimulation of the mouth or throat (no oral airway, no suctioning). Request ALS, and provide rapid but gentle transport.
Airway obstruction (partial)	Information learned from the history of the present incident will likely lead the EMT to be suspicious of an airway obstruction. The patient may have stridor, hoarseness, drooling, and dyspnea and be reluctant to swallow.	If air exchange is good, provide high-flow oxygen and transport. If air exchange is poor, assist ventilations, request ALS, and provide rapid transport. Be prepared to perform complete airway obstruction relief maneuvers.
Trauma to the neck	The history of the incident indicates an injury to the neck. The patient may present with dyspnea, hoarseness, drooling, rapid respiratory rate, and reluctance to swallow.	Immediately occlude any trauma to large neck blood vessels using direct pressure and an occlusive dressing. If air exchange is good, provide high-flow oxygen. If air exchange is poor, assist ventilations, request ALS, and provide rapid transport. Consider cervical spine immobilization.

Wheezes

DEFINITION.   High-pitched, whistling noises produced by air flowing through narrowed smaller airways. Just as pursing the lips produces a whistle, wheezes can sound musical. They are often audible without a stethoscope. Wheezing is usually louder during the expiratory phase.

Causes	Characteristics	Immediate Action
Airway obstruction (partial)	Information learned from the history of the present incident will likely lead the EMT to be suspicious of an airway obstruction. The patient may have stridor, hoarseness, drooling, and dyspnea, and be reluctant to swallow.	If air exchange is good, provide high-flow oxygen and transport. If air exchange is poor, assist ventilations, request ALS, and provide rapid transport. Be prepared to perform complete airway obstruction relief maneuvers.
Asthma	The patient has a past medical history of asthma. The onset of the acute attack is usually rapid. Dyspnea and prolonged expiration with quick inspiration are seen. The patient may have attempted to gain relief with home meds without success.	Provide low flow oxygen (humidified if available) initially. Place the patient in a sitting position. Project an attitude of calmness and reassurance.
CHF/pulmonary edema	The patient usually has a past cardiac history. Rales, frothy cough, dyspnea, and a nocturnal onset are characteristic signs. The patient's breathing will be positionally dependent (orthopnea).	Place the patient in an upright, sitting position. Provide high-flow oxygen. Assist ventilations if necessary. Monitor for patient exhaustion and respiratory failure.
Pulmonary embolism	The onset of symptoms is sudden. There may be a history of recent inactivity (such as postsurgery), pregnancy, inflamed veins, heart valve surgery, or birth control pill use. Signs include pink sputum (hemoptysis), dyspnea, wheezes (audible near the pain source), and tachycardia. Progression to cardiovascular collapse and shock may occur.	Provide high-flow oxygen. Treat for shock if hypotensive. Request ALS and provide rapid transport.
Anaphylaxis	The patient often has a past medical history of hypersensitivity (allergic reaction) and a present history of exposure. Signs and symptoms include itching, swelling, rash, hives, hoarseness, difficulty swallowing, stridor, hypotension, dyspnea, and tachycardia.	Provide high-flow oxygen. If hypotensive, position flat with legs elevated. Consider antishock trousers (MAST), preferably inflating legs only. Request ALS and provide rapid transport.

Rales and Rhonchi

DEFINITION.   *Rales* are fine crackling sounds much like the sound produced by rolling strands of hair between the fingers, next to your ear. They originate from fluid in the alveoli. The greater the amount of fluid, the louder and more bubbly the sound. Significant amounts of fluid may result in quiet lung bases. *Rhonchi* originate from fluid or mucus in the bronchioles or bronchi, and are louder, coarser, and wetter than rales.

Causes	Characteristics	Immediate Action
CHF/pulmonary edema	The patient usually has a past cardiac history. Rales, frothy cough, dyspnea, and a nocturnal onset are characteristic signs. The patient's breathing will be positionally dependent (orthopnea).	Place the patient in an upright, sitting position. Provide high-flow oxygen. Assist ventilations if necessary. Monitor for patient exhaustion and respiratory failure.
COPD	The patient most likely has a past history of lung disease and a recent history of yellow-green sputum. He/she may present with pursed lip breathing and dyspnea and be in a sitting position. All lung fields may be silent in severe cases.	Low-flow oxygen should be used initially. High-flow oxygen should be given only if respiratory distress does not improve. Monitor for patient exhaustion and respiratory failure. Prepare to assist ventilations if needed. Project an attitude of calmness and reassurance.
Pneumonia	Signs and symptoms include fever, shaking chills, chest pain on inspiration, productive cough with dark sputum, and rales or rhonchi usually involving only one lung.	Provide oxygen. If respiratory distress is present, provide high-flow oxygen. Place the patient in a position of comfort (usually a sitting position). Provide transport.

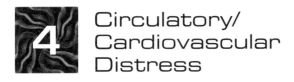

Circulatory/ Cardiovascular Distress

■ **CHEST PAIN**

DEFINITION. Subjective sensation, often described as "heavy," "squeezing," "crushing," "tight," or the like. Ask the patient about onset, pain/provocation, quality, radiation, severity, time of onset, location, and alleviation (OPQRST). Also ask about associated symptoms such as nausea, dyspnea, and diaphoresis. Obtain a SAMPLE history.

Causes	Characteristics	Immediate Action
CARDIAC		
Myocardial infarction (MI) (heart attack)	The patient complains of substernal chest pain, which is almost never sharp or knife-like, that may radiate to the arms, neck, shoulders, or jaw; weakness; dizziness; palpitations; nausea; and a sense of doom. Signs include dyspnea, tachycardia, pallor, and diaphoresis. An irregular pulse is sometimes present, and some types of MIs result in a slow pulse.	Begin with low-flow oxygen. Provide high-flow oxygen if respiratory distress, altered mental status, or shock is present. Handle the patient gently, and minimize all exertion or anxiety. Place in a semireclining position. Monitor the patient closely for possible onset of cardiogenic shock, pulmonary edema, or cardiac arrest. If one is available and you are authorized to use it, have an automated external defibrillator (AED) nearby. Project an attitude of calmness and reassurance. Request ALS and provide rapid transport.

Causes	Characteristics	Immediate Action
Angina	The patient often has a history of angina. He/she may complain of substernal chest pain that radiates to the arms, shoulders, neck, or jaw. Onset may be with exertion, cold, meals, or emotional stress. Angina is often relieved by rest and nitroglycerin. Duration should be less than 20 minutes.	Provide low-flow oxygen. Avoid exertion or anxiety. Assist with nitroglycerin if you are trained and authorized. Project an attitude of calmness and reassurance.
Pericarditis	The patient may complain of continuous substernal or precordial pain. The pain may be positional in nature. Dyspnea, fever, and tachycardia may be present.	Provide oxygen. Place the patient in a position of comfort.

PULMONARY

Causes	Characteristics	Immediate Action
Dyspnea	See Chapter 3	
Pulmonary embolism	The patient may complain of a sharp chest pain with a sudden onset. There may be a history of recent inactivity (such as postsurgery), pregnancy, inflamed lower extremity veins, heart valve surgery, or birth control pill use. Signs and symptoms include pink sputum, wheezes (may be audible near the pain source), dyspnea, and tachycardia. Signs may progress to cardiovascular collapse.	Provide high-flow oxygen. Treat for shock if hypotensive. Assure airway control and provide ventilatory assistance if needed. Request ALS and provide rapid transport.

Causes	Characteristics	Immediate Action
Simple pneumothorax	The patient may complain of sharp, unilateral chest pain with a sudden onset. There may be a history of some precipitating incident such as trauma or vigorous coughing. This often occurs in thin, young men. Dyspnea and unilaterally decreased lung sounds are noted.	Provide high-flow oxygen. Avoid positive pressure ventilation if possible. Place the patient in a position of comfort or, if lying, with affected side down (this may occasionally help). Monitor for progression to a tension pneumothorax.
Tension pneumothorax	There is a history of a simple pneumothorax or a traumatic chest injury. Unilaterally decreased lung sounds, tachycardia, and hypotension are characteristic. The trachea may shift in the late stages.	Provide high-flow oxygen. Examine for a sucking chest wound. Provide bag-valve mask ventilations if necessary. Treat for shock. Request ALS and provide rapid transport.
Pleurisy (pleuritis)	There is localized pain that increases with deep inspiration or coughing. It may be associated with a pulmonary embolism or infection.	Provide low-flow oxygen. Place the patient in a position of comfort.

OTHER CAUSES

Causes	Characteristics	Immediate Action
Chest wall muscles	There is unilateral pain that is aggravated by movement (twisting, bending, deep inspiration) or palpation. The patient may be splinting the chest wall with his/her arm.	Provide low-flow oxygen. Examine to rule out traumatic injury such as pneumothorax, cardiac tamponade, rib fracture, or lacerated liver or spleen. Transport in a position of comfort.
Aortic aneurysm	The patient often has a history of hypertension. Aortic aneurysm is often associated with syncope. Pain may radiate to the abdomen, back, one leg, or groin. A pulsatile abdominal mass is noted on palpation above the umbilicus.	Provide low-flow oxygen. If dyspneic, hypotensive, or showing signs of shock, provide high-flow oxygen. Position flat with legs elevated if needed. Request ALS and provide rapid transport.

Causes	Characteristics	Immediate Action
Esophagitis	This often follows eating. The patient may complain of a substernal burning pain, often located along the vertical aspect of the sternum. The "burning" is often relieved by antacids.	Place in a sitting position. Provide low-flow oxygen.
Gallbladder inflammation (cholecystitis)	The pain is usually in the right lower chest, right upper abdominal quadrant, or midepigastric area. Radiation to the right scapula or directly posterior to the epigastrium is common. The onset is often after eating.	No immediate action is necessary. Because of the sometimes severe pain, project an attitude of calmness and reassurance.
Anxiety	The patient may be hyperventilating and often notes peripheral numbness and tingling. The lung sounds are normal. The patient may have a high systolic pressure with a normal diastolic pressure.	Provide low-flow oxygen. Project an attitude of calmness and reassurance. Use a paper bag or rebreather mask if the symptoms persist (*use with caution*).

■ TACHYCARDIA

DEFINITION.   An increased heart rate (adults: over 100 beats/min; infants: over 140 beats/min).

Causes	Characteristics	Immediate Action
Shock	Characterized by signs of an adrenaline response: tachycardia, pallor, diaphoresis, and nausea. It results in hypotension, which may be from hypovolemia, cardiac pump failure, or vasodilation.	Provide high-flow oxygen. Position flat with legs elevated. Consider antishock trousers (MAST) for hypovolemic shock at the direction of medical control (inflate legs only for neurogenic or anaphylactic shock). Request ALS and provide rapid transport.

Causes	Characteristics	Immediate Action
MI (heart attack)	The patient complains of substernal chest pain, which is almost never sharp or knife-like, that may radiate to the arms, neck, shoulders, or jaw; weakness; dizziness; palpitations; nausea; and a sense of doom. Signs include dyspnea, tachycardia, pallor, and diaphoresis. An irregular pulse is sometimes present and some types of MIs result in a slow pulse.	Begin with low-flow oxygen. Provide high-flow oxygen if respiratory distress, altered mental status, or shock is present. Handle the patient gently, and minimize all exertion or anxiety. Place in a semireclining position. Monitor the patient closely for possible onset of cardiogenic shock, pulmonary edema, or cardiac arrest. If one is available and you are authorized to use it, have an AED nearby. Project an attitude of calmness and reassurance. Request ALS and provide rapid transport.
Pain or fear	Often caused by an injury.	Treat the underlying cause (the injury). Place the patient in a position of comfort. Project an attitude of calmness and reassurance.
Anxiety	The patient may be hyperventilating and often notes peripheral numbness and tingling. The lung sounds are normal. The patient may have a high systolic pressure with a normal diastolic pressure.	Provide low-flow oxygen. Project an attitude of calmness and reassurance. Use a paper bag or rebreather mask if the symptoms persist (*use with caution*).
Drugs (stimulants)	There may be a history of past or present abuse of stimulant drugs. This can include cola drinks, coffee, or tea in addition to recreational stimulant drugs. The patient may be hyperventilating and tachycardic.	Provide low-flow oxygen. Call the local poison control center for assistance. Project an attitude of calmness and reassurance.

Causes	Characteristics	Immediate Action
Electrical conduction abnormality	The patient may have a known history of tachycardia with a sudden onset. The tachycardia may result in hypotension and/or chest pain.	Provide low-flow oxygen. Provide high-flow oxygen if associated with hypotension, respiratory distress, or an altered mental status. Attach an ECG monitor if you are trained and authorized. Request ALS.

■ BRADYCARDIA

DEFINITION.   A decreased heart rate (adults: less than 60 beats/min). Well-trained athletes may have resting rates as low as 40 beats/min without adverse effects.

IMMEDIATE ACTION.   **Oxygen therapy.**

Causes	Characteristics	Immediate Action
Head injury	Injury may be caused by trauma or have a medical cause. The patient may be hypoventilating and hypertensive.	Provide high-flow oxygen. Assure airway control and provide ventilatory assistance if needed. Position with head slightly elevated. Request ALS and provide rapid transport.
Pacemaker failure	There is a past cardiac history and a palpable pacemaker implanted under the skin in the upper chest. The patient may have a pacemaker ID card in his/her wallet or on a medical alert tag.	Provide low-flow oxygen. Provide high-flow oxygen if associated with hypotension, respiratory distress, or an altered mental status. Monitor closely; be prepared for cardiac arrest. Attach an ECG monitor if you are trained and authorized. Request ALS and provide rapid transport.

Causes	Characteristics	Immediate Action
Drugs (depressants)	There is often a history of opiate or sedative use. The patient may be hypoventilating.	Provide low-flow oxygen initially. Increase to high-flow oxygen if hypotensive, dyspneic, or with an altered mental status. Assure airway control and provide ventilatory assistance if needed. Call the local poison control center for assistance. Request ALS if the patient has an altered mental status, inadequate ventilations or signs of shock. Transport.
Shock (terminal stage)	In this stage, hypotension from hypovolemia, cardiac pump failure, or vasodilation is uncompensated. The patient is near cardiovascular collapse.	Provide high-flow oxygen. Position flat with legs elevated. Maintain body heat. Provide ventilatory assistance if needed. Consider antishock trousers (MAST) for hypovolemic shock (inflate legs only for neurogenic and anaphylactic shock). Request ALS and provide rapid transport.
Hypoxemia (terminal stage)	The patient has a massive injury (injuries) or a severe illness.	Provide high-flow oxygen. Treat for shock. Request ALS and provide rapid transport.

■ HYPOTENSION

DEFINITION.   Systolic blood pressure less than 90 mm Hg. Postural hypotension exists when there is an increase in pulse rate of 20 beats/min or more, or a decrease in systolic pressure of 20 mm Hg or more, when the patient is moved from a lying to a standing position.

Causes	Characteristics	Immediate Action
Hypovolemia	Fluid loss may be from external hemorrhage; internal hemorrhage (dissecting or ruptured aortic aneurysm, ruptured ectopic pregnancy, gastrointestinal bleeding); or plasma volume loss (burns, ascites, dehydration, hyperglycemia). Signs and symptoms are specific to the cause. Signs of adrenaline response are present, including tachycardia, pallor, diaphoresis, and nausea.	Provide high-flow oxygen. Position flat with legs elevated. Maintain body heat. Consider antishock trousers (MAST). Request ALS and provide rapid transport.
Cardiogenic shock	The patient may have cardiac pump failure from a heart attack, heart failure, or trauma (cardiac tamponade, tension pneumothorax). Signs and symptoms are specific to the cause. Signs of right heart failure include distended neck veins and peripheral edema. Signs of left heart failure include pulmonary edema and dyspnea. Signs of an adrenaline response are also noted.	Provide high-flow oxygen. Position flat. Monitor closely for the development of pulmonary edema. Be prepared to provide ventilatory assistance. Request ALS and provide rapid transport.
Vasodilation	May be caused by peripheral pooling of the blood from sepsis, anaphylaxis, or neurogenesis (central nervous system (CNS) injury, overdose). Signs and symptoms are specific to the cause but include tachycardia, diaphoresis, and nausea with warm, pink skin.	Provide high-flow oxygen. Position flat with legs elevated. Maintain body heat. Consider antishock trousers (MAST), preferably legs only inflated. Request ALS and provide rapid transport.

■ HYPERTENSION

DEFINITION. Systolic blood pressure of over 140 mm Hg or diastolic pressure of over 90 mm Hg. Malignant hypertension exists when the blood pressure is dangerously high, often 200/140 mm Hg or higher. Hypertension can be associated with (although it is not caused by) CVA, aortic aneurysm, CHF/pulmonary edema, or angina.

Causes	Characteristics	Immediate Action
Head injury	Injury may be caused by trauma or have a medical cause. The patient may be hypoventilating and bradycardic.	Provide high-flow oxygen. Assure airway control and provide ventilatory assistance if needed. Position with head slightly elevated. Request ALS and provide rapid transport.
Essential hypertension (cause unknown)	The patient has a past medical history of hypertension.	Provide oxygen. Keep head slightly elevated.
Toxemia of pregnancy	Toxemia is often associated with the first pregnancy. The patient may complain of a headache. Signs include edema, seizures, and an altered mental status.	Provide high-flow oxygen. Assure airway control and provide ventilatory support if needed. Minimize external stimulation. Request ALS and provide rapid transport.
Anxiety	The patient may be hyperventilating and often notes peripheral numbness and tingling. The lung sounds are normal. The patient may have a high systolic pressure with a normal diastolic pressure.	Provide low-flow oxygen. Project an attitude of calmness and reassurance. Use a paper bag or rebreather mask if the symptoms persist (*use with caution*).

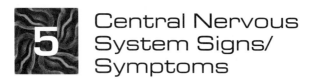

Central Nervous System Signs/ Symptoms

■ HEADACHE

DEFINITION.   A subjective sensation of pain in the head. Headache can be seen in a wide variety of medical conditions. Its onset can be gradual or very sudden. This section is only concerned with the headache of sudden, acute onset.

Causes	Characteristics	Immediate Action
Stroke (CVA): hemorrhage	Signs and symptoms of CVA include a severe, localized headache of sudden onset; stiff neck or neck pain; a history of hypertension; and present hypertension. Rapid progression to coma may occur.	Provide high-flow oxygen. Assure airway control and provide ventilatory assistance if needed. Position the patient with the head slightly elevated. Perform a focused exam. Request ALS and provide rapid transport.
Toxemia of pregnancy (eclampsia)	Toxemia is often associated with the first pregnancy. It is characterized by edema, hypertension, seizures, and an altered mental status.	Provide high-flow oxygen. Assure airway control and provide ventilatory assistance if needed. Minimize external stimulation. Perform a focused exam. Request ALS and provide rapid transport.
Chemical agent: carbon monoxide	There is a history of a toxic environment. The patient may complain of lethargy, nausea, and vomiting. Confusion and an altered mental status may occur with higher exposures.	Safely remove the patient from the toxic environment. Provide high-flow oxygen. Assure airway control and provide ventilatory assistance if needed.
Hypertension	The patient may have a past medical history of hypertension. Nosebleeds are often associated with hypertension. Diastolic pressures are >120 mm Hg.	Provide oxygen. Assure airway control and provide ventilatory assistance if needed. Position the patient with the head slightly elevated.

Causes	Characteristics	Immediate Action
Meningitis	The onset of symptoms may be sudden or progress over hours. The patient may complain of a stiff neck. Fever, rash, and an altered mental status may be noted in the exam.	Take appropriate communicable disease precautions (mask, etc.). Provide oxygen. Assure airway control and provide ventilatory assistance if needed.

■ Paralysis

DEFINITION. A reduction or complete loss of the ability to move. Partial paralysis may appear as subtle weakness or lack of coordination.

Causes	Characteristics	Immediate Action
Stroke (CVA)	Signs and symptoms include a headache, unilateral paralysis, difficulty with swallowing and speech, a history of hypertension, present hypertension, and a history of atherosclerosis. The patient may have an altered mental status.	Provide oxygen. Increase oxygen to high flow if mental status is altered. Assure airway control and provide ventilatory assistance if needed. Position the patient with the head slightly elevated. Perform a focused exam.
Head injury: trauma	The patient has a history of a traumatic mechanism of injury. The patient may present with bradycardia, hypertension, and hypoventilation. An altered mental status may be noted. Rapid progression to coma may occur.	Maintain cervical spine immobilization. Provide high-flow oxygen. Assure airway control and provide ventilatory assistance if needed. Secure patient to a backboard with the head of the board slightly elevated if possible. Request ALS and provide rapid transport.
Cervical spine injury: trauma	There is a history of a traumatic mechanism of injury. The patient may experience paralysis below the clavicles. Diaphragmatic breathing may be noted.	Maintain cervical spine immobilization. Provide high-flow oxygen. Assure airway control and provide ventilatory assistance if needed. Secure patient to a backboard. Request ALS and provide rapid transport.

Causes	Characteristics	Immediate Action
Thoracic spine injury: trauma	There is a history of a traumatic mechanism of injury. The patient may experience paralysis below the chest or waist. The lower extremities may be cool.	Maintain cervical spine immobilization. Provide high-flow oxygen. Assure airway control and provide ventilatory assistance if needed. Secure patient to a backboard. Request ALS and provide rapid transport.
Chemical agent: poisoning, snakebite, insect bite	There is a history of exposure to a poisonous agent. Full bilateral paralysis may be present.	Safely remove the patient from the cause. Treat for the cause. Isolate the exposure site. Provide high-flow oxygen. Attempt to safely identify the source of poison if possible.

■ COMA

DEFINITION.   Unresponsiveness to both verbal and painful stimuli. Because injury or illness in any of the body's systems may lead to coma, it is important not to rely on one major clue and ignore other important findings. For example, the injured patient may have a medical problem that led to the injury. Likewise, the comatose patient who smells of alcohol may have a head injury or a diabetic emergency.

IMMEDIATE ACTION.   High-flow oxygen, airway control, and ventilatory support. Thorough exam. Careful monitoring. Position patient on his/her side to protect the airway.

Causes	Characteristics	Immediate Action
ANATOMIC/STRUCTURAL		
Trauma: head injury	The patient has a history of a traumatic mechanism of injury. The patient may present with bradycardia, hypertension, and hypoventilation. An altered mental status may be noted. Rapid progression to coma may occur.	Maintain cervical spine immobilization. Provide high-flow oxygen. Assure airway control and provide ventilatory assistance if needed. Secure patient to a backboard with the head of the board slightly elevated if possible. Request ALS and provide rapid transport.

Causes	Characteristics	Immediate Action
CVA: ischemia/ hemorrhage	Signs and symptoms of CVA include a headache, unilateral paralysis, difficulty with swallowing and speech, a history of hypertension, present hypertension, and a history of atherosclerosis. The patient may have an altered mental status and progress to coma.	Provide high-flow oxygen when mental status is altered. Assure airway control and provide ventilatory assistance if needed. Position the patient with the head slightly elevated. Perform a focused exam. Request ALS and provide rapid transport.
Shock: insufficient cerebral circulation	Hypotension may result from hypovolemia, cardiac pump failure, or vasodilation. Signs of adrenaline response, including tachycardia, pallor, and diaphoresis, may be present.	Provide high-flow oxygen. Assure airway control and provide ventilatory assistance if needed. If patient is hypotensive, position flat with legs elevated. Maintain body heat. Consider antishock trousers (MAST) for hypovolemic, neurogenic, or anaphylactic shock. Request ALS and provide rapid transport.
Seizure: postictal (see also Seizures [Convulsions])	The patient may have a history of convulsions.	Protect the patient from injury. Provide high-flow oxygen initially. Assure airway control and provide ventilatory assistance if needed. Once convulsion has stopped, perform focused history and physical exam.

METABOLIC

Hypoglycemia (low blood sugar)	The patient may have a history of diabetes. Onset is relatively sudden. The patient may be drooling and have an adrenaline response characterized by tachycardia, pallor, and diaphoresis.	Provide high-flow oxygen. Assure airway control, and suction if needed. Perform a focused exam, including blood sugar level if available. Provide sugar (40% dextrose in oral liquid preparation placed inside the cheek in small amounts) only if the patient is able to control his/her own airway. For patients who remain comatose or have an altered mental status (without airway control), request ALS.

Causes	Characteristics	Immediate Action
Hyperglycemia (high blood sugar)	The patient may or may not have a history of diabetes. The onset is gradual, often with a history of a recent infection or illness. The patient presents with hyperventilation, ketone-smelling breath, fever, dehydration, and tachycardia.	Provide high-flow oxygen. Assure airway control and provide ventilatory assistance if needed. Perform blood sugar level check if available. If in doubt whether the patient has low or high blood sugar, give 40% dextrose orally as for hypoglycemia for the noncomatose patient. Request ALS and provide rapid transport.
Oxygen deficit: hypoxia	There often is a history of exposure to a toxic environment (asphyxia, toxic gas). There is obvious respiratory distress (see Chapter 3). The patient may have an altered mental status and tachycardia.	Safely remove the patient from the harmful environment. Provide high-flow oxygen. Assure airway control and provide ventilatory assistance if needed. Request ALS and provide rapid transport.
Drug/alcohol overdose	There is usually a history of drug or alcohol abuse. The patient may have respiratory depression.	Provide high-flow oxygen. Assure airway control and provide ventilatory assistance if needed. Perform a focused exam. Attempt to identify the drug or substance of abuse. Save any vomitus if possible.
Infection (septicemia, meningitis, etc.)	The patient has a history of a recent illness, usually with fever. Complaints may also include a stiff neck, rash, or febrile seizures in children.	Provide high-flow oxygen. Assure airway control. Perform a focused exam. Provide slow cooling for a febrile seizure if needed. Consider communicable disease precautions (mask, etc.).

Causes	Characteristics	Immediate Action
Heat stroke	The patient will have hot, red skin (see Chapter 7). Signs and symptoms include nausea, headache, abnormal behavior, seizure, syncope, and altered mental status.	Safely remove patient from the hot environment. Provide high-flow oxygen. Assure airway control and provide ventilatory assistance if needed. Rapidly cool using ice packs at groin, armpits, and neck. Request ALS and provide rapid transport.
Other: imbalance of the body chemistry; failure of organ systems (liver, kidney, thyroid, adrenal); or CO_2 narcosis (COPD)	Signs and symptoms are specific to the cause; for example, jaundice and distended abdomen (ascites) in a known alcoholic suggest hepatic coma.	Provide high-flow oxygen. Assure airway control and provide ventilatory support if needed. Attempt to gain as much history as possible. Request ALS and provide rapid transport.

PSYCHIATRIC

Causes	Characteristics	Immediate Action
Psychogenic ("pseudo-coma")	The history of the incident usually provides sufficient information to characterize this form of coma.	Handle patient cautiously. Project an attitude of calmness and reassurance.

■ SYNCOPE (FAINTING)

DEFINITION. A transient state of unconsciousness from which the victim has recovered. A patient who is unresponsive for longer than 3 minutes in the supine position is considered to be in a coma (see previous section).

Causes	Characteristics	Immediate Action
Cardiac rhythm disturbance (Stokes-Adams)	The patient is typically elderly and is found with an irregular, slow pulse.	Position patient flat with legs elevated. Provide high-flow oxygen. Attach ECG monitor if you are trained and so authorized. Document the ECG. Request ALS.

Causes	Characteristics	Immediate Action
Postural hypotension	Hypotension may be from hypovolemia, cardiac pump failure, or vasodilation.	Position patient flat with legs elevated. Provide high-flow oxygen. Assure airway control. Perform a thorough exam and assessment. Request ALS and provide rapid transport.
Venous pooling (orthostatic)	The patient may have a history of prolonged standing, especially in the heat, or sudden standing after prolonged sitting or lying.	Position patient flat with legs elevated. Provide oxygen.
Vasovagal (vasodepressor)	The patient may have a history consistent with stimulation of the vagus nerve: neck manipulation (such as sudden turning or a tight collar), straining to urinate or defecate, or coughing. This may occur while sitting or lying. The patient may also be bradycardic.	Position patient flat with legs elevated. Provide oxygen. Loosen tight clothing.
Psychogenic (anxiety, fear, pain)	The patient may have a history of sudden pain or fear with this incident. He/she may experience hyperventilation. It may also be a staged faint ("pseudosyncope").	Position patient flat with legs elevated. Project an attitude of calmness and reassurance.
Cerebrovascular insufficiency (transient ischemic attack [TIA])	The patient often has a history of atherosclerosis, hypertension, and headache. Signs include unilateral weakness or numbness, temporary loss of speech or vision, and temporary unawareness of surroundings.	Provide oxygen. Monitor progression of symptoms and return to normal function. Project an attitude of calmness and reassurance.
Drug overdose (common prescription medicines)	The patient may have a history of taking medications such as propranolol (Inderal), insulin, diuretics (Lasix), nitroglycerin, or narcotics (Tylenol No. 3).	Position patient flat with legs elevated. Provide high-flow oxygen. Perform a focused history and physical exam. Contact local poison control center if needed.

■ SEIZURES (CONVULSIONS)

DEFINITION. A seizure is a sudden episode of involuntary muscular contraction and relaxation. It may involve generalized tonic-clonic activity (grand mal), followed by postictal unconsciousness and then confusion, or may be focal, with localized twitching or jerking. *Status epilepticus* exists when there is a rapid succession of repeated seizures without regaining of consciousness during the intervals.

IMMEDIATE ACTION. **Protect patient from injury, provide oxygen and suction, position on his/her side (recovery position) after the seizure is complete.**

Causes	Characteristics	Immediate Action
Epilepsy	The patient may have a history of this or of generalized seizures. Some patients experience an aura (visual disturbance, dizziness, etc.) prior to the seizure. The patient may be found to be incontinent, postictal, drooling, hyperventilating, and tachycardic.	Protect the patient from further injury. Provide high-flow oxygen initially. Position on his/her side (recovery position). After the patient awakens, perform a focused history and physical exam to determine if any injuries occurred.
Head injury: trauma	The patient has a history of a traumatic mechanism of injury. The patient may present with bradycardia, hypertension, and hypoventilation. An altered mental status may be noted. Rapid progression to coma may occur.	Maintain cervical spine immobilization. Provide high-flow oxygen. Assure airway control and provide ventilatory assistance if needed. Secure patient to a backboard with the head of the board slightly elevated if possible. Request ALS and provide rapid transport.
Stroke (CVA): ischemia, hemorrhage	Signs and symptoms include a headache, unilateral paralysis, difficulty with swallowing and speech, a history of hypertension, present hypertension, and a history of atherosclerosis. The patient may have an altered mental status.	Provide oxygen. Increase oxygen to high flow if mental status is altered. Assure airway control and provide ventilatory assistance if needed. Position patient with the head slightly elevated. Perform a focused exam.

Causes	Characteristics	Immediate Action
Drug/alcohol overdose or withdrawal	The patient has a history of alcohol or substance abuse. He/she may also have recently stopped his/her intake of the substance.	Provide high-flow oxygen. Assure airway control and provide ventilatory assistance if needed. Identify the substance of abuse and determine the patient's history. Position on his/her side (recovery position). Save any vomitus if possible.
Oxygen deficit: hypoxia	There often is a history of exposure to a toxic environment (asphyxia, toxic gas). There is obvious respiratory distress (see Chapter 3). The patient may have an altered mental status and tachycardia.	Safely remove the pastient from the harmful environment. Provide high-flow oxygen. Assure airway control and provide ventilatory assistance if needed. Request ALS and provide rapid transport.
Hypoglycemia (low blood sugar)	The patient may have a history of diabetes. Onset is relatively sudden. The patient may be drooling and may have an adrenaline response characterized by tachycardia, pallor, and diaphoresis.	Provide high-flow oxygen. Assure airway control, and suction if needed. Perform a focused exam, including blood sugar level if available. Provide sugar (40% dextrose in oral liquid preparation placed inside the cheek in small amounts) only if the patient is able to control his/her own airway. For patients who remain comatose or have an altered mental status (without airway control), request ALS.

Causes	Characteristics	Immediate Action
Infection: childhood febrile seizures	There is a history of a febrile illness. The child may also have a stiff neck. Check for a stiff neck while the child is in the postictal state by flexing the head forward, chest to chin.	Provide high-flow oxygen initially. Assure airway control. Perform a focused history and physical exam. Slowly cool patient by removing clothing and using tepid sponging. If the neck is stiff, use communicable disease precautions (masks, etc.) and transport.
Heat exhaustion: sodium depletion	The patient has a history of exposure and/or exertion in a hot environment. He/she may complain of heat cramps, headache, and nausea. Signs include pale, moist skin; orthostatic syncope; and tachycardia.	Safely remove patient from the hot environment. Position flat with legs elevated. Provide high-flow oxygen. Assure airway control. Cool slowly. Slowly rehydrate with oral fluids (preferably balanced electrolyte solutions) if airway control is intact.
Toxemia of pregnancy (eclampsia)	Toxemia is often associated with the first pregnancy. It is characterized by edema, hypertension, seizures, and an altered mental status.	Provide high-flow oxygen. Assure airway control and provide ventilatory assistance if needed. Minimize external stimulation. Perform a focused exam. Request ALS and provide rapid transport.
Psychogenic: "hysterical seizures"	This is characterized by bizarre random thrashing inconsistent with the tonic-clonic activity of generalized seizures.	Handle patient cautiously. Project an attitude of calmness and reassurance.

■ Pupillary Status (Table 5–1)

Definition. The pupil is the opening in the colored iris, which contracts when exposed to bright light. Both pupils should react

Table 5-1   Pupillary Status Chart

PUPIL	EQUAL		UNEQUAL	
	Reactive	Unreactive	Reactive	Unreactive

Dilated	Hypoxia
	Pain
	Drugs
	  Alcohol
	  Stimulants
	Dim light
	  (normal)
		Anoxia
		Seizures
		Drugs
		  Glutethimide
		  (Doriden)
		  Belladonna
		  (atropine)
		  Psychodelics
				CVA
				Head injury
				Eye trauma

Mid	Normal	Hypothermia Methanol	Normal in 4% of population	Glass eye

Constricted
 	
to
Pinpoint
	Bright light
	  (normal)
		Drugs
		  Opiates
		  Barbiturates
		Brain stem
		  injury		

equally even if the light source is focused into only one pupil. Nystagmus—rapid, repetitive eye movements—can occur with overdoses of sedatives, phenytoin (Dilantin), or alcohol.

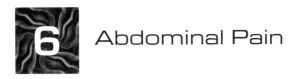

Abdominal Pain

■ DEFINITION

Abdominal pain may be due to a variety of reasons. EMTs are typically called to see patients with complaints of abdominal pain resulting from disease or nontraumatically induced disorders of the gastrointestinal (GI), cardiovascular, or genitourinary systems. The most significant causes, in terms of the need for emergent care, are

- Aneurysm (abdominal and thoracic)
- Acute MI
- GI bleeding (ulcers, colitis, etc.)
- Appendicitis
- Bowel obstruction
- Ectopic pregnancy

This chapter focuses on the "acute abdomen." Other significant causes of severe abdominal pain are discussed in Chapters 12 and 15.

The term "acute abdomen" refers to conditions in which the abdominal lining is inflamed and painful. Symptoms typically have a sudden onset. Pain is often extremely severe. The pain can be characterized by location, radiation, onset/duration, constancy, and associated symptoms or signs. Use the "OPQRST" mnemonic to assess the pain. Related signs include abdominal distention, nausea, vomiting of bloody or "coffee grounds" material (hematemesis), and bloody or tarry black stools. Physical exam may reveal abdominal rigidity, tenderness, or a pulsating abdominal mass (aortic aneurysm).

Causes	Characteristics	Immediate Action
In the field, it is often difficult to assess the specific cause of abdominal pain, such as from blood, acids, feces, or diseased or damaged organs.	An inflamed abdominal lining (peritonitis) can often be rapidly diagnosed by performing palpation and quickly removing the palpating hand from the abdominal surface (rebound tenderness). Perform this exam technique only after gentle palpation. If gentle palpation results in evidence of extreme tenderness or pain, do not perform a rebound tenderness exam. Guarding may also be observed.	Place the patient in a position of comfort. Provide high-flow oxygen. Monitor the vital signs closely for signs of impending shock. Do not allow the patient to eat or drink. Request ALS if your impression yields possible aneurysm, significant bleeding, or signs of shock. Provide rapid transport.

Skin Signs/Symptoms

■ DEFINITIONS

The assessment of the most likely condition of a patient through examination of the skin focuses on three aspects: color, temperature, and moistness (see Table 7–1).

- *Color:*—normal skin (mucous membranes in non-Caucasians) is pink because of oxygenated blood in capillaries of normal size. Dilated skin vessels cause red skin; constricted skin vessels cause pale skin.
- *Temperature:*—normal skin is warm because of warm blood in the capillaries. When the skin vessels are constricted, the peripheral temperature may be cool while the patient's trunk is warm.
- *Moistness:*—normal skin is dry.

Some medical conditions are notable for other skin findings: *edema* (swelling) can be seen in injury, heart failure, or anaphylaxis; *subcutaneous emphysema* (air crackling beneath the skin) can be seen in tracheal injury or pneumothorax.

■ PALE, COOL SKIN

Causes	Characteristics	Immediate Action
MOIST SKIN		
Adrenaline response	A compensatory response to acute illness or injury that usually presents with a fast pulse, pallor, diaphoresis, and nausea.	Identify and treat the underlying cause if possible.
Fear/fright	A psychogenic adrenaline response that improves once the cause is eliminated.	Identify and eliminate the underlying cause if possible. Provide reassurance in a calming manner.
Hypovolemia	An adrenaline response due to hypotension.	Position the patient flat with legs elevated. Provide treatment for shock, including maintaining an open airway and body heat, high-flow oxygen, and consideration of antishock trousers (MAST). Request ALS and provide rapid transport.

Table 7-1 Skin Color, Temperature, and Moistness

| TEMPERATURE | PALE | | PINK/RED | | BLUE (CYANOSIS) | YELLOW (JAUNDICE) |
	Moist	Dry	Moist	Dry		
Cool	Adrenaline response Fear/fright Shock Low blood sugar Heat exhaustion	Normal reaction to cold exposure Hypothermia				
Normal		Anemia		Anaphylaxis (with rash) Carbon monoxide High blood sugar	Hypoxemia	Liver disease Gallbladder disease
Hot			Normal reaction to heat exposure Exertional heat stroke	Infection (fever) Classic heat stroke		

Causes	Characteristics	Immediate Action
Cardiovascular collapse: pump failure	The patient often has a history of heart disease and may present with cardiac-related symptoms. An adrenaline response due to hypotension is likely in addition to orthostatic syncope.	Position the patient flat. Provide high-flow oxygen. Maintain body heat. Request ALS and provide rapid transport.
Heat exhaustion: sodium and water depletion	Characterized by a history of exposure to extreme heat or exertion, heat cramps, and orthostatic syncope.	Position the patient flat with the legs elevated. Slowly cool by removing from the hot environment. Provide oral fluids slowly (preferably balanced electrolyte-containing) to drink if the patient is able to control his/her airway.

DRY SKIN

Causes	Characteristics	Immediate Action
Normal reaction to cold exposure	The patient typically has a normal compensatory response, including fast pulse rate, and may begin shivering.	No immediate action is normally required unless exposure is prolonged. Remove from the cold exposure and prevent hypothermia.
Hypothermia	If mild to moderate, the patient may have an altered level of consciousness and CNS dysfunction (motor, sensory, judgment). If severe, the patient may be unconscious or in cardiac arrest.	For mild to moderate hypothermia, protect the patient from the environment, remove wet clothing, rewarm the core before extremities (heated oxygen or hot packs to chest and neck), provide carbohydrate intake (if patient can protect his/her airway), request ALS, and begin focused exam. For severe hypothermia, handle gently, provide high-flow oxygen, begin gradual rewarming of the core, request ALS, and provide rapid transport.

Causes	Characteristics	Immediate Action
Vasodilation: trauma to spinal cord	The patient has a history or there is a mechanism of traumatic injury. A normal adrenaline response is absent, although the patient is hypotensive. The abnormal skin is inferior to the spinal injury. Paralysis is present and symmetrical.	Provide spinal precautions. Position flat on backboard. Elevate the foot of the backboard. Provide high-flow oxygen, airway control, and ventilatory assistance if needed. Perform a rapid trauma exam and request ALS. Provide rapid transport.

■ RED, HOT SKIN

Causes	Characteristics	Immediate Action
MOIST SKIN		
Normal reaction to heat exposure	This is a normal compensatory response to heat exposure.	No immediate action is needed. Take action (remove from heat) to prevent heat exhaustion or heat stroke if exposure is prolonged.
Exertional heat stroke	This typically occurs in a hot, humid environment and/or during athletic exertion. Hypotension, an altered mental status, and body temperature over 41°C (106°F) are likely to occur.	Immediately remove the patient from the hot environment. Position the patient flat. Begin rapid cooling. Provide high-flow oxygen and maintain airway control. Request ALS and provide rapid transport.
DRY SKIN		
Infection (fever)	The patient most likely has a history of a recent illness. He/she may complain of a stiff neck. The patient may experience febrile seizures or have an altered level of consciousness.	Provide high-flow oxygen if the mental status is altered. Maintain airway control. Remove extra layers of clothing and cool the patient with tepid sponging. If the neck is stiff, exercise communicable disease precautions (gloves, mask, airborne pathogen respirator).

Causes	Characteristics	Immediate Action
Classic heat stroke	The patient is usually in a hot, humid environment. This is commonly seen in the elderly and those with chronic disease. Signs of an altered mental status or coma, dehydration, vasodilation, seizures, and body temperature >106°F may be observed.	Immediately move the patient to a cooler environment. Place the patient in a flat position. Begin rapid cooling. Provide high-flow oxygen and maintain airway control. Request ALS and provide rapid transport.
Dehydration	The skin often has poor turgor ("tenting"). The exam findings include sunken eyes, dry mucous membranes, rapid pulse, and hypotension. The patient may complain of nausea, vomiting, or diarrhea.	Provide a thorough exam and assessment to identify the cause (diabetic ketoacidosis, hyperglycemia, diarrhea, vomiting, or ascites). Provide high-flow oxygen. Request ALS and transport.

■ NORMAL TEMPERATURE

Causes	Characteristics	Immediate Action

PALE, DRY SKIN

Anemia	The patient may have a history of chronic anemia. The exam may indicate external or internal bleeding. The patient may complain of lethargy.	Provide high-flow oxygen. Control external bleeding. Position the patient flat with legs elevated if anemia is not chronic. Provide transport.

RED, DRY SKIN

Anaphylaxis (with rash)	The patient may have a history of hypersensitivity to and may have had a recent exposure to a substance (antigen). Signs of itching, swelling, hives (chest, abdomen, back, face, or neck), hoarseness, dyspnea, hypotension, and tachycardia are present in the exam.	Provide high-flow oxygen. Remove insect stinger if visible. If hypotensive, position flat with legs raised. Assist patient with his/her anaphylaxis kit if trained and authorized to do so. Consider applying antishock trousers (MAST), preferably inflating legs only. Request ALS and provide rapid transport.

Causes	Characteristics	Immediate Action
Carbon monoxide (CO) poisoning	There is a history or a suspicion of exposure to a toxic environment. The patient may have an altered mental status and be vomiting. The patient may complain of a headache or nausea.	Safely remove the patient from the toxic environment. Provide high-flow oxygen, maintain an open airway, and assist ventilations if needed. Request ALS and provide rapid transport.

Blue Skin (Cyanosis)

Hypoxemia	The discoloration is due to inadequate oxygenation of the tissues from respiratory or cardiac failure or dysfunction. The patient may exhibit signs of shock and have a decreased level of consciousness.	Provide high-flow oxygen, maintain an open airway, and assist ventilations if needed. Request ALS and provide rapid transport.

Yellow Skin (Jaundice)

Liver disease	The patient may have a history of chronic alcohol abuse or hepatitis B or C. The abdomen may be distended (ascites). An altered mental status may occur if liver disease is causing hepatic coma.	No immediate action is required. If an altered mental status or coma are present, provide high-flow oxygen. Request ALS and provide rapid transport.
Gallbladder inflammation (cholecystitis)	The patient may complain of right lower chest pain or right upper quadrant abdominal pain radiating to the right scapula. The pain is often sharp and crampy. Abdominal guarding is apparent.	No immediate action is required. Provide reassurance in a calming manner, because the pain is often extreme.

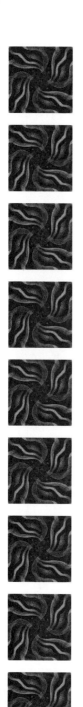

SECTION III

SPECIFIC EMERGENCIES

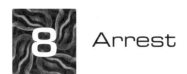

Arrest

■ AIRWAY OBSTRUCTION AND CHOKING

Foreign body obstruction of the airway commonly occurs during eating. Meat is the most common cause of obstruction in adults. Various other foods and foreign bodies cause choking in children. Factors associated with choking on food include large, poorly chewed pieces of food; elevated blood alcohol and other intoxications; laughing, talking, or playing while food is in the mouth; and upper and lower dentures. Choking may also be caused by infections of the upper airway or anaphylactic reactions that result in swelling. While this occurs most often with children, it is an emergent situation that may affect adults as well. Choking emergencies occurring in restaurants have been mistaken for heart attacks, giving rise to the name "café coronary."

When the airway is obstructed, the EMT must open it as rapidly as possible. The following information summarizes the methods for opening an obstructed airway as suggested by the American Heart Association. ALS assistance should also be requested, if available.

EMT Treatment of Conscious Patient, Sitting or Standing (Adult and Child)

■ Establish the presence of complete obstruction. Identify complete airway obstruction by asking patient, "Can you speak?" Look, listen, and feel for breathing. Look for diaphragmatic movement without air exchange.

■ Encourage the victim to cough. If the victim is still able to move some air past the obstruction, his/her efforts will be more effective than yours. Be prepared, however, to immediately perform obstructed airway techniques if needed.

■ If there is no air moving past the obstruction, perform abdominal thrusts (Fig. 8–1) until the airway is cleared or the patient becomes unconscious. Stand behind the patient and wrap your arms around his/her waist. Grasp one fist with your other hand and place the thumb side of your fist between the breastbone and navel. Press your fist into the abdomen with quick upward thrusts. Each new thrust should be a separate and distinct motion. Repeat this sequence as often as necessary until the obstruction is relieved or the victim becomes unconscious.

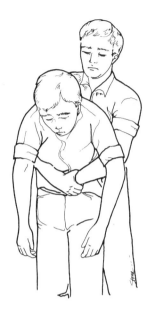

Figure 8-1

Abdominal thrusts: patient in standing position.

An alternative to abdominal thrusts is the use of chest thrusts (Fig. 8-2). Chest thrusts should only be used for markedly obese individuals or for women with far-advanced pregnancies. Stand behind the patient and place your arms under the patient's armpits to encircle the chest. Grasp one fist with the other hand and place the thumb side of your fist on the breastbone. Press with quick backward thrusts. As with abdominal thrusts, perform chest thrusts until the airway is cleared or the patient becomes unconscious.

EMT Treatment of Unconscious Victim, Supine (Adult and Child)

Establish unresponsiveness. Shake shoulder and shout, "Are you okay?" Call for additional resources as required.

Open the airway. Establish breathlessness. Look, listen, and feel with patient lying on back, face up.

■ Tilt the head back with one hand on the patient's forehead and lift the chin up with the other hand.

Attempt ventilation. If the airway remains obstructed, reposition the patient's head and reattempt ventilation.

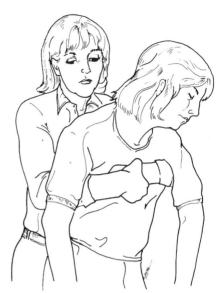

Figure 8-2

Chest thrusts: conscious patient in standing position.

If the airway remains obstructed, give five abdominal thrusts (Fig. 8–3). Position yourself by straddling the patient at the patient's thighs. Place the heel of one hand between the lower breastbone (xiphoid process) and the navel, and the second hand on top of the first. Press into the abdomen with quick upward thrusts.

Check for a foreign body. Open the mouth with the jaw-lift technique, and probe deeply into the mouth along the cheek with a hooked finger. In the child, perform the finger sweep only if an object is seen.

- A dislodged foreign body may now be manually accessible if it has not been expelled.
- Exercise extreme caution when performing the finger sweep because a reflex action of the jaw may cause injury to your fingers. An appropriate bite block or oral airway should be used to prevent injury during the finger sweep.

Attempt to ventilate. Reposition the patient's head and ventilate the patient, if possible.

If the obstruction remains, repeat this sequence as often as necessary until the obstruction is relieved.

- The longer the patient remains comatose, the more relaxed the muscles become; this may make it easier to remove the obstruction.

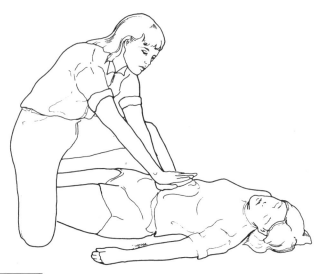

Figure 8-3

Abdominal thrusts: unconscious patient in supine position.

■ After the obstruction has been removed, reassess the patient's ABCDs. If CPR is not needed, continue to provide ventilations with 100% oxygen or high-flow oxygen (if breathing adequately) until the patient has been seen by advanced medical care providers.

EMT Treatment of Conscious Victim (Infant)

■ Confirm complete airway obstruction. Listen and observe for significant difficulty breathing and the absence of effective crying or coughing.

■ If there is no air moving past the obstruction, perform up to five back blows and five chest thrusts.

■ Perform back blows by placing the infant face down over your arm with the head slightly lower than the body. Support the infant on your thigh. Deliver the back blows between the shoulder blades using the heel of one hand.

■ Perform chest thrusts by turning the infant face up over your arm with the head slightly lower than the body. Support the infant on your thigh. Deliver the chest thrusts on the sternum in the same location as with CPR. Chest thrusts are performed at a slower rate than CPR compressions, but each should be distinct.

Repeat the back blows and chest thrusts until the airway is cleared or the patient becomes unconscious.

EMT Treatment of Unconscious Victim (Infant)

Establish unresponsiveness. Gently shake the shoulder or tap the soles of the feet. Request additional resources as required.

Position the infant on a large flat surface (large table or floor). Open the airway. Establish breathlessness. Look, listen, and feel for breathing.

- Tilt the head back with one hand on the patient's forehead and lift the chin up with the other hand.

Attempt ventilation. If the airway remains obstructed, reposition the patient's head and reattempt ventilation.

If the airway remains obstructed:

- Deliver up to five back blows
- Deliver up to five chest thrusts

Using the tongue-jaw lift, check the mouth for a visible object. If an object is seen, immediately remove it. Do not perform blind finger sweeps.

Attempt ventilation. If the airway remains obstructed, repeat back blows and chest thrusts followed by mouth visualization and ventilation attempts until the airway is cleared.

Once the airway is cleared, reassess ABCs. If CPR is not needed, continue to provide ventilations with 100% oxygen or high-flow oxygen (if breathing adequately) until the patient has been seen by advanced medical care providers.

■ CARDIORESPIRATORY ARREST

Cardiac arrest is the sudden cessation of effective cardiac output that will result in permanent organ damage or death if not treated. Respiratory arrest is the equally sudden inability to oxygenate blood and thereby maintain tissue metabolism. Although cardiac and respiratory arrest may have independent causes, they produce the same result and are often difficult to tell apart. Therefore, the combined term "cardiorespiratory" or "cardiopulmonary" arrest is frequently preferable.

Cardiorespiratory arrest is the most common mode of death in American adults, representing the final catastrophic manifestation of many underlying disorders. The most common of these disorders is ischemic heart disease, which is also known as atherosclerotic cardiovascular disease or coronary artery disease. Some 650,000 Americans die each year of ischemic heart disease; two thirds of these deaths take place outside the hospital and within 2 hours of the onset of symptoms.

Cardiopulmonary resuscitation (CPR) is the initial treatment for cardiorespiratory arrest. Although this term implies that the heart and lungs are resuscitated, CPR should be called "cardiopulmonary-cerebral resuscitation" to remind us that the brain is the organ most vulnerable to hypoxia and therefore should be the focus of CPR. Cerebral function is impaired if the brain is deprived of oxygenated blood for more than 4 to 6 minutes, so CPR must be performed immediately to be effective. In Seattle, where basic life support has been taught to about one third of the residents, 43% of patients who received bystander-initiated CPR survived an episode of ventricular fibrillation and ultimately left the hospital, compared with 21% for whom resuscitation was delayed until the arrival of EMTs and paramedics. Patients receiving CPR from bystanders also had a lesser incidence of subsequent shock, coma, and dysrhythmias. Both groups of patients did better than similar patients in cities lacking both basic life support training and community-wide rapid response systems. The superior outcome of patients in Seattle suggests that all adults should understand the pathophysiology of cardiorespiratory arrest, the mechanism of CPR, and its application.*

As defined by the American Heart Association, basic life support is a technique that externally supports the circulation and respiration of a victim of cardiac or respiratory arrest through CPR. It uses the ABCs of CPR: *a*irway, *b*reathing, and *c*irculation. This sequence is chosen because even an adequate cardiac output cannot nourish the brain if blood is unoxygenated. The following protocol is based on current American Heart Association recommendations for treating unwitnessed cardiorespiratory arrest outside the hospital that can be adapted to most circumstances. The steps designed to aid respiration can be omitted in patients with spontaneous ventilation, just as the steps designed to aid the circulation can be omitted if circulation is adequate. However, if the situation is unclear, the protocol should be followed precisely as described. It is important to keep in mind that this protocol continues to change as advances are made in out-of-hospital resuscitation techniques. Out-of-hospital defibrillation is an example of rapidly changing resuscitation technique improvements. General AED use may soon be included in basic CPR training. Additional detail regarding the use of defibrillators by first responders and EMTs may be found in Chapter 22.

---

*Community-Based CPR: What have we learned? Cobb LA, Hallstrom AP. Annals of the New York Academy of Science, 1982.

American Heart Association CPR Protocol

Establish unresponsiveness by tapping or gently shaking the patient or by shouting at him/her. Avoid cervical spine injury by sudden movement or displacement of the neck.

Position the patient, preferably on his/her back, to perform artificial ventilation and closed chest compression. Take care to avoid cervical spinal cord injury; use a logrolling technique, if possible, when moving the patient.

Open the airway. The tongue is the most common cause of upper airway obstruction in unconscious persons because it falls posteriorly when its muscles are relaxed. To overcome this obstruction, the head should be tilted backward. Open the airway by using the chin lift. This is accomplished by placing the tips of the fingers of one hand under the lower jaw on the bony part near the chin and pulling upward. The other hand presses on the patient's forehead to tilt the head back. The chin should be lifted so the teeth are nearly brought together, but the rescuer should avoid closing the mouth entirely. Loose dentures should be held in position to facilitate creation of an effective mask seal. If the dentures cannot be managed in place, they should be removed.

Establish breathlessness by positioning the ear over the patient's nose and mouth, looking toward his/her chest, and observing its rise and fall while listening and feeling for airflow during exhalation. If the patient is breathing, make sure the airway is not obstructed. If it is, or if he/she is not breathing, breathe twice for him/her.

Rescue breathing is performed with the patient's nostrils pinched shut by the thumb and fingers of the rescuer's hand, with the palm on the forehead. Initially, the rescuer blows deeply two times into the patient's mouth. Each breath should be 1.5 to 2 seconds in length (1 to 1.5 seconds for infants). The rescuer should watch out of the corner of his/her eyes to see if the chest is rising and falling. Some resistance should be encountered during inhalation (blowing into mouth), and air should be felt and seen to leave the lungs during exhalation. Ventilation may be facilitated by mask-to-nose or mask-to-stoma breaths in some patients. An artificial airway may be inserted at this point, but ventilation should not be delayed to obtain or apply adjunctive devices.

Recognize upper airway obstruction by the signs and symptoms discussed previously. Patients with partial obstruction should be encouraged to breathe on their own as long as air exchange appears to be adequate. However, if severe stridor, cyanosis, or depressed consciousness are initially present or develop, the EMT must be prepared to perform obstructed airway procedures should the patient's airway become completely obstructed.

Establish circulatory inadequacy by palpating the carotid pulse in
■ adults and children, or the brachial pulse in infants. Take a full 5
seconds in an effort to feel the pulse.

Begin closed chest compression if indicated (see Table 8–1 for guide-
■ lines). Even during properly performed CPR, blood flow to the
brain is prevented or reduced by gravity if the head is elevated above the
level of the heart. Thus, the patient should be placed in a supine position.
The EMT should position himself/herself close to the side of the patient's
chest (preferably the right side if a defibrillator is available) and locate
the lower margin of the rib cage on the side nearest to him/her. He/she
moves his/her fingers across the rib cage until they reach the xiphoid
process, selects a site two fingerbreadths up the sternum toward the
head, and places the heel of the other hand on the lower half of the
sternum above the fingers of the sternum placement hand. He/she then
extends his/her fingers to prevent their tips from lying on the chest, locks
his/her elbows, and delivers closed chest compression from his/her
shoulders.

■ This should be done with enough force to depress the sternum 1.5 to 2
inches in the adult.

■ In children, the sternum is depressed 1 to 1.5 inches (about one third to
one half the depth of the chest) using the heel of only one hand.

■ In infants, the EMT rescuer should depress the sternum 0.5 to 1 inch (about
one third to one half the depth of the chest) with two fingertips placed one
fingertip below an imaginary line drawn between the nipples.

Pressure should be released after each compression to let the sternum
■ return to its original position.

■ *Coordinate rescue breathing and closed chest compression.*

■ Fifteen compressions are delivered for every two ventilations when one
EMT is performing adult CPR. Five compressions are delivered for every
one ventilation in children and infants (one- and two-person CPR).

Table 8–1   CPR: Chest Compression and Ventilation Guidelines

	INFANTS	CHILDREN	ADULTS
Depth	0.5–1 inch	1–1.5 inches	1.5–2 inches
Use	Fingertips	Heel of one hand	Both hands
Rate	At least 100/min	100/min	80–100/min
Ratio (compressions to ventilations)	5:1	5:1	1-person: 15:2 2-person: 5:1
Ventilation length	1–1.5 sec	1–1.5 sec	1.5–2 sec

- The rate of compression when one EMT is performing adult CPR is 80 to 100/min (15 compressions/9 to 11 seconds). Five compressions for each one ventilation should be used in two-rescuer CPR.

- When two people are performing CPR, the person giving the chest compressions should pause for each ventilation. The rate of compressions is 100/min in a child and at least 100/min (at least five compressions per 3 seconds) in an infant.

If two people are performing CPR, they should switch positions periodically to avoid exhaustion. The patient should not be moved until he/she improves or until other arrangements have been made. Basic life support should not be discontinued until advanced cardiac life support can be initiated, a physician or other legally authorized health professional calls a halt, or the rescuers are too tired to do more. It is highly unlikely that EMS responders will be unable to continue CPR until ALS personnel arrive or the EMT's medical control may be contacted.

Reassess the pulse after 1 minute and then again every few minutes. If a pulse is present, ensure that the airway is open and reassess breathing. Continue ventilations with 100% oxygen (if the patient is not breathing) or provide high-flow oxygen (if breathing effectively) until ALS personnel arrive.

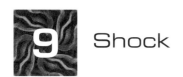

9   Shock

Shock refers to a lack of adequate tissue perfusion because of insufficient blood flow or oxygen delivery to vital organs. It can be caused by hypovolemia, inadequate cardiac function, or vasodilation (relative hypovolemia). Additionally, respiratory failure may lead to inadequate cardiac function and/or vasodilation. For example, a patient who becomes acutely hypoxic as a result of a respiratory condition will have difficulty providing adequate oxygenation to the heart, brain, and blood vessels. This in turn will decrease the ability of the heart to pump well and the ability of the body to compensate for these changes. Initial physiologic changes will be those associated with shock.

■ HYPOVOLEMIC SHOCK

Definition

Hypovolemic shock occurs when there is a loss of circulating blood volume or oxygen delivery capacity resulting in inadequate tissue perfusion. Blood losses not only create a volume insufficiency through plasma loss but also reduce the oxygen delivery capacity of the body through loss of red blood cells. In either case, the ability to adequately perfuse tissue is impaired.

Causes

EXTERNAL FLUID LOSS.

- Hemorrhage (any obvious external source)
- GI tract (vomiting, diarrhea)
- Kidneys (hyperglycemia, diuretics)
- Skin (burns, sweating)

INTERNAL FLUID LOSS.

- Closed fracture
- Ascites (peritonitis, pancreatitis, cirrhosis)
- Intestinal obstruction
- Internal bleeding (hemothorax, rupture of organ or great vessels into abdomen, rupture of ectopic pregnancy, ulceration or rupture of smaller vessels of the GI tract)

History: Subjective Reports

External hemorrhage or fluid loss is usually obvious. Internal losses may be more difficult to determine. A history of abdominal pain or related complaints with postural hypotension, fainting, and/or light-headedness in an upright posture suggests acute abdominal hemorrhage. Alcoholics, patients with liver disease, and chronic users of aspirin are particularly prone to GI bleeding. A rapid but thorough physical exam and history are needed to quickly identify the patient who may have blood volume losses as a result of internal fluid loss.

Examination: Objective Physical Findings

In the initial approach to the patient, observe the skin and general patient appearance for obvious signs of hypovolemia. Determine the postural blood pressure (not necessary when the patient has a supine systolic blood pressure of 80 mm Hg or less) and the heart rate. Return the patient to a supine position immediately if the patient becomes faint in an upright position.

Shock is often classified into mild, moderate, or severe types. In *mild shock* (often referred to as "compensated shock")

- There is a postural pulse increase of less than 20 beats/min.
- There is a postural systolic blood pressure drop of less than 20 mm Hg.
- The neck veins are flat while the patient is supine.
- The skin may be slightly pale and cool. Other vital signs are relatively normal.
- The history may reveal recent episodes of vomiting, diarrhea, or excessive sweating. Symptoms may include dark tarry stools, "coffee grounds" emesis, fatigue, decreased fluid intake, or headache.

In *moderate shock* (often referred to as the early stage of "uncompensated shock")

- There is a postural pulse increase of 20 or more beats/min.
- There is a postural systolic blood pressure drop of 20 mm Hg or more.
- The patient appears pale, sweaty, anxious, and agitated.
- The physical exam may reveal a fast heart rate, increased respiratory rate, and confused mental state. Symptoms may progress to falling blood pressure, lethargy, unconsciousness, rapid respiratory rate, and decreased or absent peripheral pulses.
- The patient may complain of thirst and nausea.

In *severe shock* (often referred to as the end stage of "uncompensated shock")

- The blood pressure is nonrecordable or difficult to obtain in any position.
- The patient is pale, cyanotic, sweating (or may be dry in final stages), tachycardic (bradycardic at final stages), and confused or comatose.
- There is a high probability of development of organ failure (kidneys, liver, and heart) and cardiac arrest.

A convenient way to categorize shock resulting from acute hemorrhage is that proposed by the American College of Surgeons. Acute hemorrhage is divided into four classes (Table 9–1). The classification is valid only for acute hemorrhage and is intended only as a guide. Tachycardia may not be seen in the elderly. Alcohol intoxication may alter the anticipated clinical signs of acute blood loss.

The EMT should continue to monitor the patient with frequent reassessment.

EMT Management

■ Improve oxygenation.

- Open airway and keep clear
- Provide high-flow oxygen.
- Provide positive pressure ventilation as needed
- Treat chest injuries (flail segment, sucking chest wound)

■ Control external hemorrhage and prevent further injury.

- Apply direct pressure to external hemorrhage sites
- Apply cervical spine and full spine immobilization if needed because of mechanism of injury
- Time permitting, splint/stabilize fractures
- Maintain body heat

■ Consider (and anticipate early) the use of antishock trousers (MAST), if you are trained and authorized to do so. Although controversial, the most applicable uses include

- Bilateral or severe lower extremity hemorrhage or fractures
- Pelvic fractures
- As an option when transport times are extended and/or when ALS services are not readily available

Anticipate MAST use early and apply without inflating (until criteria for inflation are met). Be mindful of contraindications, particularly when chest and/or head trauma is suspected.

- Position and package the patient.
- Place in supine position; elevate lower extremities (if patient is on a backboard, raise foot of board)
- Prepare and package the patient for immediate transport

■ Anticipate the need for (request early) additional resources, including ALS and aeromedical transport if appropriate.

Table 9-1 Classes of Acute Hemorrhage*

	Class I	Class II	Class III	Class IV
Blood loss (ml)	Up to 750 ml	1000–1250 ml	1500–1800 ml	2000–2500 ml
Blood loss (%)[†]	Up to 15%	20–25%	30–35%	40–50%
Pulse rate[‡]	72–84 beats/min	100 beats/min	120 beats/min	140 beats/min, or greater
Blood pressure[§]	118/82 mm Hg	110/80 mm Hg	70–90/50–60 mm Hg	50–60 mm Hg
Pulse pressure (mm Hg)[‖]	36 mm Hg	30 mm Hg	20–30 mm Hg	10–20 mm Hg
Capillary blanch test	Normal	Positive	Positive	Positive
Respiratory rate	14–20	20–30	30–40	35
CNS mental status	Slightly anxious	Mildly anxious	Anxious and confused	Confused, lethargic

*Adapted from Committee on Trauma, American College of Surgeons: Advanced Trauma Life Support Course. Chicago, American College of Surgeons, 1981, p. 45, with permission.

[†]% of blood volume in an average 70-kg male.

[‡]Assume normal rate of 72 beats/min.

[§]Assume normal pressure of 120/80 mm Hg.

[‖]Difference between systolic and diastolic.

Rapidly transport the major trauma patient to an appropriate hospital. Severe, ongoing hemorrhage is definitively managed in an operating room.

EMT Special Considerations

Patients experiencing blood loss require volume replacement with whole blood or other fluids. Often, surgical intervention is required. Rapid recognition of the shock condition, control of external hemorrhage, and rapid delivery to an appropriate hospital are the key ingredients in patient survival.

■ Cardiogenic Shock

Definition

In cardiogenic shock, there is inadequate tissue perfusion resulting from circulatory failure secondary to the inability of the heart to pump blood adequately.

Causes

Myocardial infarction is the most common cause of cardiogenic shock. Other causes include

- Arrhythmias
- Severe congestive heart failure
- Acute valvular damage (trauma or infection)
- Pulmonary embolism
- Dissecting aortic aneurysm
- Acute pericardial tamponade (bleeding into the sac around the heart, causing a squeezing effect on the heart)
- Tension pneumothorax

History: Subjective Reports

The most common complaint is chest pain, suggesting MI. Often the patient has had pain for many hours without seeking assistance. Other symptoms and history associated with MI may also be present:

- Shortness of breath
- Nausea
- Radiating pain
- Fatigue, generalized weakness
- History of coronary artery disease, past cardiac events, and/or risk factors for heart disease

Examination: Objective Physical Findings

- Low or difficult-to-obtain blood pressure, particularly with the patient upright
- Heart rate may be fast, slow, irregular, or normal
- Anxiety, agitation, decreased level of consciousness, or unconsciousness
- Pale, cool, diaphoretic skin
- Evidence of cardiac failure, distended neck veins, pulmonary edema
- Cardiogenic shock may lead to cardiac arrest.

EMT Management

- Improve oxygenation.
  - Open airway and keep clear
  - Provide high-flow oxygen; provide positive pressure ventilation, if needed
  - Assess lung sounds for pulmonary edema

- Position the patient to improve perfusion.
  - Place in supine position if blood pressure is low or absent
  - Maintain body heat
  - Minimize exertion; calm and reassure

- Reassess and monitor.
  - Frequently reassess ABCDs, vital signs, and patient complaints
  - Attach cardiac monitor, if available and you are trained to do so; document cardiac rhythm for ALS personnel and receiving hospital

- Request resources and transport.
  - Request ALS immediately
  - Rapidly transport patient to ALS services and/or appropriate hospital

EMT Special Considerations

This is a life-threatening emergency. The patient requires definitive medical care as rapidly as possible. The mortality rate is 80 to 90%.

■ ANAPHYLACTIC SHOCK

Definition

Anaphylactic shock is circulatory failure resulting from a severe allergic reaction that occurs after exposure to a foreign substance (antigen) in a patient made hypersensitive as a result of a past exposure.

Causes

Causes are generally related to antigen exposure via ingestion, bites and stings, intravenous administration, skin exposure, and inhalation. Common antigens include

- Medications (penicillin, sulfa-based antibiotics, aspirin)
- Diagnostic agents (radiographic contrast agents)
- Insect venom (bees, wasps)
- Foreign sera (immunizations, antitoxins)
- Desensitizing antigens (extracts of pollen, mold, peanuts)

History: Subjective Reports

Patients with known allergies will likely inform the EMT of this condition. Information regarding past allergic reactions and anaphylactic episodes can be valuable to the health care providers. The EMT must look for medical alert tags, bracelets, ankle bracelets, and necklaces if the patient is unable to provide information.

Examination: Objective Physical Findings

The respiratory, cardiovascular, soft tissue, and GI systems may all be involved (see Table 9–2). Commonly seen characteristics include

- Shortness of breath with a sensation of upper airway swelling
- Dizziness with possible syncope

Table 9-2 Clinical Features of Anaphylactic Shock

SYSTEM	REACTION	SYMPTOMS	SIGNS
Respiratory	Laryngeal edema, bronchospasm	Dyspnea, wheezing, cough	Stridor, respiratory distress
Cardiovascular	Vascular pooling, arrhythmias	Faintness, apprehension	Hypotension, loss of consciousness
Skin	Hives, facial swelling	Itching	Raised, red rash; edema of soft tissue, lips, tongue, posterior pharynx, eyelids, hands
Gastrointestinal	Smooth muscle contractions	Nausea, abdominal cramps	Vomiting, diarrhea

- Rapid heart rate with hypotension
- Generalized warmth with flushing red skin
- Rash or hives, often appearing on abdomen, chest, back, and face

Lower airway obstruction is characterized by wheezing as a result of pulmonary edema. Convulsions and unconsciousness may be seen in severe cases.

EMT Treatment

Identify the antigen, if possible. Remove any source of remaining antigen, including insect stingers if present.

Improve oxygenation.

- Provide high-flow oxygen
- Provide positive pressure ventilation, if necessary

Improve perfusion.

- With vascular collapse, place patient in supine position; elevate legs
- Consider antishock trousers (MAST), if you are trained in their use and authorized to do so (legs-only inflation recommended)
- Assist patient with anaphylaxis kit medications if you are trained and authorized to do so

Reassess and monitor.

- Apply cardiac monitor, if available and you are authorized to do so
- Frequently reassess ABCs, vital signs, and patient complaints

Request resources and transport.

- Immediately request ALS
- Prepare for rapid transport

EMT Special Considerations

In severe cases of anaphylactic shock, death may occur in minutes, usually from respiratory obstruction and vascular collapse. All patients, regardless of response to treatment, should be transported to the hospital.

■ SEPTIC SHOCK

Definition

Septic shock is vascular collapse brought about by severe systemic infection. It is usually seen in elderly, debilitated, or alcoholic patients.

Causes

Septic shock can occur with severe infection from any source, such as a ruptured appendix, ruptured bowel with peritonitis, severe pneumonia, or pyelonephritis. It is commonly seen as a result of a bacterial infection.

History: Subjective Reports

The history will include a recent acute localized infection, which becomes generalized to involve the whole body. Usual sites of infection are the lung and urinary tract (kidney). The patient may currently be treating the infection with antibiotics.

Examination: Objective Physical Findings

The findings of the exam and assessment may vary. Common findings include

- Low blood pressure, rapid pulse
- Confusion, altered level of consciousness
- Warm skin that may be dry or sweaty; fever
- Rapid, shallow respirations
- Signs and symptoms associated with an ongoing infection (cough, generalized weakness, fatigue, loss of appetite, rash)

The source of infection may or may not be obvious.

EMT Treatment

- Improve oxygenation.
  - Provide open airway and keep clear
  - Provide high-flow oxygen
  - Provide positive pressure ventilation, if needed

- Improve perfusion
  - Position supine with lower extremities elevated as needed to support blood pressure
  - Avoid overheating

- Reassess and transport.
  - Reassess ABCs and vital signs frequently
  - Attach cardiac monitor, if available and you are authorized to do so

- Request resources and transport.
  - Request ALS.
  - Rapidly transport to hospital.

10 Trauma Management

This chapter on trauma is a continuation of that part of Chapter 2 dealing with examination of the trauma patient. Specific field management of injuries found during the focused physical examination is also contained in this chapter.

Many of the trauma patients seen by the EMT will be noncritical, having only minor, non-life-threatening injuries. In evaluating trauma, the EMT's responsibility is to quickly identify the critical trauma patient. When major or multisystem trauma is suspected, emphasis must be placed on the management of airway, breathing, circulation, and disability/defibrillation (the ABCDs). In caring for the trauma victim, time becomes the next critical factor to consider. Because time is critical, the EMT must never become involved with obvious, non-life-threatening injuries while neglecting a more serious problem of management of the ABCDs. All necessary manpower and effort must be focused on treating disorders in airway, breathing, circulation and disability/defibrillation. At present, the only oxygen-carrying substance is whole blood, available only at major treatment facilities. Therefore, it is imperative that trauma patients, particularly those with potential for severe hemorrhage, be extricated and moved to appropriate facilities as rapidly as is practical. Picture-perfect extrications can be counterproductive if they become too lengthy and the patient progresses into hypovolemic shock.

■ INITIAL SIZE-UP

As the first EMTs are arriving, the EMT in charge must quickly assess the scene and the need for specific resources. The assessment must be done quickly during the approach to the scene and should involve the following elements.

SAFETY.   Assess the scene for potential hazards (examples include fire hazards from a fuel spill, downed power lines, unstable vehicles, nondeployed airbags, confined spaces, hazardous material cargo, and, if weapons are involved, the location and security of these weapons). The EMT must ensure that EMS personnel are adequately protected from recognized hazards.

MECHANISM.   Assess the scene for evidence of rapid deceleration (car vs. pole, motorcycle vs. tree), vehicle speeds, use of protective devices (seat belts, air bag deployed, helmet), significant vehicle damage, number of vehicles involved, and the potential for multiple patients. When a weapon is involved, attempt to determine the type of weapon (handgun, rifle, gun caliber; knife, size of knife; baseball bat; fists only), and the position of the assailant relative to the patient.

RESOURCES.   Quickly determine if any special resources may be required (extrication tools, rescue teams, additional manpower, additional ground transport vehicles, heavy equipment, fire suppression, haz mat teams, ALS, aeromedical transport, or additional command officers). If multiple patients are identified, implement procedures for managing multiple casualty incidents. Additional resources are most helpful when they are requested early.

OTHER INJURY RISK FACTORS.   Quickly determine if there are other factors contributing to the accident or injury that may affect the patient's condition (alcohol or drugs involved, ejected patients, dead patient from same vehicle, history of chronic disease, advanced pregnancy, extremely hot or cold ambient temperature).

■ TRIAGE AND RAPID EXTRICATION

Because time is crucial to the critical trauma patient, the EMT must quickly identify such patients (see Table 10–1). In an incident involving only a few patients, triage is useful in that it provides a means of determining the focus of the initial manpower resources. These "smaller" incidents also provide a means of triage practice in preparation for larger scale multiple casualty incidents. Once the initial triage is complete, additional resource requirements can be better defined and patient care can begin. When critical trauma patients are identified, rapid extrication so that assessment and patient management can effectively occur is paramount. Since the majority of trauma patients who die do so because of airway or breathing compromise, severe hemorrhage, and/or significant cerebral insult, the principles of START triage outlined in Chapter 2 may be utilized in other settings of trauma triage.

■ INITIAL MANAGEMENT

In the trauma setting, one EMT must become the leader and maintain control of the overall scene and patient management. This EMT will perform the initial size-up and also assess the circumstances surrounding the trauma scene to determine the mechanism involved. Once protection from identified hazards has been achieved, patient management may begin. The EMT in charge should direct his/her partner to begin triage when multiple patients are involved. When only one critical patient is identified, the EMT team should focus on this patient. Later arriving manpower can be directed to attend to the less seriously injured patients.

In managing the care of the critically injured patient, all efforts must be made to support airway/breathing/circulation and to control bleeding before continuing with a more detailed patient examination.

Table 10-1 Critical Trauma Patient Examples by Injury Types

TYPES OF INJURIES	SPECIFIC PATIENT EXAMPLES
Significant injury to the airway	Major facial trauma Injury to the anterior neck Inhalation burn injuries
Significant injury to the chest or breathing mechanism	Flail chest Inhalation burn injuries Trauma with respiratory distress Sucking chest wound
Significant injury to the cardiovascular system	Major hemorrhage from anywhere Penetrating injury to the chest or back Trauma with shock
Significant mechanism of trauma	Penetrating wound to the "box" (from the top of head to the groin) Trauma resulting in two or more long bone fractures Trauma accompanied by burns Falls greater than 2.5 times the patient's height or >10 feet Multisystem trauma Pediatric, geriatric, and advanced pregnancy patients with significant mechanism
Significant injury to the CNS or spinal cord	Trauma with an altered level of consciousness Significant head injury Spinal cord injury, particularly when neurogenic shock or paralysis is present

INITIAL IMPRESSION

- While approaching the patient, take a quick look to determine if the patient appears to be critically injured.

- Attempt to determine if the patient appears unconscious, is breathing with difficulty, is severely bleeding or has severe obvious injuries. This process should take a few seconds and be done simultaneously with other actions.

- Upon arrival at the patient, immediately perform or direct manual cervical spine immobilization.

AIRWAY AND BREATHING

Immediately determine the quality and volume of respirations as well as the patient's ability to breathe adequately.

- Check for obvious obstructions. Pay special attention to the comatose patient's ability to avoid choking on blood, secretions, and vomit. Provide suctioning if needed.
- Check for the presence and symmetry of lung sounds by listening just below the clavicles.
- Be alert for stridor (raspy, noisy respirations) secondary to trauma to the trachea.
- Use a bag-valve mask to assist or provide ventilations if patient's respirations are slow, labored, or absent.
- Provide high-flow oxygen to patients who do not require assisted ventilations.

CIRCULATION

- Assess the presence, rate, and quality of the pulse.
- CPR is of little value if the patient is in an upright position. Rapid extrication of pulseless patients is therefore essential. Immediately begin CPR.
- Check for obvious gross hemorrhage and immediately treat as required if severe.
- As quickly as possible, direct another team member to obtain the first complete set of vital signs. This should be complete by the time the primary survey is completed.

DISABILITY

A natural by-product of the primary survey is an understanding of the patient's state and level of consciousness. A simple means of assessing the level of consciousness is by using the AVPU system:

- A—*Alert* (awake and aware of surroundings)
- V—Responds to *verbal* stimulus (note whether the response is appropriate)
- P—Responds to *painful* stimulus (note the type of response)
- U—*Unresponsive* (the patient is not awake and does not respond to any stimulus)

Anticipate reasons for an altered level of consciousness (hypoxia, shock, brain injury, intoxicant use, underlying medical condition, purposeful behavior).

Patients found unconscious or with injury to the face or head, or who have been involved with a mechanism that could have caused trauma to the head or neck, should have a firm cervical collar applied before extrication, if possible. Manually stabilize the head and neck in the normal anatomic position until mechanical stabilization (cervical immobilizing device, etc.) is provided.

DEFIBRILLATION

Although ventricular fibrillation is rarely caused by severe trauma, it is not uncommon for trauma to be caused by sudden cardiac arrest. When circumstances and information indicate the possibility of sudden cardiac arrest prior to the traumatic event, the EMT should consider assessing for ventricular fibrillation utilizing an AED.

■ FOCUSED HISTORY AND PHYSICAL EXAMINATION

Once the initial assessment has been completed and life-threatening problems managed, and after the patient has been extricated from any dangerous location, a more thorough physical exam to identify less potentially life-threatening injuries is performed. In addition to the neck/head-to-toe exam, the EMT must simultaneously ensure that the following tasks are accomplished:

- ■ If life-threatening problems continue, resources must be focused on managing these problems and preparing for rapid transport. A detailed physical exam of the critical trauma patient would then be performed during transport, if time permits.
- ■ Frequently obtain the patient's vital signs, especially if there is multiple system trauma, because internal hemorrhage may not be apparent.
- ■ Reassess the flow and delivery mechanism of oxygen provided and readjust as required.
- ■ If time permits, direct the treatment of lesser injuries, beginning with those injuries that have the greatest potential to further affect the patient's ABCDs.
- ■ Be aware that the patient may have chronic illnesses that are not readily apparent. Obtain a SAMPLE history. If the patient is conscious, question him/her about medical history, medicines, alcohol, and street drugs. Alcohol or sedatives can mask severe injury.

Neck

- ■ Assume that a potential cervical spine injury is present in any patient experiencing significant forces (acceleration, deceleration, blunt) to the neck or head.
  - – Examples include diving accidents, falls from significant heights, and motor vehicle accidents.
  - – Spinal (neurogenic) shock may be present in association with low cervical or high thoracic injury. Treat by providing high-flow oxygen, placing the patient supine on a backboard with the legs elevated, and considering antishock trousers (MAST) (inflate legs only).

- ■ With manual head stabilization continuing, assess the anterior and posterior aspects of the neck, the base of the neck, and the lower aspects of the head so that a cervical collar could be applied soon afterward.
  - – Palpate the posterior aspect of the neck for deformity, tenderness or other obvious injury.
  - – Inspect and palpate the anterior aspect of the neck for deformity, tenderness, subcutaneous emphysema, obvious injury, neck vein distention, and trachea location.
  - – Inspect and palpate the clavicles for deformity, subcutaneous emphysema, crepitus, tenderness, or obvious injury. Note the use of neck muscles for respiration or retractions below the clavicles.
  - – Inspect and palpate the chin and lower jaw for deformity, obvious injury, or tenderness.

- ■ When a penetrating injury to the neck is identified, immediately treat with an occlusive dressing and head-down position.

■ Use the jaw thrust or chin lift methods to open the airway in the patient with a potential cervical spine injury. If minimal manpower exists and the airway is compromised, the EMT must make every effort to minimize neck and head movement while managing the airway.

■ Maintain manual stabilization of the cervical spine and head until a cervical collar has been applied and the patient is secured to a backboard using a cervical immobilization device.

■ Patients wearing a motorcycle or other similar tight-fitting helmet should have the helmet removed. This is done for two reasons: (1) the helmet must be off to adequately manage the compromised airway, and (2) the helmet will cause neck flexion when the patient is placed on the backboard. See Appendix H for helmet removal procedures.

Head

Figures 10–1 and 10–2 illustrate the anatomy of the head.

■ Always assume that patients who have sustained serious head trauma may have injuries to the cervical spine. Manually stabilize the head and neck until a firm cervical collar may be applied.

■ Inspect the scalp for obvious lacerations, open injuries, or deformities.
  – Scalp lacerations, even with arterial bleeding, can be controlled with direct pressure and direct pressure bandages.
  – Injured areas of the skull should be palpated carefully, because hematomas can hide underneath fragmented skull fractures.
  – Open skull fractures with exposed brain tissue should be covered with a sterile dressing. *Do not push tissue back into the skull.*

■ Recall that head trauma alone does not cause shock unless it is serious enough to cause death. Look for other sources, such as bleeding or injury, if shock is present.

■ Patients with isolated head injuries who are not exhibiting signs of shock should be transported with the head and upper body elevated (elevate the head of the backboard).

■ Consider the possibility of a significant head injury. Table 10–2 describes the characteristics of lateral hematoma (Fig. 10–3), superior (supratentorial) hematoma (Fig. 10–4), basilar skull fracture, and concussion.

■ Record findings of all neurologic checks on all head-injured patients (see Appendix G).

■ Watch for signs of increasing intracranial pressure. Changes in vital signs can be used to differentiate shock from increasing intracranial pressure (see Table 10–3).

Face

Upper Face

■ Inspect and palpate the upper face for deformity, obvious injury, bleeding, swelling, and tenderness.

■ Control bleeding with direct pressure.

■ Blunt trauma to the forehead may produce significant trauma to the frontal lobes of the brain. Such an injury may cause behavioral changes such as

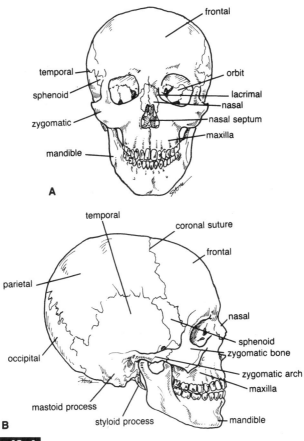

Figure 10-1

Anatomy of the skull. *A*, Frontal view. *B*, Side view.

agitation (yelling, attempting to refuse treatment, repetitive questioning, or combativeness) or occasionally seizures. Note all changes in behavior, and state levels of consciousness.

Eyes

■ Note pupillary size and reactivity to light. Dilated, slowly reactive pupils in alert patients may indicate trauma to the eye(s) and may not necessarily indicate brain damage.

■ Note position of the eyes. A fixed eye that cannot be moved laterally or down, with an orbit sunken into the skull or a globe bulging outward, implies orbit fracture. Cover both eyes to prevent undue movement. Both pupils should move together and in the same direction.

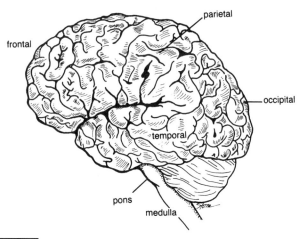

Figure 10-2

Areas of the brain and brain stem.

- Test visual acuity. Have the patient identify the number of fingers held before him/her. Test each eye individually. Do not do this when the globe is lacerated or has been impaled by a foreign object. *Stabilize the object—never remove it.* Cover the uninjured eye also.

- Lacerations of the lid may be controlled with gentle direct pressure. Lacerations preventing lid closure should be treated with moistened eye patches to protect the cornea from damage.

- Hemorrhagic discoloration of soft tissue around the eyes (raccoon's eyes) in the presence of head trauma implies basilar skull fracture. Be alert for changes in patient's neurologic status.

- When a small foreign body is lodged under the eyelid, attempt to rinse it out with sterile saline. If it cannot be rinsed free, bandage the eyes.

- Stabilize an impaled object in place, and bandage both eyes.

- The eyeball avulsed from its socket should be protected in the same fashion as one impaled by an object.

- Chemical burns to the eyes should be rinsed for 20 minutes with sterile water (irrigating fluid). Thermal burns are dressed and bandaged. Ultraviolet light burns, from a welding arc or snow blindness, feel like sand in the eye. Treat with cool compresses over closed eyelids.

- Contact lenses should be left in place until the patient reaches the emergency department, unless they must be removed during irrigation of chemical splash or foreign bodies.

Midface: Nose

- Inspect the nose for deformity, bleeding, or discharge.
  - Clear fluid draining from the nose is a sign of serious trauma to the skull. The fluid should be allowed to drain freely.

Table 10-2 Characteristics of Lateral Hematoma, Superior Hematoma, Basilar Skull Fracture, and Concussion

CAUSE	PUPILLARY SIZE	RESPIRATORY PATTERN	REMARKS
Lateral Hematoma Injury to temporal area of skull with bleeding into temporal area of brain. Bleeding causes brain to shift to one side and down, affecting basic brain functions. 	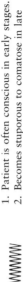 Dilated, unreactive pupil on same side as injury. Drooping eyelid.	WWWWWWWWWWW Sustained hyperventilation.	1. Patient is often conscious in early stages. 2. Becomes stuporous to comatose in late stages. 3. Patient paralyzed on same side as injury to skull. 4. Important to recognize this condition early, because bleeding may stop, patient may apparently return to normal, and a second, fatal bleeding may occur, usually within 30 minutes. 5. Problem can be resolved only in hospital by twist drilling of skull to relieve pressure. 6. Patient may have projectile vomiting, yawning, hiccups.

Table continued on following page

113

Table 10-2 (Continued)

CAUSE	PUPILLARY SIZE	RESPIRATORY PATTERN	REMARKS
Superior Hematoma Injury to top (parietal) area of skull with bleeding across top of brain. Bleeding causes both sides of brain to compress downward. 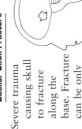	Pupils are small and sluggish reaction to light initially; become fixed in midposition as bleeding progresses and compression of brain stem causes different levels of brain to stop functioning.	⋀⋀⋀—⋀⋀⋀ Cheyne-Stokes respiration early in injury, to sustained hyperventilation, to slow, ⋀⋀⋀⋀⋀⋀⋀⋀ irregular, and finally respiratory arrest as medulla (respiratory center) is affected.	1. Patient is often conscious in early stages. 2. Becomes stuporous to comatose in late stages. 3. Patient will display decorticate* rigidity early with noxious stimulus. 4. Progresses to decerebrate‡ rigidity when brain stem is affected. 5. Becomes flaccid without response to noxious stimuli in late stages (medulla affected). 6. May have projectile vomiting, yawning, hiccups.
Basilar Skull Fracture Severe trauma causing skull to fracture along the base. Fracture can be only on one side.	Pupillary response is same as in superior hematoma, depending on area of brain affected. Discoloration of soft tissue around the eyes (periorbital ecchymosis, or "raccoon eyes").	Respiratory patterns will depend on the level of brain damage, as in superior hematoma.	1. Patient usually has decreased level of consciousness. 2. Blood or cerebrospinal fluid from ear(s), nose is common sign. 3. Discoloration of mastoid behind ear(s) (Battle sign). 4. May have projectile vomiting, yawning, hiccups.

Concussion

Period of being "knocked out" or unconscious with related period of amnesia, lasting from seconds to several minutes. Can be thought of as bruise, as opposed to severe bleeding. Injury may be at impact site or on opposite side of brain, because of rebound force.

Not specific.

Not specific.

1. Patient unconscious because of interruption of the portion of the brain that maintains wakefulness (reticular activating system). Unconsciousness is not caused by bleeding inside the skull.
2. The longer the patient is unconscious, the more severe the damage.
3. Normal side effects: headache, dizziness, fatigue.
4. Patient must be carefully monitored to determine whether injury is more serious (e.g., subdural bleeding).

---

* Patient is supine with one or both arms bent at elbows, fists clenched, hands on chest, and toes pointed down. Extremities rigid.
‡ Patient is supine with one or both arms extended down along chest, fists clenched, and toes point down. Extremities rigid.

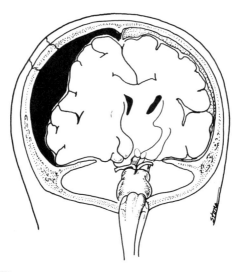

Figure 10-3

Lateral hematoma.

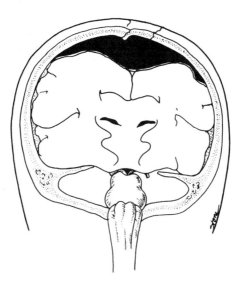

Figure 10-4

Superior hematoma.

Table 10-3   Signs of Shock and Increasing Intracranial Pressure

VITAL SIGNS	SHOCK	INCREASING INTRACRANIAL PRESSURE
Pulse	Fast	Slow
Blood Pressure	Low	High

–Bleeding from the nostril(s) without obvious deformity or swelling of the nose may be a sign of basilar skull fracture.

■ Unstable zygomatic or maxillary bones with soft tissue swelling of the face (pumpkin face) may progress to complete airway obstruction. The patient requires immediate airway control.

■ Foreign bodies in the nose, if they have not been removed by the child or parent, will not be removable by the EMT.

Lower Face: Mouth, Jaw

■ Inspect the jaw for deformity, bleeding, or swelling.

■ Inspect the mouth for bleeding, dentures, loose or broken teeth, vomit, foreign objects, and odors (e.g., alcohol). Teeth are a common lower airway obstruction following aspiration.

■ Lacerations of the tongue or oral soft tissue may require direct pressure to stop bleeding. Use suction as necessary.

■ Severe trauma to area around the mouth may cause soft tissue swelling and can progress to complete airway obstruction.

■ Fractures of both sides of the jaw (known as "bucket handle" fractures) may allow the tongue to fall downward and occlude the airway.

■ Because bleeding from an object impaled in the cheek can present airway problems, the object may be removed. Suction as necessary. Pack the inside of the cheek with dressings, apply pressure dressings to the outside of the cheek, and monitor the airway carefully.

Ears

■ Inspect the ears for blood, fluid, or foreign objects (e.g., broken glass).

■ Bloody or clear fluid leaking from the ear(s) indicates a basilar skull fracture.

■ Complete or partial avulsions of the ear should be packed in sterile dressing. Unattached portions should be wrapped in a sterile dressing and brought to the hospital with the patient.

■ Ruptured or punctured eardrums require no special treatment. Cover the ear lightly with a sterile dressing.

■ Foreign bodies lodged in the ear should be left in place.

Spine

Figure 10–5 illustrates the anatomy of the spine.

■ Using both hands, palpate the spine for deformity, tenderness, and open injuries. Minimize patient movement during this process.

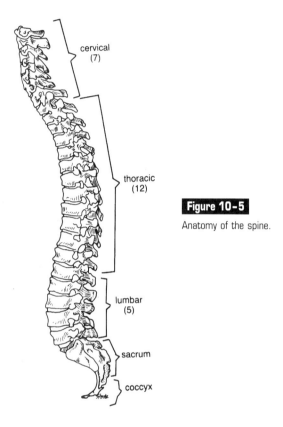

cervical
(7)

thoracic
(12)

Figure 10-5

Anatomy of the spine.

lumbar
(5)

sacrum

coccyx

■ Palpate the entire spine, starting at the neck and moving toward the buttocks.

Chest

■ The first step in the management of chest trauma is the assessment of air movement by evaluation of the breath sounds.
  - The EMT should listen to both anterior and posterior as well as upper and lower portions of the chest, if possible. At a minimum, assess breath sounds under the clavicles and in the upper chest at the midaxillary line.
  - Examination of the trauma patient should include comparing the bilateral presence and symmetry of breath sounds.
  - The primary consideration is to establish an accurate baseline for later comparisons.

■ Assess the chest by inspection and palpation.
  - Look for obvious injury or deformity, including bruising, lacerations, and penetrating injuries.
  - Observe the chest during inspiration for symmetrical movement.

–Palpate the chest by placing one hand on each side of the chest and firmly pressing inward (one hand toward the other).

■ Significant trauma to the clavicle(s) and the body region under the clavicle(s) (the first rib) is correlated with major vessel injury. The aortic arch, subclavian arteries, and veins are located in this region.
  –Blood pressures should be determined in both arms. Look for significant differences (systolic difference >10 mm Hg).
  –Assess the equality of both radial pulses for unequal palpable pressure.

■ The presence of a flail chest or flail sternum (sternum moving inward with inspiration and outward with expiration) may require ventilatory assistance with a bag-valve mask. The flail segment may be splinted using a hand or bulky dressings (see Figs. 10–6 and 10–7). Blunt trauma, without obvious chest wall injury, may cause cardiac damage. There is also a high correlation of cardiac damage with a flail sternum.

■ A simple rib fracture is recognized by point tenderness and localized pain aggravated by deep breathing. EMT treatment consists of manual stabilization with a pillow, sitting position, and administration of high-flow oxygen.

■ Damage to the aorta or large vessels or to the heart may cause cardiac tamponade or immediate shock. Signs of cardiac tamponade include
  –Hypotension (especially with narrow pulse pressure—the gap between systolic and diastolic pressures)
  –Distended neck veins
  –Muffled heart sounds

This is a life-threatening emergency and requires rapid definitive treatment
■ A penetrating injury to the chest may result in a sucking chest wound. EMT treatment consists of an occlusive dressing using a three-sided seal, high-

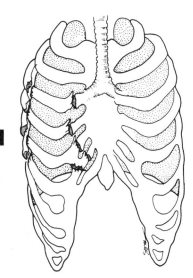

Figure 10-6

Flail chest.

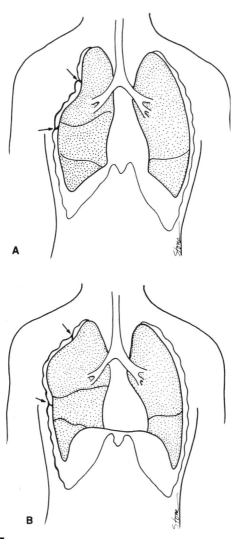

Figure 10-7

Flail chest. Notice the paradoxical movement of the flail segment. *A,* Inspiration. *B,* Expiration.

flow oxygen, very careful monitoring of respiratory status, and rapid transport. Transport with injured side down, if possible.

■ Anticipate the possibility of the development of a tension pneumothorax (Fig. 10-8). Check lung sounds on the injured side frequently. Signs of tension pneumothorax include
 – Absence of breath sounds on the affected side
 – Subcutaneous air or blood (tissue swelling, feels like breakfast cereal under the skin if air, or spongy if blood)
 – Hypotension and shock that worsens with loss of breath sounds
 – Increased heart rate and respiratory rate
 – Distended neck veins

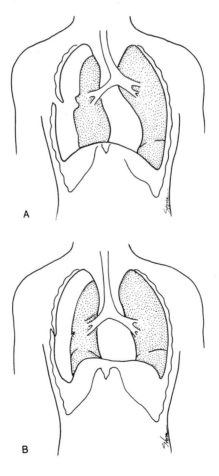

Figure 10-8

Tension pneumothorax. *A*, Inspiration. Notice the shift of the trachea. *B*, Expiration.

–Deviation of the trachea away from the injured side (grasp fingers around trachea just above suprasternal notch to locate position relative to midline of neck; *note* that this is typically a very late sign)

This is a life-threatening emergency and requires rapid treatment. An occlusive dressing should be opened briefly to see if air under pressure escapes. Provide high-flow oxygen and transport rapidly with injured side down, if possible. Call for ALS services, if available.

■ Blunt or penetrating trauma to the lower chest may also cause damage to the contents of the upper abdomen: the liver, spleen, and kidney(s). All three organs are susceptible to deceleration-type injuries without obvious gross injury to the surface of the thorax.
  –When possible, postural blood pressure should be determined to check for hypovolemia.
  –Distention of the abdomen may be a clue to internal hemorrhage.
  –Treat for hypovolemia as required with high-flow oxygen and elevation of extremities. The patient requires volume replacement and surgical care as soon as possible.

Penetrating injuries are usually obvious—treat with an occlusive dressing. *Do not remove objects impaled in the chest, even if in or near the heart.* Stabilize with gauze packing prior to transport.

Abdomen

As with chest trauma, the two factors dictating management of blunt or penetrating injury to the abdomen are the mechanism and the signs and symptoms of hypovolemic shock.

■ Assess the abdomen by inspection and palpation.
  –Look for obvious injuries, bulging, distention, bruising, or guarding by the patient.
  –Palpate each quadrant, feeling for distention, tenderness, or a pulsating mass in the upper quadrants.
  –Observe the abdomen for paradoxical movement with respirations.

■ Re-examine the abdomen frequently.

■ *Do not return bowel or viscera back to abdomen.* Cover with sterile, moist (if sterile solution is available) dressings, then cover completely with occlusive dressings.

■ *Do not remove objects impaled in the abdomen.* Stabilize with gauze packing.

■ Treat for shock
  –Provide high-flow oxygen
  –Elevate extremities
  –Maintain body heat

■ Shock may be treated with antishock trousers (MAST). They should not be used, however, with penetrating trauma above the umbilicus. With pregnant patients, do not inflate the abdominal segment.

Back

■ Some patients require spinal immobilization even though there is no potential for cervical spine injury.

 –Patients with penetrating injuries to the back (gunshot wound, stab wound) near the spinal column should receive spinal immobilization.
 –Patients with blunt traumatic injury to the lower thoracic or lumbar spine should receive spinal immobilization.

■ Patients placed on a backboard should be secured for minimal movement. The EMT should pad the space at the lower back and behind the knees and ankles. A folded blanket should also be placed between the legs from groin to ankles, and at the sides from armpit to heels.

■ Motor and sensory neurologic checks should be performed before and after the patient is placed on a backboard. Make note of any changes.

■ Try to understand the mechanism of injury. The spine may be fractured even if the patient does not have signs/symptoms of injury initially.

Pelvis

■ Inspect and palpate the pelvis for deformity, tenderness, crepitus, and open injuries.
 –Begin by looking for symmetry.
 –Provide firm downward pressure on each side of the pelvis. Then, apply firm inward compression using one hand on each side of the pelvis.
 –Assess femoral pulses for equal strength.

■ Pelvic fractures and penetrating wounds in the pelvic area may injure large blood vessels, bladder, bowel, or uterus, causing severe hemorrhage without obvious external signs. Therefore, treatment for patients with suspected pelvic injuries is directed at stabilization and the anticipation of shock.
 –Provide high-flow oxygen.
 –Place the patient supine on a backboard with the foot of the board elevated if treating for shock. For less severe, non-multisystem trauma patients, place the patient on the backboard in the position of greatest comfort. Secure the patient firmly to the board with padding on both sides of the pelvis.
 –Antishock trousers (MAST) may be considered for pelvic fractures. They may be particularly useful as a splinting device.

■ It is often difficult to distinguish between fractures of the pelvis and fractures of the head or neck of the femur(s). If in doubt, do not use a traction splint on a leg that may have a fracture of the head or neck of the femur. Consider using antishock trousers (MAST) as a splinting device.

Genitalia

■ Maintain privacy during treatment and examinations. Explain to patients what you are doing at all times, because they often will be unable to see the examination or treatment procedures.

■ Control bleeding with direct pressure. Vaginal bleeding can be treated by placing pads or dressings over the vaginal opening. *Never perform a direct internal examination of the vagina.*

■ Injuries to the testicles should be stabilized and the testes supported during transport.

Extremities

Figures 10–9, 10–10, and 10–11 show the bones of the extremities.

- Assess the extremities by inspecting and palpating each portion of the extremity.
  - Look at each extremity for obvious injuries (open or closed), bleeding, or deformity.
  - Palpate each extremity for obvious deformity, crepitus, tenderness, and skin temperature.

- Assess gross movement and sensation of the extremities.
  - Have the patient wiggle his/her feet and toes.
  - Lightly pinch the top of each foot and have the patient identify the foot being touched.
  - Have the patient grasp your fingers and squeeze. Assess the strength and symmetry.
  - If the patient displays a lack of movement or sensation during this evaluation, perform a more specific sensation evaluation by pinching various body surface areas, starting with the feet and moving upward, until pain is noted by the patient. Note the level at which pain was experienced.

- If the patient does not have severe life-threatening injuries, take time to assess the full extent of the injury (e.g., extremity fractures only) and to

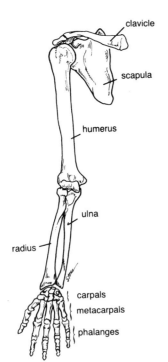

clavicle

scapula

humerus

ulna

radius

carpals
metacarpals
phalanges

Figure 10-9

Bones of the shoulder, arms, and hand.

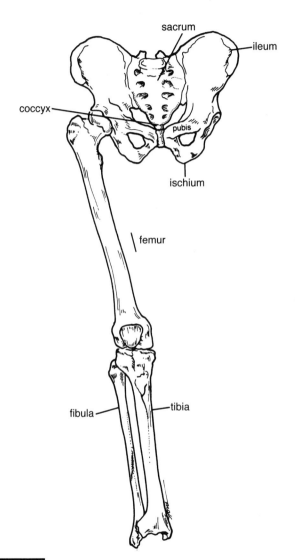

Figure 10-10

Bones of the pelvis, hip, and leg.

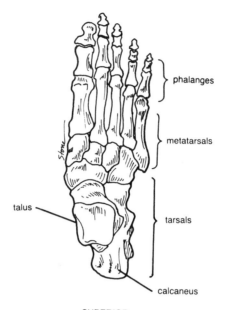

phalanges

metatarsals

talus

tarsals

calcaneus

SUPERIOR

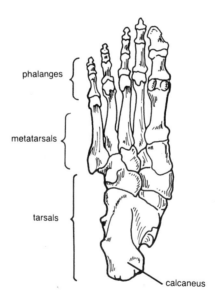

phalanges

metatarsals

tarsals

calcaneus

PLANTAR

Figure 10-11

Bones of the feet.

determine the precise location of the injury on the extremity (see Table 10–4).
– Use direct pressure to control bleeding; supplement with pressure dressings once major bleeding is controlled.
– Before and after treatment for fractures, check
  a. Distal pulses (pulse is present distal to the injury)
  b. Motor function (the injured extremity has normal motor function)
  c. Sensation (the patient can feel the extremity distal to the injury and has no tingling)

■ Fractured limbs should be realigned as nearly as possible to anatomic position. Types of fractures are shown in Figure 10–12.
– Apply traction in the direction in which the limb is found at the scene, and gently attempt to move the limb to its correct anatomic position.
– Support joints and the limb below the fracture site during realignment and splinting.
– Bones protruding from open fractures may be pulled back into the skin once gross impurities are removed.
– *Do not attempt to realign bones end to end.* It is only necessary to place them near their normal position to relieve pain and allow nerves and vessels to return to normal positions.
– Maintain traction until splinting is completed, with a minimum of movement once limb is aligned.
– Use sterile dressings to cover open wounds at the fracture site.
– When possible, elevate the injured extremity after splinting. Place a cold pack near the fracture site.

■ *Splint all injured joints as they are found.* Do not attempt to realign the limb.

■ Save bone fragments and pack in sterile dressing. Moisten with sterile solution, when available.

■ It is possible to damage or sever major blood vessels, especially in the thigh or groin areas and the knee, causing significant hemorrhage. Watch for shock signs/symptoms.

Table 10-4   Injuries to the Extremities

CHARACTERISTICS	DISLOCATION	SPRAIN	STRAIN	FRACTURE
Location	Joint	Joint	Between joints	Either
Symptoms				
Pain	Yes	Yes	Yes	Yes
Loss of function	Yes	No	No	Usually
Signs				
Deformity	Yes	No	No	Usually
Swelling	Yes	Yes	No	Yes
Bruising	Occasionally	Usually	No	Yes

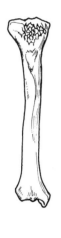

impacted

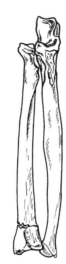

greenstick

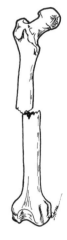

transverse

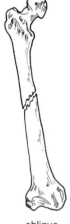

oblique

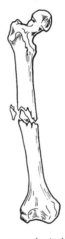

comminuted

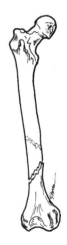

spiral

Figure 10-12

Types of fractures.

Hip

- ■ Fractures and/or dislocations of the hip may be associated with pelvic fractures.
  - –Observe the legs for symmetry. Note if one leg appears shorter than the other or is rotated compared to the other.
  - –Inspect the upper leg for swelling or bulging.

- ■ Check distal pulses and perform a simple motor and sensory examination.
  - –*Motor*: Have the patient wiggle his/her toes and flex his/her foot.
  - –*Sensory*: Lightly pinch the patient's skin at the lower extremity and top of foot.

- ■ If in doubt whether the injury is to the femoral neck or the pelvis, do not use a traction splint.
  - –Place the patient on a backboard using a position that is most comfortable. A patient with a posterior dislocation may prefer the affected leg to remain toward the uninjured side.
  - –Use plenty of heavy padding (i.e., blankets) to stabilize the extremity and pelvic area.
  - –Check for distal pulses after splinting or moving.

Amputation

- ■ Direct pressure at the amputation site will normally control bleeding. Use tourniquets only as a last resort.
- ■ Partial amputations should be placed in normal anatomic alignment.
  - –Wrap with bulky pressure dressings to control bleeding.
  - –When possible, elevate the extremity after bleeding is controlled.

- ■ Completely amputated portions should be wrapped in sterile dressings and placed in a closed plastic bag. The plastic bag with the amputated extremity is then placed in a second plastic bag before being placed on ice and sent with the patient in the same transporting vehicle. (*Use caution to avoid frostbite of the severed part.*)
- ■ Treat for shock as required. Amputations of toes and fingers do not normally require ALS services unless the patient has lost a large volume of blood.

■ SPECIAL TRAUMA PATIENTS

Trauma patients who are pregnant, elderly, or young often require a slightly modified approach. These patients have special considerations, when faced with trauma, that may not apply to the typical adult population. Additional information regarding these patients may be found in Chapters 15, 16, and 18.

Trauma in Pregnant Patients

- ■ All pregnant patients involved with trauma are to be evaluated by a physician in a hospital. While the injury to the mother may appear minor, physiologic changes resulting from pregnancy may mask the early signs of shock.

– Lap safety belts can easily cause trauma to the fetus or uterus, particularly if worn incorrectly.

– The prominence of the abdomen increases the susceptibility to blunt as well as penetrating trauma.

Give oxygen to all pregnant patients involved with trauma.

■ If time permits, check for fetal heart sounds and continue to monitor during treatment and transport. Do not delay rapid transport of the critically injured pregnant trauma patient. (*Note:* The EMT may not be able to hear fetal heart sounds with a regular stethoscope. Use a fetal stethoscope or Doppler, if available.)

■ Penetrating abdominal trauma, vaginal bleeding, or fetal heart rate of less than 100 beats/min should be considered critical. Use ALS assistance, if available, or rapid transport to facility with emergency obstetric personnel.

■ Keep in mind that the best way to care for an unborn baby in distress is to provide the best care possible when treating the mother.

Trauma in Pediatric Patients

Trauma is the most common cause of death in pediatric patients. Motor vehicle accidents and falls remain the most likely causes of accidental death in children from birth to 14 years of age, with head injuries being the most common type of traumatic injury. The failure to provide rapid resuscitation remains a major cause of preventable trauma death in children. While much of the trauma care provided to the child is similar to that provided to the adult, the EMT must maintain awareness of the subtle differences between adult and pediatric patients. Additional details on pediatric care are included in Chapter 16.

■ Cervical spine immobilization is particularly critical in the infant. Because of the infant's large head compared to the body, sudden deceleration events (fall, motor vehicle accident, violent assault) can exert tremendous forces to the neck resulting from momentum.

■ The protuberant occiput of the infant and small child creates neck flexion when the child is placed supine on a flat board. This flexion not only causes undesirable cervical spine movement, but may also interfere with the child's airway.

■ The relatively small airway of the pediatric patient may be easily obstructed by foreign bodies (toys, food, vomitus) or edema. The airway must be completely open and clear.

■ With head injury being a common type of pediatric trauma injury, airway obstruction and/or respiratory arrest are likely to occur. As a result, the EMT must diligently attend to the child's airway and breathing.

■ Significant gastric distention during bag-valve mask ventilations can occur quickly. This will subsequently interfere with the ability of the diaphragm to move without restriction and will increase the risk of vomiting.

■ Hypotension is a very late sign of hypovolemia in the pediatric patient. Pediatric patients quickly attempt to compensate for volume loss. They are likely to exhibit signs of compensation, including rapid heart rate, rapid respiratory rate, decreased pulse quality, prolonged capillary refill, and cool peripheral skin (extremities).

■ Because the pediatric patient may be incapable of communicating or unwilling to openly communicate with the EMT, the assessment is largely based on the general impression, physical examination, environment, and history from older children or adults. The EMT must maintain awareness of the possibility of injury from assault (abuse) or neglect.

Trauma in Elderly Patients

Trauma continues to be a major cause of death in the elderly. Increased life expectancy and health awareness has increased the activity of this rapidly growing age group. Such activity also exposes the elderly to increased opportunities for trauma. Driving, walking, and leisure and sports activities are prime examples. As with the pediatric patient, falls and motor vehicle accidents are the leading causes of traumatic death in this age group.

Although the term "elderly" is difficult to define, the EMT should consider patients older than 65 years of age, those who appear aged, and younger persons with chronic medical conditions commonly associated with the elderly as being in this group of patients. Physiologic changes resulting from aging must be considered by the EMT in the examination and assessment of the traumatically injured elderly patient. Additional details on managing geriatric patients are contained in Chapter 18.

■ The patient may have chronic lung disease or pneumonia resulting in lower oxygen reserves. The chest muscles used in respiration may also be weak while the chest wall is more rigid. These conditions create difficulties when attempting to compensate for traumatic injuries.

■ The patient may have heart disease or previous heart muscle damage. Regardless of the cause, the elderly patient may not be able to compensate with an increased heart rate or peripheral shunting of blood. The elderly patient's cardiac output may already be poor, making this patient unable to increase cardiac output as a compensatory response to trauma.

■ The elderly patient is more prone to neurologic dysfunction and may be forgetful, easily disoriented, or suffering from dementia or Alzheimer's disease. Previous strokes may also have altered the elderly patient's neurologic status.

■ Musculoskeletal changes make the elderly patient's bones more brittle and therefore easily fractured. Multiple fractures may occur even with seemingly minimal mechanisms.

■ Sensory changes in the elderly patient, such as hearing deficits, vision impairment, slowed responses, and chronic neurologic changes, create additional challenges to the EMT's exam and assessment.

■ Chronic disease may be exacerbated by trauma. The emotional or physiologic effects of the trauma may create shortness of breath due to emphysema or cause chest pain due to angina.

■ Medications taken regularly by the patient may inhibit normal compensatory mechanisms or worsen the effects of the traumatic injuries. For example, medications that slow the heart rate will inhibit the elderly patient's ability to compensate with an adrenaline response.

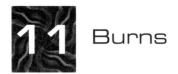

Burns

■ DEFINITION

A burn may be defined as a traumatic injury to the skin and soft tissue resulting from exposure to energy, typically in the form of thermal energy. The contact energy causing the burn can be in the form of dry heat (flame, hot gas), wet heat (steam or hot liquid), chemicals (caustics, acids), electricity (arcing), or radiation.

■ CLASSIFICATIONS

Burns may be classified in several different manners based on the source of energy, the degree of severity, or the degree of tissue involvement. Traditionally, burn classifications based upon the source of energy and degree of severity have been used by EMTs.

Source of Energy

Burns are divided into four categories based on the source of the energy causing the burn.

Thermal

Thermal burns result from contact (skin or mucous membranes) with flame, hot gases, or hot objects. The contact may also be in the form of exposure through the radiation of heat (e.g., sunlight).

- Typically, the degree of severity is based on the temperature of the contact object and the time of exposure.
- This is the most common type of burn injury.

Electrical

Electrical burns result from the conduction of an electrical current through the body or a portion of the body, including tissue and bone.

- Burns result from arcing or the heat developed as the electricity meets electrical resistance.
- The burn severity is a function of the amount of electrical current (affected by the voltage and resistance), the amount of surface resistance encountered, the path of the electricity, and the time of exposure to the electrical current.
- Additional complications, including cardiac arrhythmias, are associated with contact with electrical current.

Chemical

Chemical burns are caused by caustic or acidic substances that have made direct contact with the skin or mucous membranes.

- The burn is usually caused by a chemical reaction with the body's moisture. The reaction often produces heat.
- The severity of the burn is directly related to the type of chemical, the chemical's concentration, the degree of chemical reaction, and the time of exposure. In some cases, exposure does not result in any burn due to a lack of a chemical reaction.
- Burns from chemicals may be complicated by other systemic injuries or illnesses resulting from the chemical exposure.

Radiation

Burns may be caused by acute exposure to radioactive sources either through direct contact or close proximity exposure to a high-dose radiation source.

- As with most radiation exposure, the severity of the injury is related to the time of exposure, the distance to the source, and the amount of shielding present.
- The burned area may produce burning pain, redness, loss of hair, and persistent dryness.
- The symptoms may not completely develop for 2 weeks or more.

Degree of Severity

Burns are categorized by severity as first, second, third, and fourth degree, depending on the burn characteristics (see Table 11–1).

FIRST DEGREE.   First-degree burns are superficial, mild burns usually requiring little or no medical attention. Treatment is usually provided only to relieve pain.

SECOND DEGREE.   Second-degree burns involve the epidermis and are characterized by the presence of blisters. Moderate damage to the skin is possible. These burns will usually heal over a period of days or weeks.

THIRD DEGREE.   Third-degree burns involve the full thickness of skin through to the dermis. These burns will require skin grafting unless only a small area is affected.

FOURTH DEGREE.   Fourth-degree burns involve injury of the epidermis, dermis, and subcutaneous tissue down to the muscle and/or bone. The extent of this type of burn may not be obvious initially, because the most common source is accidental electrocution. All that may be visible is the damaged areas at the entrance and exit of the electrical source.

Table 11-1   Burn Characteristics

Classification	Damage	Examples	Appearance	Sensation
First	Superficial	Sunburn	Redness	Moderately painful
Second	Partial thickness (mostly epidermal damage)	Heat/flame	Blisters	Very painful
Third	Full thickness (epidermis and dermis)	Heat/flame	White, leathery, charred	No pain at site
Fourth	Full thickness (includes muscle and/or bone)	Electricity	Exposed muscle, bone, charred surface	No pain at site

Assessment of Burn Injury Severity

Evaluation of the burn injury is focused on determining life-threatening complications, the degree of severity, the body surface area involved, and other potential complications specific to the patient. The assessment is critical in that major and many moderate burns should be evaluated at a specialized burn care center.

Major Burns

- All inhalation injuries and burns affecting ventilation, including those causing respiratory distress
- Burns associated with shock or an altered mental status
- Burns involving the face, hands, eyes, ears, feet, and perineum
- Burns involving over 30% of the body regardless of the degree
- Electrical burns
- Second-degree burns involving more than 20% of an adult's body surface or more than 10% of a child's body surface
- Third-degree burns involving 10% or more of an adult's body surface or greater than 5% of a child's body surface
- Burns complicated by fractures, other trauma, or chronic (pre-existing) illness
- Burns in high-risk patients such as children, the elderly, and those with severe chronic illness

■ Significant chemical, electrical, and radiation burns as well as those involving the potential for significant carbon monoxide inhalation

MODERATE BURNS

■ Second-degree burns involving between 15 and 25% of an adult's body surface or 10 to 20% of a child's body surface
■ Third-degree burns of 2 to 10% of the body surface, not involving the eyes, ears, face, hands, feet, or perineum

MINOR BURNS

■ All lesser burns

■ FOCUSED HISTORY

1. Quickly determine if it is safe to approach the patient. Identify the source of injury (electrical, chemical, thermal, radiation) and take appropriate safety measures to protect the EMT team members.
2. Obtain as much information as possible concerning the mechanism or source of the burns.
   a. The electrical voltage and/or current
   b. The name of chemical or radioactive source involved
   c. The extent and location of the exposure
   d. The status of the patient immediately following the exposure (unconscious, apneic)
3. Determine if there is any additional mechanism that could cause other trauma.
   a. Did the patient experience any injury or trauma after the exposure (struck head during fall, inhaled chemical vapors or dust)?
   b. Was the patient trapped in a small environment during a fire?
   c. Does the patient still have contact with hot objects or caustic chemicals (chemical remaining on the skin, patient unconscious against a hot boiler)?
4. Determine if the patient has any chronic illness that could be complicated by the burns or that may complicate recovery from them.
   a. Diabetes, renal disease, or heart disease
   b. Immune system disorders (human immunodeficiency virus)
   c. Respiratory disease (COPD, asthma)

■ PHYSICAL EXAMINATION

■ Ensure that the patient is completely removed from the source of burns.
■ Quickly assess the ABCDs for potentially life-threatening injuries.
   – Open the airway.
   a. Look for obvious swelling of the airway (mouth and neck).

b. Inspect for soot or burns in the mouth, and for singed nasal hair.
c. Listen for hoarseness, stridor, or a raspy voice.
–Assess ventilations.
a. Assess the respiratory rate and chest expansion.
b. Look for circumferential chest burns.
c. Assess the lung sounds for wheezes, rhonchi, or rales.
–Assess the circulation.
a. Check for carotid and peripheral pulses when extremities are burned.
b. Inspect for any major bleeding.
–Assess the level of consciousness. In the event of cardiac arrest, assess for ventricular fibrillation using an AED.

- Immediately treat any life-threatening conditions found in the initial assessment before proceeding with the physical examination.
- Obtain an initial set of vital signs. If necessary, the blood pressure may be taken on a burned extremity. Before doing so, place gauze over the area to be covered by the blood pressure cuff.
- Consider the significantly burned patient as a critically injured trauma patient. Complete the physical examination as would be done on any other critically injured trauma patient.
- Determine the approximate total percentage of body surface (skin) area involved by burns. *Do not delay care in order to determine the percentage of burned body surface area.*
  –*Rule of Nines*: The rule of nines may be used to approximate the percentage of burned skin area. It is sometimes more accurate to approximate the unburned percentage of skin and subtract that percentage from 100% to determine the percentage of the skin area involved. Estimate the percentage of each classification of burn. If in doubt whether a burn is second or third degree, consider it third degree. (Body surface area percentages for adults and children are presented in Figure 11–1.)
  –*Palm Rule*: Another method of estimating the percentage of burned skin area is using the palm rule. In this method, the patient's palm surface area is considered approximately 1% of his/her body surface area. Look at the patient's palm and estimate the percentage of skin area burned.

■ EMT Treatment

■ Once it is safe to do so, remove the patient from the source of burns.

- Extinguish and remove smoldering clothes from the patient.
- Remove the patient from the electrical source. DO NOT ENDANGER RESCUERS. USE EXTREME CAUTION.
- Immediately wash chemicals off patient with copious amounts of water.
- Brush solid chemical substances (e.g., lime) off the patient before applying water.
- Remove objects that may continue to cause burns, such as hot metal objects (jewelry, eyeglasses).

■ Treat the ABCDs immediately.

- Provide oxygen to all burn patients. If respiratory system injury is suspected or respiratory distress is present, provide high-flow oxygen. Provide high-flow oxygen to all other major burn patients.

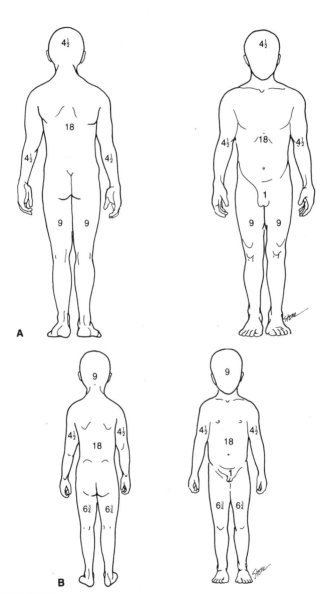

Figure 11-1

Relative percentages of body surface area. *A*, Adult. *B*, Child.

- If respiratory distress is progressively worsening (hoarseness, wheezing, cough), the patient requires ALS services and rapid transport.
- Be prepared to assist ventilations if needed.
- Control hemorrhage with direct pressure and pressure bandage.
- Treat shock and hypotension as with any trauma patient. Initial hypotension is seldom due to the burn injury. Look for other sources of injury or illness producing the shock.
- Provide high-flow oxygen if the mental status is altered. If spinal injury is suspected, stabilize the cervical spine with a cervical collar, cervical immobilization device, and backboard.
- Treat any other medical emergencies found in the initial assessment as would be done in any other circumstances.

■ Cover burns with dry dressings or sheets. Dressing/sheets should be sterile when possible, but that is not essential.

- Small burns may be cooled with moist dressings if this is done immediately after the burn occurs. In larger area burns (>9% of body surface area), the moist dressings will promote heat loss and may make the area more susceptible to infection. Moist towels applied prior to the EMT's arrival should therefore be replaced with dry dressings.
- *Do not allow the application of ointments, sprays, or creams to burns*, because the hospital burn staff will have to remove them, causing more discomfort to the patient.
- *Do not apply ice to the burn surface.*
- *Do not attempt to break blisters.* Leave them intact.
- If fingers or toes are burned, separate them whenever possible with sterile gauze pads.
- If the eyes are involved in the burn, cover both eyes.

■ Additional treatment for electrical burns may be needed.

- Monitor ventilations because the electrical current may have disrupted the function of the diaphragm and other chest muscles involved in the respiratory process.
- Apply an ECG monitor if available and you are authorized to do so. Document the ECG strip for use by ALS personnel and the receiving hospital.
- Be prepared for cardiac arrest, particularly due to ventricular fibrillation or ventricular tachycardia.
- Have an AED near the patient, if available and you are authorized to use it.

■ Conserve body heat. Once treatment is complete, cover the patient with warming blankets. Burns covering large surface areas lose great amounts of body heat from evaporation, because the protective skin layer is destroyed, thus making burn patients prime candidates for hypothermia.

■ Treat all other injuries found in the secondary survey.

■ Transport major burn patients and other appropriate burn patients to the nearest burn center or similarly suitable hospital if at all possible.

Medical Emergencies

Respiratory Distress

As discussed in Chapter 3, there are several different aspects of respiratory distress. Some are objective signs, observable by the EMT: changes in respiratory rate, diaphragmatic breathing, difficulty speaking, or abnormal breath sounds. The subjective symptom of shortness of breath is called dyspnea. What is common to all forms of respiratory distress is some interference with gas exchange. The result is either too little oxygen or too much carbon dioxide in the blood.

This section discusses the medical causes of acute respiratory distress. Other causes are covered elsewhere in this book: obstruction of the upper airway in Chapter 8, trauma to the chest in Chapter 10, respiratory burns in Chapter 11, inhaled poisons in Chapter 13, asphyxia from drowning in Chapter 14, pediatric respiratory distress in Chapter 16, and hyperventilation syndrome in Chapter 17.

■ ASTHMA

Definition

Asthma is an episodic disease manifested by bronchial constriction from smooth muscle contraction and/or excessive mucus secretions. The patient with asthma has often had similar attacks in the past and may be receiving prescribed medications such as steroids or bronchodilators. Between attacks the person is usually free of symptoms.

The term "status asthmaticus" refers to a particularly severe ongoing asthmatic attack that does not respond to the usual medications and may be fatal.

Acute Scenario

An attack is usually provoked by an outside source such as pollutants, smoke, dust, stress, exercise, pollens and other allergens, or infection. During the attack, the bronchi tend to increase in diameter with inhalation but collapse on exhalation, causing pronounced wheezing and an extended, forced expiratory phase. The difficulty in expiration may cause "air trapping." This tends to worsen the respiratory distress because inspiration then becomes difficult to achieve. Many asthmatic patients use aerosol inhalers, small-volume nebulizers, or bronchodilator pills when they feel an oncoming attack. The asthmatic patient may only call the EMS system when his/her prescribed treatment has failed to give adequate relief.

History: Subjective Reports

The chief complaint will be increasing shortness of breath (dyspnea). Patients with a known history of asthma will be able to relate whether or not the shortness of breath is due to an acute asthma attack. The patient may relate information of a recent acute allergen exposure or respiratory infection. The patient in status asthmaticus may also relate a history of the present incident of dyspnea lasting for several hours, possibly days. Patients in severe respiratory distress and status asthmaticus may also complain of fatigue and drowsiness. Usually, the patient is known to be asthmatic. The past medical history may include similar attacks and treatment in an emergency department.

It is also important to obtain a complete medication history. The types of medications being used by the patient on a regular basis have a great impact on the treatment provided by ALS personnel and the receiving hospital. Information regarding what medications the patient used to relieve the symptoms of this episode must also be obtained. Learn how many times the patient attempted to use each medication and by which method (e.g., "Used her Proventil inhaler four times and has used her home nebulizer twice today without relief"). As with all other patients, a thorough past medical history should also be obtained if possible (i.e., history of heart disease, allergic reactions).

Examination: Objective Physical Findings

The patient is usually found sitting forward and is often wheezing audibly. The patient often appears pale, diaphoretic, and tachypneic. He/she will have tachycardia, a prolonged expiratory phase, difficulty speaking except possibly in short phrases, and coughing. Most asthmatic persons in acute, severe distress are tired from the effort required to breathe, are very frightened and anxious, and may have cyanosis at the lips or nail beds.

- When approaching the patient, look for the obvious signs of respiratory distress:
  - Fear, anxiety, drowsiness, exhaustion, or agitation
  - Fast respiratory rate
  - Pale and/or cyanotic at the lips or nail beds
- Ask the patient a question (the purpose is to hear how the patient is able to speak).
  - Can the patient speak at all?
  - Are the patient's sentences short?
  - Do you hear audible wheezes or gasping?

- Look at the neck and upper chest.
  - Are the neck veins distended while the patient is in a sitting position?
  - Are there retractions at the base of the neck and inferior to the clavicles with inspiration?
- Listen to the lung sounds.
  - Listen to the lung sounds over the posterior thorax. Wheezes, often heard on expiration, may be heard over all lung fields, including during inspiration.
  - Absence of lung sounds in all or part of the lung fields ("quiet chest") is a serious indication of severe, life-threatening asthma.
- The patient with a severe asthma attack may also appear to have an extremely distended (hyperinflated) chest.
- The EMT may notice several inhalers or a nebulizer near the patient. The patient may even be attempting to use his/her medications during the EMT's arrival.

EMT Treatment

■ Provide immediate oxygen at 2 to 4 L/min by nasal cannula. Provide humidified oxygen, if possible.

■ Place the patient in a sitting position.

■ Often the patient can be comforted with a calm approach and reassurance.

■ If the patient continues to be in respiratory distress, attempt to provide high-flow oxygen. Many patients will not tolerate a mask due to a feeling of suffocation.

■ Assist the patient in taking any prescribed medications, if he/she has not already attempted to do so. If you are trained and authorized to do so, provide a bronchodilator by metered-dose inhaler or small-volume nebulizer (see Chapter 23).

■ Perform a focused physical examination of the patient to rule out other possibilities for the acute respiratory distress.

■ Be prepared to ventilate the patient with a bag-valve mask should respiratory failure occur.

■ If available, request ALS services.

■ Patients with severe asthma attacks need rapid provision of, or transport to, ALS services.

EMT Special Considerations

■ Acute asthmatic attacks can be a common problem with asthmatic children. Parents usually will not call for help unless the attack is severe or there have been many attacks in a short period of time.

■ Keep everyone at the scene calm and avoid obvious hurry. Although the patient needs rapid care, anxiety created by others at the scene will only be harmful to the patient.

■ Asthma patients many times will tolerate oxygen at a higher rate of flow per minute.

■ Be alert for respiratory arrest. The patient may experience respiratory failure as a result of exhaustion or hypoxia. He/she may even experience cardiac arrest as a result of the severe hypoxia. Be prepared to ventilate the patient.

■ When ventilating the asthmatic patient in respiratory arrest, keep in mind the concept of air trapping. Attempting to ventilate with large volumes of air or with rapid ventilations will only increase the amount of air trapping. Continuing to do so may cause a pneumothorax, which can quickly lead to a tension pneumothorax.
  – Squeeze the bag only until resistance is felt or the chest starts to rise.
  – Allow more time for expiration than for inspiration.
  – Ensure that the patient is being transported either to an ALS unit or to a hospital emergency department.

■ CHRONIC OBSTRUCTIVE PULMONARY DISEASE (COPD)

Definition

COPD is divided into two basic categories: chronic bronchitis and emphysema. Both diseases involve progressively destructive changes in the lungs, and patients will most likely give a history of longstanding disease. In some patients, the EMT may be the first to recognize the possibility of COPD in a patient who seldomly sees a physician. Most of these patients have been heavy smokers for years. Other factors are exposure to allergens, chemicals, pollutants, or repeated infections. The result of this destruction of alveoli, airways, and pulmonary blood vessels is poorly functioning gas exchange, resulting in higher than normal levels of CO_2 and lower than normal levels of O_2 in the blood. Unlike healthy persons, whose automatic impulse to breathe is regulated by the level of CO_2 in the blood, breathing in the person with COPD (who has been living with high levels of CO_2 for years) is regulated by the level of oxygen in the blood. The prevalence of COPD continues to increase in the United States, and it is now regarded as the second most common cause of hospital admissions.

Chronic bronchitis is defined as a productive cough for 3 months of a year for at least 2 consecutive years. In chronic bronchitis, the lungs produce an excess of mucus and have difficulty expelling mucus from the bronchioles. The CO_2 retained in the lungs creates pulmonary hypertension, which can lead to right heart failure.

Emphysema is characterized by a decreased elasticity of the lung tissue, resulting in distention of the alveoli, which are filled with trapped air.

Acute Scenario

The patient with COPD has little respiratory reserve to compensate for even minor demands on the respiratory system. The stress of an otherwise minor respiratory illness, such as the flu, can push this patient into acute respiratory distress. Any event that creates a demand for increased oxygen availability may cause an exacerbation of the patient's COPD. In addition to a respiratory illness, examples include exertion, stress, anxiety, and climate changes.

History: Subjective Reports

The chief complaint of the COPD patient who is experiencing difficulty will be shortness of breath (dyspnea). The history of the present episode may reveal a recent "chest cold," fever, increasing dyspnea on exertion, and a change from a persistent (but often unproductive) cough to an increasing cough productive of thick yellow-green sputum. Gather specific information about this particular episode (When did it start?, What aggravated it?, etc.). Usually, the patient has a known past medical history of COPD. As stated earlier, the patient nearly always has a history of chronic tobacco smoking. As with the asthmatic patient, the EMT must also gather information regarding the patient's medications, use of these medications with this episode, and significant past medical history.

Examination: Objective Physical Findings

The COPD patient typically will be an anxious-looking, older person with a barrel-shaped chest, sitting upright and leaning forward. The patient often is found in the tripod position (sitting upright, jaw thrust forward, hands resting on the knees). Speech will come in short phrases because the patient will be breathing rapidly through pursed lips, using the accessory muscles of the neck and chest to aid respiration. (The very acutely ill patient may actually have a decreased respiratory rate because of the very high level of CO_2 in the blood. This is called "CO_2 narcosis.") A prolonged expiratory phase will be noted. The patient may cough up infected yellow-green sputum. Auscultation of the chest may reveal rales, rhonchi, wheezes, or squeaks. These sounds may be faint and only present high up on the posterior chest.

Although it may be difficult (and unimportant) to distinguish between the two, chronic bronchitis and emphysema may present somewhat differently. The patient with *chronic bronchitis* may be markedly cyanotic and obese, giving rise to the reference to these patients as "blue bloaters." The COPD patient with chronic bronchitis who has some degree of right heart failure will have swelling of the ankles (peripheral edema) and distended neck veins. The patient with *emphysema* may be thin, may not be as cyanotic, and may be "puffing" through pursed lips. These patients are often referred to as "pink puffers." In practice, it may be difficult to tell them apart, especially when an emphysema patient's respiratory distress is acute and cyanosis is present. The EMT examination for both types of COPD patients is the same. It also closely resembles the initial exam of the patient with an acute asthmatic episode.

- When approaching the patient, look for the obvious signs of respiratory distress:
  - Fear, anxiety, drowsiness, exhaustion, or agitation
  - Fast respiratory rate
  - Pale and/or cyanotic at the lips or nail beds
  - Pursed-lip breathing

- Ask the patient a question (the purpose is to hear how the patient is able to speak).
  - Can the patient speak at all?
  - Are the patient's sentences short?
  - Do you hear audible wheezes, rhonchi, rales, or gasping?
  - Is the patient coughing? Is it productive?

- Look at the neck and upper chest.
  - Are the neck veins distended while the patient is in a sitting position?
  - Are there retractions at the base of the neck and inferior to the clavicles with inspiration?

- Listen to the lung sounds.
  - Listen to the lung sounds on the posterior thorax. Wheezes may be heard in the upper lung fields. Rhonchi (coarse moist sounds) are the most likely sounds to be heard. Rales (fine popping sounds) may also be heard.
  - Absence of lung sounds in all or part of the lung fields ("quiet chest") is a serious indication of severe, life-threatening respiratory distress.

- Look for the characteristics of COPD.
  - The patient with chronic lung disease should appear to have a barrel-shaped chest.
  - The chronic bronchitis patient may also have peripheral edema and pitting in the lower extremities.
  - The chronic smoker has tobacco stains and clubbing of the fingers.

- The EMT may notice several inhalers or a nebulizer near the patient. The patient may also be on home oxygen.

EMT Treatment

- Provide immediate oxygen at 2 L/min by nasal cannula. Provide humidified oxygen, if possible.

- Place the patient in a sitting position.

- Often the patient can be comforted with a calm approach and reassurance.

If the patient continues to be in respiratory distress, attempt to provide high-flow oxygen. Many patients will not tolerate a mask due to a feeling of suffocation.

Assist the patient in taking any prescribed medications, if he/she has not already attempted to do so. If you are trained and authorized to do so, provide a bronchodilator by small-volume nebulizer (see Chapter 23).

Perform a focused physical examination of the patient to rule out other possibilities for the acute respiratory distress, such as CHF with pulmonary edema.

Encourage the patient to cough. Provide a basin for the collection of the mucus. Take the mucus to the hospital with the patient if possible.

Be prepared to ventilate the patient with a bag-valve mask should respiratory failure occur.

If available, request ALS services.

Patients with severe exacerbation of COPD need rapid provision of, or transport to, ALS services.

EMT Special Considerations

- It is particularly important to emphasize that the COPD patient in acute respiratory distress *needs oxygen*, despite the possibility that raising the blood oxygen level could reduce the drive to breathe. *Never* withhold oxygen from the COPD patient in respiratory distress.
- As with the asthmatic patient, be alert for respiratory arrest. The patient may experience respiratory failure as a result of exhaustion or hypoxia. He/she may even experience cardiac arrest as a result of the severe hypoxia. Be prepared to ventilate the patient.
- When ventilating the COPD patient in respiratory arrest, keep in mind the concept of air trapping. Attempting to ventilate with large volumes of air or with rapid ventilations will only increase the amount of air trapping. Continuing to do so may cause a pneumothorax, which can quickly lead to a tension pneumothorax.
  – Squeeze the bag only until resistance is felt or the chest starts to rise.
  – Allow more time for expiration than for inspiration.
  – Ensure that the patient is being transported either to an ALS unit or to a hospital emergency department.

◾ PULMONARY EDEMA

Definition

Pulmonary edema is the accumulation of fluid in the lungs. The most common cause of pulmonary edema is cardiac dysfunction, typically the failure of the left side of the heart to efficiently pump out the blood that is returning from the lungs. This cardiac dysfunction is caused by acute MI or CHF. The capillaries in the lungs and other pulmonary vessels lose fluid into the alveoli, interfering with the exchange of oxygen and carbon dioxide.

Other less common causes of pulmonary edema include conditions in which the alveoli are directly damaged: smoke inhalation or other toxic inhalation, near-drowning, aspiration, pneumonia, or infection. More rarely, pulmonary edema is seen in some other conditions: narcotic overdose; high altitude (HAPE); CNS damage, such as head injury or spinal injury; or chronic conditions such as cancer or liver disease. Occasionally, the patient who is receiving IV fluids can have circulatory overload if the flow rate is not carefully monitored ("runaway IV").

Acute Scenario

Pulmonary edema can result suddenly following an MI (heart attack). However, pulmonary edema generally does not have a sudden onset. Usually, it takes several hours to develop. As a result, patients often minimize the seriousness of the problem (hoping it will go away if they ignore it) until the dyspnea becomes impossible to ignore. Therefore, the EMT is likely to encounter the patient with pulmonary edema in an advanced state of acute respiratory distress.

History: Subjective Reports

The chief complaint of the pulmonary edema patient will be shortness of breath (dyspnea). The history of the present episode will reveal dyspnea that is worse while the patient is lying flat (orthopnea) and often wakes the patient from sleep during the night with the sensation of needing air (paroxysmal noctural dyspnea). These patients often sleep with two or three pillows, in a semisitting position. Their dyspnea is often worse on exertion. Chest pain may be present. The patient may also relate symptoms he/she has attributed to the flu or a respiratory infection (shortness of breath, fatigue, and a persistent cough). Often the patient has a past medical history of heart disease or high blood pressure (hypertension).

Examination: Objective Physical Findings

The patient will be an anxious-looking person, sitting bolt upright, possibly agitated, restless, or combative. The patient may cough up frothy, pink (blood-tinged) sputum. Cyanosis may be present. Respirations are rapid and shallow, tachycardia is usually present, and the blood pressure is generally elevated (particularly the diastolic pressure). Auscultation of the chest may reveal rales, rhonchi, or wheezes. In severe cases, lung bases may be silent or may only be heard high up on the posterior chest.

The patient in CHF may have both left heart failure (leading to pulmonary edema) and right heart failure. If significant right heart failure is present, the patient will have swelling of the ankles (peripheral edema) and distended neck veins.

It can be difficult to distinguish cardiac pulmonary edema from COPD with acute respiratory failure. Because the treatment is different, Table 12–1 may help.

EMT Treatment

The following therapeutic measures should be performed *in the sequence listed below and only as necessary.*

■ Provide oxygen.

  ■ Use the condition of the patient as a guide to determine the delivery method and flow rate.
  ■ Begin with nasal prongs using low flow (2 L/min).
  ■ If the respiratory distress continues, immediately begin high-flow oxygen (non- or partial rebreather mask at a rate sufficient to maintain bag inflation).

■ Assist with ventilations.

  ■ Patients with cardiac pulmonary edema can usually ventilate adequately on their own.
  ■ Mechanical ventilation with a bag-valve or demand-valve mask may be necessary if the patient's condition is severe:
    –The respiratory distress worsens
    –The patient becomes too exhausted to breathe (respiratory failure)
    –The patient becomes drowsy or obtunded (hypoxia)
  ■ The patient may resist initial attempts at bag-valve mask ventilation assistance, but will stop resisting as breathing becomes easier.
  ■ Continued reassurance and constant explanation of the ventilatory assistance procedures will usually relieve much of the anxiety. Keep in mind that much of the patient's anxiety may be related to the hypoxia and will not be alleviated until oxygenation is improved.

■ Position the patient in an upright, sitting position with feet dangling to reduce venous return (most patients will already be doing this). Keep the patient upright with feet dangling while transporting to the hospital.

■ Minimize exertion and anxiety.

  ■ Avoid patient exertion of any type if at all possible. Even short walking distances may push the patient over the edge to severe respiratory distress.
  ■ During patient movement from the present location to the transport vehicle, the patient is often placed on a stretcher. Monitor the patient closely, because the elevated position of the legs may further exacerbate the respiratory distress.

Table 12-1 Distinguishing Characteristics of Cardiac Pulmonary Edema and COPD with Acute Respiratory Failure

	CARDIAC PULMONARY EDEMA	COPD WITH ACUTE RESPIRATORY FAILURE
History	The patient may have cardiac medications (nitroglycerin, digoxin, diltiazem) and diuretics or water pills (furosemide).	The patient may have lung medications (theophylline, albuterol) or home oxygen.
Physical Signs		
"Barrel chest"	Rare	Often present
Clubbing of fingers	Rare	Often present
Cyanosis	Less prominent	More prominent
Blood pressure	Usually elevated (particularly the diastolic)	Usually normal or only slightly elevated
Rales	More common	Less common
Wheezing	Less common	More common
Prolonged expiratory phase	Rare	Often present
Sputum	White or pink	Yellow-green

Ensure that the patient has rapid provision of, or transport to, ALS services.

■ PULMONARY EMBOLISM

Definition

An *embolism* is a blood clot or foreign body lodged in a blood vessel, blocking the circulation of blood to areas beyond the site. When an embolism lodges in a pulmonary artery or arteriole, blocking the flow of blood to part of the lungs, it is called a *pulmonary embolism.* Blood clots generally come from other parts of the body, usually from the veins of the legs or pelvis, and occasionally from around an artificial heart valve. Blood clots are formed in a number of different medical conditions or as a result of predisposing factors: inactivity (such as prolonged bed rest after surgery); inflamed veins (thrombophlebitis); or birth control pill use, particularly when associated with smoking. Foreign body embolism can be a fat particle from a broken bone end, an air bubble from a neck wound, or amniotic fluid as a complication of childbirth.

Acute Scenario

An embolus that forms or is created in a large vessel of the body is likely to be large enough to cause significant interruption of blood flow within the lung if it is dislodged and travels there. The sudden blockage of circulation to part of the lungs causes the sudden onset of respiratory distress, because the part of the lung deprived of circulation no longer participates in the exchange of gases.

History: Subjective Reports

The symptoms resulting from pulmonary embolism will vary greatly depending upon the size and location of the embolism. The chief complaint will be the sudden onset of severe shortness of breath (dyspnea). Patients may also complain of pleuritic chest pain and coughing up of blood (hemoptysis). The past medical history may include one of the predisposing conditions just discussed, such as thrombophlebitis. Some patients will provide a history of recent, less severe episodes of dyspnea. These patients may actually have been experiencing the symptoms of small pulmonary emboli (showers). When the embolism is larger or lodges in a main pulmonary vessel, the symptoms will be severe. Severe dyspnea, anxiety, and dizziness will be the primary symptoms.

Examination: Objective Physical Findings

Determination of vital signs will reveal rapid breathing, tachycardia, and possibly hypotension. Auscultation of the chest may reveal wheezes audible near the pain source. Check the lower extremities for evidence of inflammation of the veins. The obvious signs of a significant pulmonary embolism will be signs and symptoms of hypoxia and cardiovascular collapse (tachypnea, tachycardia, hypotension, and anxiety).

EMT Treatment

▓ Provide immediate high-flow oxygen.

▓ Treatment for shock may be indicated, if the patient is hypotensive or displaying other signs of shock. The EMT may be seeing the patient during the early stage of shock (compensatory stage). Antishock trousers (MAST) are not recommended for the pulmonary embolism patient.

▓ The acutely ill patient with a suspected pulmonary embolism needs the rapid provision of, or transport to, ALS services.

■ PNEUMONIA

Definition

Pneumonia is an infection in one or both lungs, which occurs when a portion of the lung is filled with fluid or pus. The most common causes are bacteria or viruses. It can also be caused by aspiration of vomitus, or be secondary to cancer.

Acute Scenario

Pneumonia causes acute respiratory distress when the inflammation interferes with the exchange of gas.

History: Subjective Reports

The symptoms resulting from pneumonia may vary depending upon the cause. When the pneumonia is from a lung infection, the chief complaint may be the sudden onset of shaking, chills and fever. Shortness of breath (dyspnea) is usually present. Chest pain, especially on inspiration, may be present. The history of the present illness may reveal a cough productive of dark sputum.

Examination: Objective Physical Findings

The patient may be any age but more commonly will be an elderly, debilitated person. The skin will be hot and dry. Respirations will be rapid. Auscultation of the chest may reveal rhonchi, usually involving one lung only, or decreased breath sounds. Abnormal lungs sounds (rhonchi or absent sounds) are often heard in only a small section or lobe of one lung (referred to as consolidation).

EMT Treatment

■ Provide oxygen.

  ■ Begin with low-flow oxygen.
  ■ If respiratory distress is severe, provide high-flow oxygen.

■ Place the patient in a position of comfort, usually sitting.

■ Consider the possibility of septic shock while performing the focused physical examination.

■ Transport the patient for physician evaluation and treatment of the underlying cause.

■ PLEURISY (PLEURITIS)

Definition

Pleurisy (pleuritis) is an inflammation of the double-layered lining of the lung (pleura). Injury or disease can cause the loss of friction-free movement of the chest wall lining (parietal pleura) against the lung covering (visceral pleura). The most common cause is infection. Less common causes include pulmonary embolism and cancer.

Acute Scenario

Severe pain can come from the friction of the inflamed lining surfaces rubbing against each other. The onset may be sudden.

History: Subjective Reports

The chief complaint will be localized pain associated with respiration (pleuritic), especially increased with deep inspiration. The patient may be short of breath if the pain is severe. Other complaints include a cough, fever, and/or chills, which are consistent with an infectious cause of the pleurisy.

Examination: Objective Physical Findings

The examination may be unremarkable, except for a possibly increased respiratory rate, fever, and coughing.

EMT Treatment

▓ Provide oxygen.

  ■ Begin with low-flow oxygen.
  ■ If respiratory distress is severe, provide high-flow oxygen.

▓ Place the patient in a position of comfort.

▓ Transport for physician evaluation and treatment of the underlying cause.

Cardiovascular Disorders

As was discussed in Chapter 4, there are several different aspects to cardiovascular distress. Some are objective signs observable by the EMT, such as changes in heart rate or blood pressure. Chest pain, in contrast, is entirely subjective. The medical causes of these signs and symptoms are the subject of this section. Other illnesses or trauma can cause similar signs and symptoms, as listed in Chapter 4.

■ HEART ATTACK (MYOCARDIAL INFARCTION)

Definition

An acute MI occurs when there is sudden blockage by a thrombus, or blood clot, of a coronary artery, which supplies blood to the heart muscle (myocardium). A portion of the myocardium dies after being deprived of oxygenated blood. An MI may also occur as a result of a disease process called atherosclerosis, which involves the narrowing and hardening of the blood vessels. Atherosclerosis in the coronary arteries is called coronary artery disease (CAD). Atherosclerosis occurs in the blood vessel walls when cholesterol deposits, scarring, and calcium deposits gradually build up over the years. CAD can start at a very early age and it takes years to progress. Thus, MIs most commonly occur in people in their 50s, 60s, and 70s but can occur in those in their 30s and 40s.

Acute Scenario

An MI is an acute medical emergency because the MI patient is at high risk for three very serious complications: sudden cardiac arrest, cardiogenic shock, and pulmonary edema. Cardiac rhythm disturbances (arrhythmias) occur with the greatest frequency in the first hour after MI, and arrhythmia can cause sudden cardiac arrest in the MI patient without warning.

History: Subjective Reports

The chief complaint of the MI patient will usually be intense, continuous chest pain, located under the sternum. The patient may report that the pain radiates down the left arm (in approximately 25% of patients) or to both arms, the jaw, neck, back, or upper abdomen. Patients may use any of several words to describe the quality of the pain, such as "crushing," "squeezing," "heavy," "tight," or "aching." The history may reveal that the pain has been present for 15 minutes or more. The onset may have occurred while the patient was at rest, sleeping or sitting quietly. The pain typically is not relieved by nitroglycerin, rest, or antacids.

Other associated symptoms may also be present: shortness of breath, weakness, nausea, vomiting, dizziness, or palpitations. Some patients may feel that, if they could only belch, the pain would go away. For some patients, the primary complaint is shortness of breath or the inability to get enough air. Often the pressure sensation is overlooked by the patient or attributed to the shortness of breath. Dyspnea in a patient at risk for CAD is a significant finding and should make the EMT suspicious of acute MI. If significant left heart failure has occurred and pulmonary edema is developing, dyspnea and cough may worsen. The past medical history may reveal some of the risk factors for MI: diabetes, hypertension, smoking, high cholesterol, and a family history of heart disease.

The MI patient is usually extremely anxious and fearful, with a feeling of impending doom. People express fear in different ways. Some become demanding and may adamantly refuse the oxygen mask. Others may have *denial* and minimize the severity of the symptoms. Still others may be fearful because they recall a heart attack experienced by their mother, father, or other family member at a similar age.

A small percentage of patients may experience a silent MI, also called "MI without tears." These patients are usually diabetics or elderly and do not complain of chest pain or discomfort. Their only complaint may be sudden shortness of breath, lightheadedness or confusion, weakness, or mild epigastric distress.

Examination: Objective Physical Findings

The MI patient will be an anxious-looking person, usually with pale, cool, clammy skin, that may appear gray in Caucasians. A rapid, irregular pulse may be present, although occasionally patients with some MIs may have a very slow pulse rate. The blood pressure may have fallen, but it may only be down to "normal" if the past medical history included hypertension. If significant pulmonary edema has occurred, the respiratory rate may be rapid, and auscultation of the chest may reveal rales or wheezes (cardiac asthma).

■ After placing the patient on oxygen, obtain a quick impression of the patient's discomfort if possible.
  – Have the patient take a deep inspiration. The pain should not change with chest wall movement.
  – Note the look of apprehension, discomfort, or writhing from the pain.

- Quickly reassess the ABCDs.
  - Determine if the patient is unconscious or lethargic.
  - Listen to the lungs.
  - Determine the respiratory rate and depth.
  - Obtain a blood pressure measurement (preferably in each arm).
  - Determine the pulse rate, quality, and regularity.
  - Take special note of an irregular pulse. The pulse can be categorized as regularly irregular (such as a dropped beat every three or four beats) or irregularly irregular (random, with no regular pattern).
- Monitor the vital signs regularly
- Look for ankle swelling (peripheral edema). Press with the thumb to see if indentation persists (pitting edema).
- Check the neck veins for distention.

EMT Treatment

If the patient is unconscious, treatment consists of assessment and management of the ABCDs: airway, breathing, circulation, and disability/defibrillation.

Once these priorities are managed, provide oxygen in high concentration. Extremely anxious and fearful patients may refuse the mask, and a nasal cannula may be better tolerated, but that is a second choice. Patients with less severe symptoms often do well with low-flow oxygen by nasal cannula.

Keep the patient calm, if conscious, and provide reassurance. Do not have the patient walk or exert himself/herself. Lift, move, or carry the patient as necessary to avoid additional demands on the heart.

Place the patient in a semireclining position. If the patient is in cardiogenic shock, place in a supine position.

Monitor the vital signs regularly.

Avoid the use of sirens unless absolutely necessary.

Assure rapid provision of, or transport to, ALS services.

NOTE. Acute MI can be treated with thrombolytic agents. These drugs can dissolve the clot causing the myocardial infarction and reduce the damage to the heart muscle. The sooner these agents are given, the more effective they are. Regardless of whether thrombolytic agents, emergent angioplasty, or other treatment regimens are preferred in your community, it is extremely important to rapidly transport patients with suspected MIs. Remember, "time is muscle" in the setting of acute MI.

■ Angina Pectoris

Definition

Angina pectoris refers to pain in the chest (literally, "choking in the chest"). Angina is a symptom of CAD and is caused by an insufficient blood supply to the heart muscle. The pain occurs when the need of the myocardium for oxygen exceeds the available supply of oxygenated blood. It is usually triggered by physical exertion or emotional stress and is relieved by rest. It is of short duration, usually less than 10 minutes. Angina differs from MI in that the flow of oxygenated blood is only reduced rather than completely blocked.

Acute Scenario

Angina occurs as a symptom of CAD, a chronic disease with which most patients learn to live. These patients may call for EMS when they are having increasing episodes of angina, the angina episode lasts longer than normal, or they are getting less relief from rest or the heart medication nitroglycerin. Increasing angina can be a sign of worsening CAD, which can lead to acute MI.

History: Subjective Reports

The chief complaint of the angina patient will usually be mild to moderate chest pain, located under the sternum. The patient may report that the pain radiates down the left arm or to both arms, the jaw, or the epigastrium. Rarely the pain only occurs at a remote site such as the left arm or jaw. Patients may use any of several words to describe the quality of the pain, such as "squeezing," "pressure," "aching," "tightness," or "discomfort." The history of the present illness may reveal that the pain has a short duration, usually 3 to 5 minutes and rarely more than 10 minutes. The onset may have occurred with physical exertion, emotional stress, cold weather, or a large meal. The pain will usually be relieved by rest or nitroglycerin tablets, and usually will not change with respiration or change of position.

Other associated symptoms may be present, including shortness of breath, weakness, nausea, or anxiety. Patients will often have a past medical history of cardiac disease and may be taking prescribed cardiac medications, such as nitroglycerin or diltiazem (cardizem).

It can be difficult to distinguish angina pectoris from acute MI (Table 12–2). When there is any doubt, treat the patient as if an MI were occurring.

Examination: Objective Physical Findings

■ The patient may look quite ill during an episode of pain, but will take on a normal appearance rapidly when the pain subsides.

Table 12-2   Distinguishing Characteristics of Angina Pectoris and Myocardial Infarction

CHARACTERISTIC	ANGINA	MYOCARDIAL INFARCTION
Pain		
Intensity	Mild to moderate	Severe, frightening
Duration	3–5 minutes (rarely over 10 minutes)	Over 15 minutes
Setting of onset	Physical exertion Emotional stress Cold weather	May occur at rest
Alleviation of pain	Rest, nitroglycerin	Not by rest or nitroglycerin
Associated symptoms	May be none	Often nausea, weakness, anxiety, sweating

- Conduct the same physical examination as for MI.
- Determine if the patient required a typical (for the patient) number of nitroglycerin tablets to relieve the pain and if the nitroglycerin produced a "bite" when used. This indicates that the medicine is still good. Moisture decreases the effectiveness of nitroglycerin, and patients who require frequent doses of their nitroglycerin will find it loses effectiveness sooner. Do not rely on the issue date on the bottle.
- Determine if the episode is the same as previous episodes with regard to the onset, intensity, and duration of pain. If the patient describes the current episode as different from previous experiences, treat as for an MI.

EMT Treatment

- If the current episode is normal, based upon previous episodes, assist with oxygen (2 to 4 L/min).

- Keep the scene calm and quiet.

- Complete the focused exam, including complete vital signs.

- Assist the patient with his/her prescribed nitroglycerin, if this episode is the same as that for which he/she would normally take nitroglycerin. Consider this assistance only if
  - The systolic blood pressure is at least 100 mm Hg
  - The patient has not taken more than a total of three nitroglycerin tablets or sprays for this episode
  - The patient is in a sitting or supine position

■ Treat the patient as having an MI if this episode of pain

- Is different than normal *or*
- Is not relieved with three nitroglycerin tablets *or*
- Lasts longer than 15 minutes, *or*
- Worsens or becomes atypical for the patient in any way

■ CONGESTIVE HEART FAILURE

Definition

Congestive heart failure (CHF) occurs when the heart muscle fails to pump effectively. This ineffectiveness leads to fluid accumulation in the tissue spaces. When the left side of the heart fails, fluid accumulates in the lungs (pulmonary edema). When the right side of the heart fails, fluid accumulates in the extremities (peripheral edema). If right heart failure exists for a long period, fluid eventually also accumulates in the abdominal organs, resulting in abdominal distention (ascites).

The most common cause of CHF is myocardial infarction. The onset of CHF may be 3 to 7 days or more after the occurrence of the MI. Other causes of CHF include cardiac rhythm disturbance; high blood pressure (hypertension); blood volume (fluid) overload from various sources, such as excess salt in the diet; and heart valve disease.

CHF may be mild or severe and life threatening. Pulmonary edema is the most extreme form of CHF. A full description of the signs, symptoms, and treatment of pulmonary edema is given in the previous section on respiratory distress.

Acute Scenario

The patient with right heart failure rarely calls for emergency medical assistance for this condition alone. Generally, right heart failure is seen in patients who are calling for some other, more urgent reason, such as COPD (chronic bronchitis) with respiratory decompensation or MI. Similarly, left heart failure can be mild, as in chronic CHF, or acute, as in acute MI with pulmonary edema.

History: Subjective Reports

Since the patient with right heart failure will usually be seen by the EMT when there is some more pressing emergency condition, the chief complaint will not be related to the right heart failure.

The chief complaint of the patient with left heart failure will be shortness of breath (dyspnea). The patient may also complain of progressive fatigue. If the left heart failure is advanced, the patient may complain of all the symptoms of pulmonary edema (see Pulmonary Edema in this chapter).

Examination: Objective Physical Findings

The patient with right heart failure will have swelling of the extremities (peripheral edema). Press with the thumb to see if indentation persists (pitting edema). Pitting edema can occur when the peripheral edema has persisted for a long time (chronic CHF). Abdominal fluid accumulation (ascites) and distended neck veins may also be seen.

The patient with left heart failure may have all or only a few of the signs of pulmonary edema: frothy, pink sputum; cyanosis; rapid, shallow respirations; tachycardia; high blood pressure; and rales or rhonchi. The patient with CHF may have both left and right heart failure at the same time and thus have signs of both.

EMT Treatment

Right heart failure requires no specific treatment by the EMT. CHF with left heart failure is treated the same as pulmonary edema.

- Provide oxygen.
  - Use the condition of the patient as a guide to determine the delivery method and flow rate.
  - Begin with nasal prongs using low flow (2 L/min).
  - If the respiratory distress continues, immediately begin high-flow oxygen (non- or partial rebreather mask at a rate sufficient to maintain bag inflation).

- Assist with ventilations.
  - Patients with cardiac pulmonary edema can usually ventilate adequately on their own.
  - Mechanical ventilation with a bag-valve or demand-valve mask may be necessary if the patient's condition is severe:
    – The respiratory distress worsens
    – The patient becomes too exhausted to breathe (respiratory failure)
    – The patient becomes drowsy or obtunded (hypoxia)
  - The patient may resist initial attempts at bag-valve mask ventilation assistance, but will stop resisting as breathing becomes easier.
  - Continued reassurance and constant explanation of the ventilatory assistance procedures will usually relieve much of the anxiety. Keep in mind that much of the patient's anxiety may be related to the hypoxia and will not be alleviated until oxygenation is improved.

- Position the patient in an upright, sitting position with feet dangling to reduce venous return (most patients will already be doing this). Keep the patient upright with feet dangling while transporting to the hospital.

- Minimize exertion and anxiety.
  - Avoid patient exertion of any type if at all possible. Even short walking distances may push the patient over the edge to severe respiratory distress.

■ During patient movement from the present location to the transport vehicle, the patient is often placed on a stretcher. Monitor the patient closely because the elevated position of the legs may further exacerbate the respiratory distress.

■ Ensure that the patient has rapid provision of, or transport to, ALS services.

EMT Special Considerations
Be aware that sudden worsening of chronic CHF is often caused by myocardial infarction.

■ Pacemaker Failure
Definition
A *cardiac pacemaker* is a device that artificially delivers an electrical impulse to the heart to control its rate and rhythm. Implanted surgically, an operation, it has two parts: the generating unit, placed under the skin near the surface; and the wires, which are sewn into the myocardium. *Pacemaker failure* occurs when something goes wrong with the device and it fails to deliver the electrical impulse to the heart. Failure is a rare event, and it is usually caused by battery failure or mechanical malfunction, not by loose wires.

Acute Scenario
The pacemaker failure may cause the heart to be unable to maintain a rate adequate for normal blood pressure. The patient is then at risk for heart failure or cardiogenic shock.

History: Subjective Reports
The chief complaint of the patient with pacemaker failure is likely to be sudden weakness or dizziness. The EMT may be called to the scene because of a decreased level of consciousness or cardiac arrest. The past medical history will indicate heart disease, pacemaker implant surgery, and cardiac medications. Most patients with pacemakers carry a card detailing the model, type, and rate setting for the unit.

Examination: Objective Physical Findings
The pulse rate in pacemaker failure will be slow: usually less than 50 beats/min and often 35 to 45 beats/min. However, it may increase initially. The rate is usually fixed and regular, although occasionally it may be irregular. Some patients may have syncopal episodes. The

patient may also exhibit signs of shock with the exception of tachycardia.

The pacemaker generating unit should be palpable under the skin, usually on the chest just below the clavicle (the left side is more common than the right).

EMT Treatment

■ Provide oxygen. If the patient's underlying heart rate is very slow, the patient will most likely require high-flow oxygen.

■ Treat for shock.

■ Anticipate and prepare for the possibility of cardiac arrest. Continuously monitor the patient's vital signs.

■ Provide rapid transport to ALS services.

EMT Special Considerations

The artificial cardiac pacemaker does not prevent heart disease, such as atherosclerosis or CAD. Therefore, it is possible for a patient with an implanted pacemaker to have angina pectoris, CHF, or even MI. Any patient with signs and symptoms of angina, CHF, or MI who also has a pacemaker is treated the same as any other patient with those signs and symptoms.

■ STOKES-ADAMS ATTACKS

Definition

Stokes-Adams attacks are cardiac rhythm disturbances in which the heart rate becomes very fast or very slow, causing a temporary reduction in cardiac output. The reduction in cardiac output results in transient hypotension, a reduction in cerebral blood flow, and often fainting.

Acute Scenario

Stokes-Adams attacks can cause fainting (syncope), during which the patient can sustain injury while falling. The syncope may even occur while seated. Stokes-Adams attacks can recur and may last long enough to cause cardiac arrest.

History: Subjective Reports

Usually, patients do not have any warning that Stokes-Adams attacks are about to occur. The chief complaint may be related to injury sustained from a fall during the syncopal episode. Patients may complain of palpitations or lightheadedness.

Examination: Objective Physical Findings

The Stokes-Adams attack patient is often an elderly person and is usually found by the EMT after the pulse has returned to normal. Patients typically return to consciousness spontaneously. Injury may be found if the patient fell during a syncopal episode.

EMT Treatment

■ Keep the patient flat, with the legs raised.

■ Provide high-flow oxygen.

■ Monitor the pulse rate closely. Document irregularities by recording the time of occurrence, duration of irregularity, and any pattern noted (regularly irregular or irregularly irregular). Record the findings.

■ Examine for possible injuries resulting from the syncope, fall, or convulsion.

EMT Special Considerations

Stokes-Adams attack is only one of many possible causes of fainting (syncope). A list of others can be found in Chapter 5.

■ Pericarditis

Definition

Pericarditis is the inflammation of the pericardial sac surrounding the heart. It is most commonly caused by a viral infection. It may also appear in post-MI patients at 2 to 6 weeks after the MI, which may be after the patient has been discharged to go home.

Acute Scenario

Severe pain can come from the friction of the inflamed lining surfaces rubbing against each other. The patient is at risk for cardiac rhythm disturbances (arrhythmia) or cardiac tamponade.

History: Subjective Reports

The chief complaint will be substernal or precordial chest pain, of variable intensity. The pain may radiate to the shoulders. The quality of pain is also variable, from a deep, dull ache to a sharp, burning pain. The patient may report that the onset of the pain was not sudden, but rather developed over hours or days. The pain may be affected by a change in position to a leaning-forward position. The pain is often not relieved by nitroglycerin. It may be aggravated by deep breathing, swallowing, or coughing. Shortness of breath (dyspnea) may be present as the patient attempts to avoid the pain of deep breathing. Past medical history may include cardiac disease and a recent MI.

Examination: Objective Physical Findings

The pericarditis patient will be anxious looking and may be breathing rapidly to avoid the pain of deep breathing. A slight fever may be present. As the pericarditis progressively worsens, the patient may become hypotensive, with a narrowing pulse pressure (difference between the systolic and diastolic blood pressures).

EMT Treatment

■ It may be difficult to distinguish pericarditis from acute MI. When in doubt, treat the patient as if an MI were occurring.

■ Provide high-flow oxygen.

■ Ensure rapid provision of, or transport to, ALS services.

■ HYPERTENSION

Definition

Hypertension simply means high blood pressure. It is defined as a systolic pressure of over 140 mm Hg or a diastolic pressure of over 90 mm Hg. The causes of hypertension, which are listed in Chapter 4, include head injury, essential hypertension (cause unknown), toxemia of pregnancy, and anxiety. Hypertension can be associated with (although it is not caused by) CVA, aortic aneurysm, CHF, pulmonary edema, or angina.

Acute Scenario

"Malignant hypertension" exists when the blood pressure is dangerously high, often 200/140 mm Hg or higher. This can cause severe vascular damage (such as CVA or dissecting aortic aneurysm), CHF with pulmonary edema, acute kidney failure, and death. In patients with known hypertension who abruptly stop therapy, hypertensive emergencies may develop.

History: Subjective Reports

The chief complaint may be headache or blurred vision. Associated symptoms include severe nosebleeds, nausea, or dyspnea. The past medical history may include hypertension, cardiac disease, vascular disease, or alcoholism.

Examination: Objective Physical Findings

High blood pressure is the hallmark finding. Other findings may depend upon the cause of the hypertension (such as toxemia in the pregnant patient) or may be the result of chronic hypertension (such as CHF). Similarly, the signs of a CVA or a dissecting aortic aneurysm will be specific to those medical conditions.

Occasionally, a severe nosebleed that does not stop after the usual treatment is associated with high blood pressure.

EMT Treatment

■ Treatment may be specific to the other medical conditions found.

■ If no other medical condition is found, place the patient in a sitting position, provide oxygen, and transport.

■ AORTIC ANEURYSM

Definition

Outpouching from weakening of the anterior wall of a blood vessel is called an aneurysm. The term *dissecting aneurysm* refers to bleeding through a tear of the arterial wall between the inner and outer linings. This creates a false channel in the arterial wall, which may result in occlusion of arteries branching off the injured artery. *Rupture of an aneurysm* is the worst complication, because the rupture will lead to massive hemorrhage. Aortic aneurysm can occur in either the thorax or the abdomen (Figs. 12–1 and 12–2). Aortic aneurysms of these locations are typically referred to as "thoracic dissecting aneurysms" and "abdominal aortic aneurysms" (AAAs), respectively.

Acute Scenario

There are no symptoms associated with the formation and development of an aneurysm. However, when an abdominal aortic aneurysm dissects, blood can leak into the abdominal cavity. Signs and symptoms of an "acute abdomen" then occur, because blood is an irritant to the abdominal lining (peritoneum). Likewise, if blood from a thoracic aortic aneurysm leaks into the thoracic cavity, chest pain occurs. When an aortic aneurysm ruptures, the rapid hemorrhage causes hypovolemic shock.

The dissecting aneurysm may also create symptoms resulting from the pressure placed on nearby structures by the bulging area of the aorta (see Figure 12–3).

History: Subjective Reports

Thoracic Aneurysm	Abdominal Aneurysm
■ Patients often have a history of hypertension.	■ Patients often have a history of arteriosclerosis.
■ The pain may begin in the chest and progress toward the legs or into the back.	■ The patient may report a previously diagnosed aneurysm.
■ The pain is often described as a tearing or "hot poker" through the chest or between the shoulder blades.	■ The pain is often described as a tearing through to the lower back.
■ The patient may have a fainting spell, with or without associated pain, which can include all the symptoms of shock.	■ The patient may have fainting, with or without associated pain, which can include all the symptoms of shock.
■ The pain is steady and unchanged with position.	■ The pain is steady and unchanged with position.
■ One or both upper extremities may be cold or numb.	■ One or both lower extremities may be cold or numb.

Examination: Objective Physical Findings

Thoracic Aneurysm	Abdominal Aneurysm
■ Palpate and compare radial pulses in both arms for presence and gross difference in amplitude.	■ Gently palpate the midline of the abdomen (above the umbilicus) for a pulsatile mass extending to one side of the aortic midline.
■ Auscultate and compare blood pressures in both arms for gross differences in readings.	■ Palpate and compare the amplitude of the femoral pulses.
■ Palpate and compare the carotid pulses for difference in amplitude. Do not check both sides at the same time.	■ Palpate the abdomen for fluid, rigidity, and increasing abdominal size.
■ Check for neurologic symptoms as a result of an occluded carotid artery or arteries.	■ Assess the vital signs frequently to monitor for shock.
■ Check for signs of cardiac tamponade –Distended neck veins –Falling blood pressure –Falling pulse pressure	■ Assess postural blood pressures if the patient's systolic blood pressure is above 90 mm Hg when supine.
■ Assess postural blood pressures if the patient's systolic blood pressure is above 90 mm Hg when supine.	■ Compare the warmth and color of the legs.

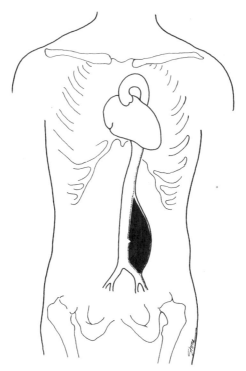

Figure 12-1

Abdominal aortic aneurysm involving a portion of the femoral artery.

EMT Treatment

▩ Provide oxygen.

- Without signs of shock, rupture, syncope, dizziness, or postural changes, provide low-flow oxygen by nasal cannula.
- When signs and symptoms of rupture or bleeding are noted, provide high-flow oxygen.
- Ventilate with bag-valve mask if needed.

▩ Place the patient supine with the lower extremities elevated to treat low blood pressure.

▩ Consider applying antishock trousers (MAST), if available. Use the abdominal section (in addition to the leg sections) for abdominal aortic aneurysm only. Request ALS services life support if available and provide rapid transport to the most appropriate receiving hospital.

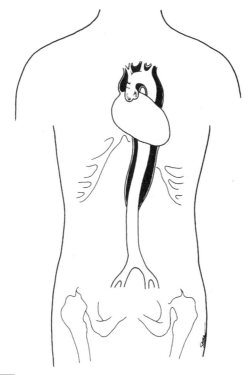

Figure 12-2

Thoracic aortic aneurysm.

■ IMPLANTABLE CARDIOVERTER DEFIBRILLATOR (ICD) EMERGENCIES

Definition

Patients who have survived an episode of sudden cardiac arrest or who have recurrent episodes of life-threatening arrhythmias may have an ICD surgically placed in their bodies. The ICD is a device that continuously senses the heart's rhythm (primarily through rate detection). If the rhythm suddenly changes to a life-threatening rhythm, the device will automatically charge and deliver an electrical current across the heart. The electricity, if successful, will convert the abnormal rhythm to a normal rhythm. Usually it takes 10 to 20 seconds for the device to sense the abnormal rhythm, charge, and deliver the shock. Most of the time the patient will lose consciousness before the shock occurs, but sometimes the patient may remain conscious. Older devices were placed beneath abdominal muscles in the left upper quadrant because of the size of the device. Today, as a

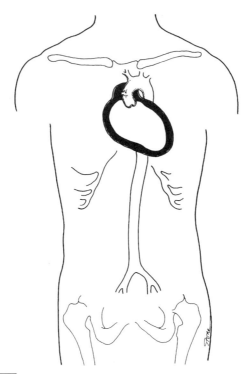

Figure 12-3

Dissecting thoracic aortic aneurysm causing cardiac tamponade.

result of technology improvements, the ICD is often placed in the left upper chest. Wires placed under the skin connect the device to patches placed on the heart. Newer ICDs are inserted like pacemakers and have wire electrodes placed within the heart. Most ICDs are "programmed" to deliver up to six shocks in sequence, if needed. Design improvements have also allowed the incorporation of pacemaker capabilities. There are 100,000 patients in the United States with ICDs.

EMT Treatment

The EMT should, in general, ignore the presence of the ICD and do whatever is necessary for the patient. In other words, if CPR is needed, CPR should be performed. There is little chance that the ICD will discharge during CPR. Even if it does, there is virtually no risk to the EMT. The most that could be felt is a small tingle in the EMT's hands if the patient's chest is touched during a discharge. With the use of universal precautions, even this is unlikely to occur.

Occasionally, patients with an ICD will request the assistance of the EMS system due to a discharge of the device. When this occurs, the EMT should assume that one of the following scenarios met the ICD's programmed criteria, which prompted the discharge:

- The ICD sensed a rapid, lethal arrhythmia (e.g., ventricular fibrillation).
- The ICD sensed a rapid, potentially harmful or possibly nonharmful arrhythmia.
- The ICD malfunctioned for some reason.

With these thoughts in mind, the EMT's examination and history should be focused on the events leading up to the discharge. Ask the patient questions about signs or symptoms noted prior to the discharge (e.g., chest pain, dizziness, shortness of breath, palpitations). Many cardiologists are now advising patients to stay home if the device discharges once or twice and if no symptoms are present after the discharge. Ask the patient when his/her cardiologist directed the patient to go to the hospital or office following an ICD discharge. The patients have usually been well educated by their physicians. When in doubt, or if the patient is symptomatic in any way, transport the patient. Treat the patient based on his/her complaints and exam findings.

Rarely, the ICD will malfunction, resulting in repeated discharges. These patients must be provided with or transported to ALS services and an appropriately equipped emergency department as rapidly as possible so that the device can be turned off.

Neurologic Disorders

As indicated in Chapter 5, there are several different aspects of problems originating in the CNS. Neurologic problems include impairments in consciousness (coma, syncope) and in involuntary control over movement (seizures, paralysis). These signs can occur as a result of problems that do not originate in the CNS and those other medical or traumatic conditions (listed in Chapter 5) are discussed in other chapters of this book. The subject of this section is neurologic disorders.

■ STROKE (CEREBROVASCULAR ACCIDENT)

Definition

A CVA is a syndrome associated with an interruption in blood supply to a portion of the brain, resulting in temporary, reversible or irreversible brain tissue ischemia. In the United States, stroke (CVA) is the third leading cause of death and continues to be a significant cause of disability. The effects depend upon which part of the brain is involved, such as the part controlling speech or the parts controlling movement of one side of the body. Three distinctly different mechanisms can cause a CVA. The most common is a clot (thrombus) that progressively blocks a cerebral artery, usually as a result of atherosclerosis. Another is a wandering blood clot (embolus) that lodges in a cerebral artery, blocking blood flow. This can result from atherosclerosis, heart valve disease, cardiac rhythm disturbance (atrial fibrillation), sickle cell disease, or rarely birth control pill use. The third possible cause of CVA is hemorrhage into brain tissue from rupture of a cerebral blood vessel, usually associated with high blood pressure (hypertension).

Acute Scenario

Strokes can vary in severity from mild, in which only a small area of the brain is affected and little difficulty is experienced by the patient, to severe, with coma, seizures, or respiratory difficulty. Although a thrombus (clot) is the most common cause of strokes, the severity of the symptoms and effects are generally much greater in hemorrhagic strokes. A stroke may resemble a transient ischemic attack (TIA) (discussed next) but have symptoms that last longer (days to weeks). The symptoms may then reverse completely or nearly completely. As with a TIA, this type of stroke is often a warning sign of an increased risk for a completed stroke (irreversible symptoms). In other strokes, the symptoms may progress slowly, resulting, however, in irreversible damage to brain tissue. Still other strokes may progress very rapidly. Hemorrhagic strokes can progress to death in a matter of hours.

Early recognition and treatment for stroke patients are crucial to the reduction of death and disability from strokes. The EMT should understand the risk factors for stroke, which include

- Hypertension; hypertension with smoking has an even greater risk
- Smoking
- Diabetes
- Elevated cholesterol levels
- Use of oral contraceptives—smoking while using oral contraceptives has a significantly increased risk
- Existing cardiac disease—valvular disease and atrial fibrillation are common cardiac conditions seen in the stroke patient
- Previous strokes—small, reversible strokes and TIAs place the patient at a clearly increased risk of a more severe stroke because these are simply stroke warning signs

The EMT can play a significant role in preventing the progression of symptoms toward a severe stroke. By recognizing the risk factors and warning signs, the EMT can ensure that the patient receives proper evaluation and treatment by a physician. It is becoming common for parallels to be drawn between strokes and MIs. This is being done not only because the causes of impaired blood supply in the brain are similar to those of impaired blood supply in the heart, but also because the urgency is similar in both. In the case of a hemorrhagic stroke, the time to definitive therapy is critical to the patient's likelihood of survival and subsequent disabilities. Just as "time is muscle" to the MI patient, the stroke patient must receive rapid assessment, care, and transport.

History: Subjective Reports

What the patient relates as the symptoms of the present problem may indicate whether the CVA is thrombotic, embolic, or hemorrhagic, as Table 12–3 illustrates. A thorough history is critical to the assessment of the stroke patient. While it may not be crucial that the EMT differentiate between a thrombotic and an embolic stroke, every effort must be made to identify the potential hemorrhagic stroke. In some communities, this differentiation may alter the destination of transport based upon the potential surgical needs of a severe hemorrhagic stroke.

In addition to the usual history taking, the EMT should ask about the following:

1. What symptoms were present immediately prior to this event?
   a. Did the patient complain of dizziness, headache, visual aura, vision difficulty, a stiff neck, or palpitations?
   b. Was the patient noted to be experiencing confusion, impaired coordination, irregular breathing, or difficulty speaking or comprehending?

2. What was the timing of the onset of symptoms?
   a. What time did the first symptoms appear?
   b. What was the patient doing at the time of onset?
   c. How quickly did other symptoms appear?

3. Has the patient experienced any similar symptoms or complained of any other symptoms recently?
   a. Has the patient had recent episodes of falling, or staring blankly?
   b. Has the patient had a recent infection, illness, or unusual difficulty with a chronic illness?

Also, the EMT should include a past medical history that identifies

- Previous strokes, TIAs, emboli, or carotid artery occlusions
- Possible risk factors for stroke or heart disease
- Family history of strokes
- Lifestyle risk factors (IV drug use, cocaine use)

Examination: Objective Physical Findings

The examination findings will vary greatly depending upon the portion of the brain involved, the cause of the stroke, and the extent of injury that has already occurred. Signs of a CVA include facial asym-

Table 12-3 Types of Cerebrovascular Accident

SYMPTOM	THROMBUS	EMBOLUS	HEMORRHAGE
Onset of symptoms	Can evolve over several hours	Sudden	Sudden
Activity at onset	Often occurs while sleeping or without activity	No association with activity	Often occurs during daytime when activity is present
Headache	Mild	Moderate	Severe
History of TIAs	Often	Occasional	None
Past medical history	Atherosclerosis	Heart valve disease, atrial fibrillation, sickle cell disease	Hypertension
Associated symptoms	One-sided weakness, dizziness	One-sided weakness, dizziness	Headache, stiff neck

metry, speech disturbance, lack of coordination, unequal pupils, unequal grip strength, unilateral paralysis, decreased level of consciousness, and seizures. It is useful to conduct a neurologic exam in order to document the level and type of dysfunction present (see Appendix G). The observations made in the field serve as useful reference observations should the dysfunction change. The physical exam report should include that the observations were made.

Assess the ABCDs

- Assess the airway. Considering that many stroke patients have an altered mental status, the assessment of the patient's ability to protect his/her airway is critical.
  - Is the patient able to maintain his/her airway open?
  - Does the patient have snoring respirations without manual manipulation of the airway?
  - Can the patient cough or speak?
- Assess the breathing. Stroke patients will often develop irregular breathing patterns. At times, the respirations may not be adequate to provide sufficient oxygenation.
  - If the breathing is very slow, irregular, or absent, immediately begin assisting ventilations.
  - If the rate and depth appear adequate, assess the breathing pattern.
  - Assess the lung sounds, particularly with an altered mental status, because the patient may easily have aspirated.
- Assess the circulation. Hypertension is often noted in the stroke patient. Hypotension is a serious sign that often results from another concurrent injury or illness other than the stroke.
  - Is the patient hypertensive or hypotensive?
  - Is the pulse rapid or irregular?
- Assess disability.
  - Is the patient unconscious or with an altered mental status?
  - Is the alteration of mental status improving, remaining the same, or progressively worsening?
  - Assess the level of consciousness using
    a. Orientation to person, place, and/or time
    b. The Glascow coma scale
    c. Response to verbal and painful stimuli

Continue Focused Physical Examination

- Frequently obtain and record the vital signs.
  - Pulse—rate, regularity, symmetry
  - Respirations—rate, pattern, breath sounds
  - Blood pressure—systolic and diastolic measurements
  - Pupillary responses—size, reaction to light, symmetry, deviated gaze
  Monitor the vital signs for progressive changes. Increasing blood pressure with decreasing heart rate are signs of a serious brain injury.
- Conduct multiple neurologic assessments (see Appendix G for a neurologic checklist).
  - Ability to speak and comprehend
  - Ability to follow commands
  - Motor function—ability to move all limbs, grip strength, symmetry of motor function

Be alert for changes in the neurologic assessment. Progressive worsening of neurologic functions may indicate progression of the stroke.

■ Observe the patient for other possible signs of stroke:
  – Facial droop
  – Seizures—generalized or focal
  – Vomiting
  – Hemiplegia

■ Examine for other injuries or illnesses.
  – Trauma, particularly head trauma, may exhibit signs and symptoms similar to stroke. Examine for traumatic injuries and inquire about recent traumatic mechanisms (fall, assault, and motor vehicle accident).
  – Some medical conditions may also exhibit signs and symptoms that resemble those of stroke. Look for signs or history of
    a. Alcohol or drug abuse or intoxication
    b. Diabetes complications
    c. Seizure disorders
    d. Infectious diseases of the nervous system (e.g., meningitis)

EMT Treatment

■ Provide supplemental oxygen.

  ■ At a minimum, low-flow oxygen should be administered to all stroke patients.
  ■ Patients with irregular or erratic respiratory patterns as well as those with altered mental status should be provided with high flow oxygen.
  ■ Provide ventilatory assistance to patients whose respirations are slow, absent, or inadequate.

■ Monitor vital signs and neurologic status frequently.

  ■ Be alert for respiratory difficulty that may require ventilatory assistance.
  ■ Be especially alert for a rising blood pressure with a falling pulse rate.
  ■ Monitor the patient for a declining mental status.
  ■ These conditions indicate a need for rapid provision of, or transport to, ALS services and an emergency department.

■ Transport the supine patient with the head slightly elevated if the blood pressure is high.

■ Emotional support to the patient is very important, especially if he/she is conscious and understands what is happening. Explain to the patient that he/she may be having a stroke and it is impossible to say what the final outcome will be, but there is hope that the problem is temporary and that much function will return. Always try to be reassuring to the patient, but do not make exaggerated claims that everything will be all right.

■ Protect paralyzed extremities from injury.

■ Give nothing by mouth.

EMT Special Considerations

Be aware that the inability to speak can occur in a patient otherwise quite capable of hearing, thinking, and feeling. The EMT may be able to communicate *to* the patient, even when the CVA patient is not able to communicate back to the EMT. Avoid thoughtless comments that an apparently unconscious patient could misinterpret and find upsetting. Remember that these patients may be able to follow simple commands, such as "squeeze my hand." There are many studies currently underway to identify improved therapies for stroke patients. Significant research is being directed toward the use of thrombolytic agents (clot-dissolving drugs) in thrombotic or embolic strokes. Advances in these areas may alter the treatment and/or transport destination for stroke patients in the future.

■ TRANSIENT ISCHEMIC ATTACK (TIA)

Definition

TIAs refer to symptoms of stroke that subside completely within 24 hours and usually within 6 hours. TIAs (also called "mini strokes") are caused by temporary reduction in blood supply to a portion of the brain. The relationship between TIA and CVA is very similar to the relationship between angina and MI. In fact, the underlying disease is the same: atherosclerosis. TIAs vary in frequency, and affected persons are normal between attacks. The diagnosis can be made only after rapid recovery has occurred; it cannot be made prior to complete recovery from the symptoms.

Acute Scenario

The sudden changes in behavior, speech, or motor function result from cerebral vascular insufficiency. A TIA can present as a syncopal episode.

History: Subjective Reports

The symptoms experienced by the patient will vary depending upon the portion of the brain affected. The most common episode described by family members or bystanders is that the patient suddenly became unresponsive, staring blankly while remaining awake. Associated symptoms include headache, dizziness, unilateral weakness or numbness, and loss of speech or vision. Some TIA patients will not have any symptoms other than the episode of unresponsiveness while awake. The past medical history will often reveal recurrent episodes of similar symptoms. As with the stroke patient, it is important for the EMT to obtain a complete history, including potential risk factors for stroke. The patient experiencing a TIA is now at greater risk for stroke, and therefore needs to be evaluated by a physician. This evaluation and treatment may prevent a future stroke.

Examination: Objective Physical Findings

The most common presentation is a short-lived neurologic loss. The loss depends upon the portion of the brain involved: speech disturbance, lack of coordination, unilateral paralysis, and so on. Because it may not be possible in the field to tell a TIA from a CVA, a thorough hospital neurologic examination is indicated. Often, the symptoms of a TIA are resolved by the time EMS responders arrive at the scene. In this case, most of the physical assessment results in normal findings. Regardless of the symptoms, the physical examination should be conducted in the same manner as for stroke patients.

EMT Treatment

■ If the signs and symptoms are not completely resolved, treat as if a CVA were occurring.

■ If the signs and symptoms have completely resolved, monitor the progression of symptoms or return of function. Transport for physician evaluation, even if the symptoms have cleared.

■ EPILEPSY

Definition

Epilepsy is a chronic disease characterized by seizures. It can be caused by an old brain injury with scarring, a birth injury, or genetic predisposition. In a large number of adults, the cause is unknown (idiopathic). Epilepsy is usually easily controlled by medication. *Seizures* (convulsions) are sudden episodes of involuntary muscle contraction and relaxation, caused by excessive brain cell electrical activity. Seizures have many other causes in addition to epilepsy, as listed in Chapter 5.

Seizures can involve generalized tonic-clonic activity ("grand mal") followed by unconsciousness and then confusion (postictal state). In other cases, seizures may be partial (focal) and limited to certain body parts. Partial seizures include such activity as localized muscle jerking, fleeting localized painful sensations, or involuntary repetitive behavior. Some partial seizures progress to generalized muscular activity. Generalized seizures include full-body convulsions or brief lapses of awareness ("petit mal"). *Status epilepticus* exists when there is a rapid succession of repeated seizures without regaining of consciousness during the intervals.

Acute Scenario

Seizures are the acute manifestation of epilepsy. As stated earlier, the actual cause of the epilepsy may or may not be identifiable. Medications keep the disease under control, but occasionally patients forget to take them or the dose is not sufficient. Status epilepticus is an acute medical emergency because the patient could die of hypoxia or aspiration during the episode.

History: Subjective Reports

The patient may report an aura—a sensation of light, color, or smell—before a seizure occurs.

The postictal patient may complain of a headache. Postseizure confusion and amnesia for the seizure and preceding events may occur. Occasionally, the postictal phase is prolonged. However, the patient generally demonstrates some progressive improvement in orientation. The history obtained from family members or close friends is often useful in determining if the seizure activity and postictal phase experienced by the patient are normal for him/her. History taking should also include recent illnesses and medication changes.

Examination: Objective Physical Findings

In some patients, a generalized seizure begins with focal signs or deviation of the eyes. The actual beginning of a generalized seizure is sudden unconsciousness with a short (30-second) period of tonic stiffening. This leads into the thrashing tonic-clonic activity, which generally lasts about 2 minutes. During this period, three things can occur. First, loss of control over the bowels and bladder is common, resulting in staining of clothing. Second, contraction of the chest muscles interferes with respiration, resulting in temporary cyanosis, which usually resolves rapidly after the seizure is over. Third, contraction of the jaw muscles can occasionally cause biting of the tongue or lips.

During the postictal period, seizure patients need to be examined for injuries of the extremities caused by the thrashing. The EMT must use extreme caution because many seizure patients are not only disoriented but also combative when they awaken. Other signs in the postictal period include slow return to consciousness, disorientation, drooling, fatigue, rapid pulse, or rapid respirations. The patient should be searched for a medical ID tag and seizure medications.

EMT Treatment

Protect the patient from injury during the seizure. Do not attempt rigid restraint of the patient.

If the jaws have not yet clenched, a padded tongue blade (bite block) should be placed between the patient's back teeth. *Do not force this into place during an active seizure. Do not use the front teeth. Do not insert fingers into the patient's mouth. Do not allow the bite block to slip into the mouth and obstruct the airway.*

Provide high-flow oxygen until the patient awakens, and suction as necessary. During transportation, low-flow oxygen (2 L/min) should be administered if the patient is awake and merely confused.

In the postictal period, examine the patient and turn on his/her side to prevent aspiration.

Provide emotional support and reassurance to the confused postictal patient. Be alert for combative behavior.

Transport all seizure patients to the hospital. Bring the patient's medications if possible.

For *status epilepticus*, provide

- High-flow oxygen
- Airway control and ventilatory assistance
- Rapid provision of, or transport to, ALS services and the emergency department

Diabetes

Diabetes mellitus is a disease in which the body is unable to efficiently utilize glucose (sugar) for energy. It is caused by a decrease in insulin, a hormone produced by the pancreas. There are two types of diabetes: a milder form, usually appearing in adulthood; and a more severe form, usually appearing in childhood, in which the diabetic is dependent upon insulin injections. Diabetes is controllable through diet, oral pills that stimulate insulin production, or insulin injections. Diabetic persons need to balance their food intake with the amount of insulin used.

■ Low Blood Glucose (Hypoglycemia)

Definition

Low blood glucose (hypoglycemia) occurs when the diabetic has taken too much insulin, has not eaten enough food, has had too much exercise, or has some combination of these factors. This condition is also called "insulin shock."

Acute Scenario

In hypoglycemia, the glucose is taken up by the body cells faster than it appears in the bloodstream. The brain is the most quickly affected organ.

History: Subjective Reports

Hypoglycemia generally occurs only in the diabetic who receives daily insulin injections. It may also occur in the patient who has taken too many oral diabetes medications (accidental or intentional ingestion). The onset of hypoglycemia is generally rapid, although it may be gradual if a long-acting insulin is used. The patient will be a known diabetic, often with a medical ID tag. If conscious, the patient will often relate a history of taking the normal amount of insulin, but exercising particularly strenuously, having a recent illness, or not eating. Common symptoms are headache, dizziness, confusion, weakness, and hunger. If the patient is alert and oriented, ask the following questions:

1. Are you a diabetic?
   a. How do you control your diabetes (diet, pills, or insulin)?
   b. How long have you been a diabetic? Patients with newly diagnosed diabetes may be less familiar with their disease and make errors in their eating, activity, or medication regulation.
   c. Are you being treated by a physician for your diabetes? Although a prescription is generally required for insulin, some patients may be able to get insulin without being under a physician's care.

2. Did you eat today?
   a. What did you eat and when? High-sugar and low-protein foods will be used very quickly and result in hypoglycemia later in the day if insulin is also taken.
   b. Is this a normal meal or snack for you? Many patients alter their meal routine because of lifestyle factors such as traveling, a busy schedule, or other commitments.

3. When did you last take your insulin?
   a. Did you take the normal dosage?
   b. What type of insulin did you take?

4. Have you been able to regularly control your blood sugar lately?
   a. Some patients may be having difficulty with extreme fluctuations in blood sugar levels, and therefore are prone to hypoglycemia.
   b. Recent or current illnesses, particularly infections, will alter the blood glucose requirements, and thus may make the patient susceptible to hypoglycemia.

If the patient did not eat adequately and took insulin, the patient probably has low blood glucose. If the patient ate and did not take the insulin, the patient probably has high blood glucose (discussed in the next part of this section).

Examination: Objective Physical Findings

If conscious, the patient may exhibit various disturbances in behavior: disorientation, lack of coordination, confusion, irritability, or hostility. The exam findings include an altered mental status, shaking or tremors, slightly elevated heart rate, and sweatiness.

If the patient is unconscious, the history may be difficult to obtain. Usually the only information from bystanders that is reliable is whether the onset of symptoms was sudden (over minutes) or gradual (over hours or days). Assessment of the patient then depends upon physical findings. Signs of low blood sugar include drooling; pale, cool, moist skin; full, rapid pulse; normal blood pressure and respirations; and convulsions in late stages. The examination must include a search for medical alert tags, diabetes medications, or other indicators of a past history of diabetes.

It can be difficult to distinguish low blood glucose from high blood glucose (see Table 12–4). When there is any doubt, treat the patient as if low blood glucose were present.

EMT Treatment

■ If the patient is conscious and able to protect his/her own airway, administer sugar by mouth in the form of candy, sweetened fruit juice, sugar cubes, or prepared dextrose solution tubes.

■ If the patient is unconscious, first attend to the ABCDs: airway, breathing, circulation, and disability. Provide high-flow oxygen and suction, as necessary. Without a history of a rapid onset of symptoms, the EMT must assess the patient for other possible causes of unconsciousness.

■ Ensure rapid provision of, or transport to, ALS services.

■ Often, family members are experienced in checking the patient's blood sugar level. Provided the equipment is available, have the family member check the patient's blood sugar. The normal range of blood sugar for the adult is 80 to 120 mg/100 ml of blood. Family members may also be equipped with and trained to provide a glucagon injection. The EMT may also find that this has been done prior to the arrival of the first EMS responders.

■ Once the patient is awake and oriented, he/she needs to eat. The sugar provided initially may not last long. The patient needs to eat a meal, preferably including protein-containing foods (peanut butter, eggs, sandwich, etc.).

EMT Special Considerations

Alcoholism presents two special problems in the management of diabetic emergencies. The first is the problem of misidentification. Police and others have been known to assume that a person acting

Table 12-4	Distinguishing Characteristics of Low Blood Glucose (Hypoglycemia) and High Blood Glucose (Hyperglycemia)	
	LOW BLOOD GLUCOSE	HIGH BLOOD GLUCOSE
The Three Most Reliable Signals		
Onset	Rapid—minutes	Gradual—hours to days
Skin moistness	Wet, drooling	Dry
Respirations	Normal or shallow	Rapid, deep
History		
Food intake adequate	No	Yes
Insulin	Excessive	Insufficient
Strenuous exercise	Often	Rare
Associated symptoms	Hunger	Thirst
	Headache	Abdominal pain
	Dizziness	Nausea, vomiting
		Infection, fever
Physical Findings		
Blood pressure		May be decreased, with postural signs
Breath odor (acetone)	None	Sweet, fruity
Skin: temperature, color	Cool, pale	Warm, flushed
Behavior	May be uncoordinated, confused, combative	Restlessness
Seizures	In late stages	Rare
Improvement with sugar	Rapid: 1–2 minutes	No response

oddly who has a breath odor is drunk, when in fact the person is a diabetic. When that person needs treatment for hypoglycemia and receives a jail cell instead, death is the probable result. When there is reasonable doubt, treat as if the patient is a diabetic.

The second problem alcoholism presents is in the patient who simultaneously is acutely intoxicated and has a diabetic emergency. It is too easy to assume that an inebriated person (or an unconscious person smelling strongly of alcohol) has only one problem. Physical examination of every patient needs to be thorough enough to uncover *all* likely conditions. Medical ID tags can be very useful, but only if they are looked for and read. Again, when in doubt, opt in favor of the patient and treat as if diabetic.

■ High Blood Glucose (Hyperglycemia)

Definition

High blood glucose (hyperglycemia) occurs when glucose accumulates in the body because it is not being efficiently utilized. This inefficient utilization of glucose occurs when the amount of insulin in the body is not adequate. When the body cells are not able to utilize glucose for energy, fat is broken down and waste products of ketones and acids are produced. For this reason, this condition is also called *ketoacidosis*. It can occur when a diabetic person fails to take insulin or when the body is challenged by some unusual stress, such as infection. Since there are varying degrees of hyperglycemia, the symptoms will vary greatly and may not always lead to true diabetic ketoacidosis.

Acute Scenario

With an insufficient amount of insulin, the glucose taken in by the patient tends to remain in the blood. This excess blood glucose creates a physiologic response that explains the common signs and symptoms of hyperglycemia. The body produces extra urine in an attempt to eliminate the extra sugar circulating in the blood. This fluid loss, combined with the acidosis, causes coma (also called "diabetic coma"). The dehydration can also cause hypovolemia and hypotension. In an attempt to correct the acidosis, hyperventilation occurs (Kussmaul respirations).

History: Subjective Reports

The onset of hyperglycemia is generally gradual, over 12 to 48 hours. The chief complaint will often be abdominal pain, with nausea and vomiting. The history of the present illness may reveal intense thirst (polydipsia), increased appetite (polyphagia), increased urination (polyuria), a recent infection, or fever. Hyperglycemia and its associated symptoms are often the first clues to the undiagnosed diabetic patient. As with hypoglycemia, a thorough history must be obtained. The following questions should be asked:

1. Are you a diabetic?
    a. How do you control your diabetes (diet, pills, or insulin)?
    b. How long have you been a diabetic? Patients with newly diagnosed diabetes may be less familiar with their disease and make errors in their eating, activity, or medication regulation.
    c. Are you being treated by a physician for your diabetes? Some patients do not completely understand the importance of accurate medication dosing and scheduling as well as strict dietary controls.

2. Did you eat today?
   a. What did you eat and when? High-sugar and high-protein foods will provide an increased blood glucose level. Without sufficient insulin, blood glucose continues to increase.
   b. Is this a normal meal or snack for you? Some patients will have their diet and/or meal schedule altered as a result of an illness or stress.

3. When did you last take your insulin?
   a. Did you take the normal dosage?
   b. Why haven't you been taking your diabetes medication?

4. Have you been able to regularly control your blood sugar lately?
   a. Some patients fail to adequately monitor their blood sugar levels. As a result, an elevated level may not be detected.
   b. Recent or current illnesses, particularly infections, will alter the blood glucose requirements, and thus may make the patient susceptible to hyperglycemia.

If the patient ate and did not take his/her insulin, the problem is probably high blood glucose. When this process continues over days, the blood sugar level increases, creating the condition of hyperglycemia.

Examination: Objective Physical Findings

If the patient is unconscious, the history may be difficult to obtain. Assessment of the patient then depends upon physical findings. Signs of high blood sugar include warm, dry skin; rapid, deep respirations; rapid, weak pulse; possibly lowered blood pressure with postural hypotension; and possibly a sweet, fruity breath odor (acetone), which smells like nail polish remover.

It can sometimes be difficult to distinguish high blood glucose from low blood glucose (see Table 12–4). When there is any doubt, treat as if low blood glucose were present.

EMT Treatment

■ Assess the ABCDs

   ■ Ensure that the airway is protected, particularly in the patient with an altered mental status or who is unconscious. Be alert for vomiting.
   ■ Provide oxygen even though the patient appears to be hyperventilating.
   ■ If the patient is hypotensive or exhibiting signs of dehydration, place him/her in the supine position with the legs elevated.

■ Ensure rapid provision of, or transport to, ALS services.

■ As with hypoglycemia, family members may be equipped and trained to check the patient's blood sugar level. This may be done only if the patient is not seriously ill (e.g., conscious, not hypotensive, not showing signs of ketoacidosis). Do not delay care and transport to check the blood sugar level unless ALS services are responding.

Abdominal and Gastrointestinal Disorders

■ Acute Abdomen

Definition

The term "acute abdomen" refers to a wide variety of medical conditions that result in irritation or inflammation of the abdominal lining (peritoneum), causing abdominal pain. An acute abdomen can originate from problems in the gastrointestinal system, cardiovascular system, or genitourinary system.

The major reasons for abdominal pain are listed in Table 12–5 based upon the most common location of associated abdominal pain (Fig. 12–4). Additional causes, generally with no unique localization, include the following:

- Intestinal obstruction
- Mononucleosis
- Uremia
- Sickle cell anemia
- Food poisoning
- Diabetic ketoacidosis (high blood glucose)
- Intoxication (lead, methyl alcohol, various drug overdoses, narcotic withdrawal)

Table 12-5   Causes of Abdominal Pain by Location

Right Upper Quadrant	Epigastrium	Left Upper Quadrant
Acute cholecystitis	MI	Ruptured spleen
Pneumonia with pleural reaction	Duodenal ulcer	Pyelonephritis
	Esophagitis	Pneumonia with pleural reaction
Hepatitis	Pancreatitis	
Pyelonephritis (inflamed kidney)		

Right Lower Quadrant	Periumbilicus	Left Lower Quadrant
Appendicitis	Abdominal aortic aneurysm	Ectopic pregnancy
Ectopic pregnancy	Appendicitis	Ovarian cyst
Ovarian cyst	Pancreatitis	Incarcerated hernia
Incarcerated hernia		Diverticulitis
Kidney stone		Kidney stone

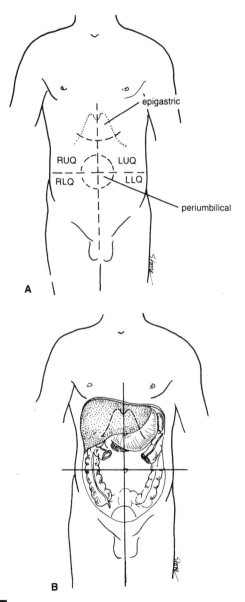

Figure 12-4

A, Surface anatomy of the abdomen. *B,* Major underlying organs.

Acute Scenario

The abdominal organs are separated into two categories: hollow and solid. Hollow organs are the esophagus, stomach, gallbladder, bile ducts, small intestine, large intestine (including the rectum), appendix, ureters, urinary bladder, fallopian tubes, uterus, vagina, and inferior vena cava. Solid organs are the liver, spleen, pancreas, ovaries, and kidneys.

Abdominal disorders fall into five main pathologic categories, which affect both hollow and solid organs and produce similar symptoms in both types of organs.

- *Inflammation* is the reaction of tissue to injury. Usually it has a history of slow onset over hours or days. The pain is usually steady. Often, there is a history of fever or chills. Inflammation can be life threatening.

- *Hemorrhage* may occur acutely or chronically, usually with steady pain. Fever is seldom present. The pain can radiate to one or both shoulders if the diaphragm is irritated. Signs and symptoms of hypovolemia may be exhibited.

- *Perforation* is a hole in a hollow organ. Steady pain of sudden onset is often felt. It is always a severe problem. Fever develops several hours following perforation.

- *Obstruction* is blockage in a hollow organ. The pain is usually crampy as the organ attempts to work against the obstructed area. It is moderately rapid in onset, without fever. Nausea and vomiting are common.

- *Ischemia* is a complete or temporary lack of blood, and therefore oxygen, to an organ. Steady pain occurs that is sudden in onset, unchanging, and often very severe.

History: Subjective Reports

The patient's history should include the onset of the pain; the severity, quality, and location of the pain; radiation of the pain; any associated symptoms; and anything that has been done to relieve the pain. As with all patients, the significant past medical history must be obtained.

Onset, Severity and Quality

Steady pain indicates inflammation whereas intermittent or colicky pain indicates obstruction.

- Pancreatitis pain is often steady and boring.
- Sudden, extremely severe pain is common with acute pancreatitis, ruptured aneurysm, ruptured ectopic pregnancy, and perforated ulcer.

Location and Radiation

- Acute appendicitis usually begins as periumbilical pain that later localizes in the right lower quadrant.
- Pancreatitis, posterior penetrating ulcer, or abdominal aortic aneurysm often radiates straight through to the back.

■ MI, pneumonia, diaphragm irritation, and inflamed gallbladder (cholecystitis) pain may radiate to the shoulder.

ASSOCIATED SYMPTOMS

■ Prolonged vomiting may suggest obstruction.

■ Nausea and vomiting are common with appendicitis and pancreatitis.

■ The patient with an abdominal aortic aneurysm may complain of pain radiating down one leg.

AGGRAVATION AND/OR RELIEF OF SYMPTOMS

■ Pain from a duodenal ulcer may be relieved with eating or antacids.

■ Symptoms of acute cholecystitis often occur after eating a greasy or fatty meal.

■ The pain of esophagitis may worsen at night or when supine, but may improve with antacids.

■ Pancreatitis pain is often worsened by rapid movement, coughing, and deep breathing.

■ Constipation and abdominal cramps may occur with bowel obstruction.

■ The patient with acute peritonitis will want to lie still because movement dramatically increases the pain.

PAST HISTORY AND RISK FACTORS

■ A past abdominal surgery may result in adhesions, which increase the likelihood of an intestinal obstruction.

■ For many patients, the symptoms may be chronic such that the patient has a history of ulcers, diverticulosis, sickle cell disease, or ovarian cysts.

■ Patients may relate a recent history of similar events, such as recurrent episodes of colicky lower abdominal pain found with kidney stones.

■ The history may reveal risk factors for specific abdominal conditions such as hypertension or Marfan syndrome with abdominal aortic aneurysm; chronic alcohol abuse with pancreatitis or ulcer; and elevated cholesterol levels with kidney stones.

■ Cholecystitis is commonly seen in overweight women who are in their late 30s or 40s.

■ In the female patient, the history must include the possibility of pregnancy or a known pregnancy. Left or right lower abdominal pain in a woman of child-bearing age must be assumed to be an ectopic pregnancy until proven otherwise.

Examination: Objective Physical Findings

Assess the ABCDs

■ Respiratory difficulty is often associated with splinting of respirations. The patient breathes shallowly and slowly to minimize worsening of the abdominal pain.

■ Effects on the cardiovascular system noted in the exam typically are limited to heart rate changes and shock. Shock indicates a rapidly progressing condition such as peritonitis, ruptured aneurysm, ruptured ectopic pregnancy, or perforation of the diverticula.

■ Consciousness may be altered if the abdominal condition has progressed to a shock state.

Perform Focused Physical Examination

■ Obtain and record the vital signs.
  – A decreased blood pressure or signs of shock indicate a potential surgical emergency.
  – The heart rate may be increased as a result of the pain, fever, or bleeding. The pain may also lower the heart rate in some patients as a result of vagal stimulation.
  – The respiratory rate may be increased as a result of splinted, shallow respirations.
  – Lung sounds may reveal rhonchi, rales, or a localized quiet lung field in the pneumonia patient.
  – Fever may be present, suggesting appendicitis or cholecystitis.
■ Examine the abdomen.
  – Visually determine whether distention is present.
  – Gently palpate all quadrants looking for rigidity, tenderness, or a pulsating mass (particularly in the upper quadrants).
  – Testing for rebound tenderness generally does not benefit the EMT. The intense pain created by this test will likely create additional anxiety and reluctance to allow any other form of abdominal exam for fear of further pain. Extensive physical examination in the field is not warranted, because the exam will have to be repeated in the hospital.
  – Assess the equality of femoral pulses when an abdominal aortic aneurysm is suspected.

EMT Treatment

■ Provide treatment for the ABCs.

  ■ At a minimum, provide low-flow oxygen.
  ■ Patients with shortness of breath, signs of shock, an altered mental status, or signs of peritonitis should be provided with high-flow oxygen.
  ■ Be prepared to assist in airway control should vomiting occur.

■ Position the patient.

  ■ In most cases, place the patient in a position most comfortable for him/her. Many patients will not be able to find a comfortable position and may be writhing around on the bed or floor.
  ■ If there is evidence of volume depletion (hypotension, postural changes in pulse rate or blood pressure), place the patient in a supine position and elevate the lower extremities.

■ Abdominal pain should always be evaluated in the hospital.

■ Do not allow the patient to eat or drink.

■ GASTROINTESTINAL BLEEDING

Definition

Bleeding can occur in either the upper or the lower portions of the GI tract. It can occur very suddenly, at a rapid rate, or it can occur slowly over a prolonged period. Common reasons for upper GI tract bleeding include peptic ulcer, esophageal varices, and gastritis. Upper GI bleeding is often alcohol related. Lower GI bleeding seldom presents acutely. *Peptic ulcer* produces bleeding in the stomach, often when lack of food intake allows gastric acid to damage the stomach lining. *Esophageal varices* occur when chronic alcohol abuse causes cirrhosis of the liver. The cirrhosis causes shunting of the blood flow into the blood vessels of the stomach and esophagus, resulting in distended esophageal veins (varices). These distended veins are fragile and can rupture, causing profuse vomiting of blood. *Gastritis* (inflammation of the stomach) can be caused by overuse of aspirin or alcohol or by stress.

Acute Scenario

The sudden vomiting of blood can be both frightening and life threatening. These patients are in obvious danger of hypovolemic shock. What is less obvious is that hypovolemia can also develop in the patient who is bleeding in the GI tract at a slow rate.

History: Subjective Reports

The chief complaint of patients with GI bleeding will vary depending upon the rate of the bleeding. A loss of 4 liters over several weeks may produce only mild weakness. The rapid loss of 1 liter may produce dizziness and other symptoms of shock. When blood leaks into the stomach at a slow rate, the gastric acid turns it to brown material with a "coffee grounds" appearance, and this may be what a patient will report vomiting. Abdominal pain may be reported in the epigastrium or left upper quadrant. The past medical history may include alcohol abuse and liver disease, and the history of the present incident may reveal an alcohol "binge." Pertinent questions to ask when obtaining the history include the following:

1. What symptoms are present now? What is the patient's chief complaint?
   a. Does the patient have abdominal pain or discomfort?
   b. Where is the pain or discomfort located?
   c. When did the symptoms begin?

2. Has the patient had any vomiting or unusual stools recently?
   a. What did the emesis look like? Did it have a "coffee grounds" appearance?

   b. Did the patient forcefully dry heave before the symptoms began?
   c. Has the patient noticed any unusual-appearing stools? Have they been dark, tarry, or sticky?

3. Has the patient ever had similar symptoms in the past?
   a. Does the patient have a history of GI bleeding?
   b. Have these symptoms been recurrent? Over what period of time have they been occurring?
   c. What was done to relieve the symptoms in the past?
4. Does the patient have any risk factors for GI bleeding?
   a. Does the patient drink a significant amount of alcohol on a regular basis?
   b. Does the patient frequently take any of the following medications: aspirin, prednisone, or antacids?

Examination: Objective Physical Findings

Assess the ABCDs

- Significant vomiting, particularly with an altered mental status, poses a great risk to the airway. Monitor the airway closely.
- The patient in shock may have an increased respiratory rate.
- Assess the lung sounds for possible aspiration of vomitus, particularly in the lethargic or unconscious patient.
- Occasionally, GI bleeding may mask other medical conditions. The alcohol abuse patient experiencing a GI bleed may also be lethargic as a result of hypoglycemia, or he/she may be short of breath because of COPD exacerbation.

Perform Quick Focused Physical Examination

- Assess the vital signs.
  - Determine the postural pulse and blood pressure unless the patient's blood pressure is 80 mm Hg or less with the patient supine.
  - Determine the heart rate, skin temperature and color, and the respiratory rate. The patient will likely be exhibiting signs of an adrenaline response (tachycardia; cool, pale, moist skin; tachypnea). The skin may also be yellow (jaundice) if liver disease is present.
- Examine the abdomen for tenderness on palpation and signs of peritoneal inflammation, distention, or ascites (fluid in the abdomen).
- The patient's environment (usually the bathroom) may provide clues to the extent and type of bleeding. Note any evidence of GI bleeding. Look for:
  - "Coffee grounds" emesis
  - Bright red blood passing from the rectum
  - Melena (dark stools)

On occasion, it may be difficult to distinguish GI bleeding with vomiting (hematemesis) from coughing of blood from the lung (hemoptysis). Table 12–6 compares hemoptysis with hematemesis.

Table 12-6   Comparison of Hemoptysis and Hematemesis

	HEMOPTYSIS (BLOOD FROM LUNGS)	HEMATEMESIS (BLOOD FROM GI TRACT)
Initial symptoms	Coughing	Nausea and vomiting
Character of blood	Frothy or stringy, mixed with sputum	Never frothy, mixed with gastric contents
Subsequent sputum	Blood streaked	Usually no sputum
Color of blood	Bright red	Dark red or brown, coffee grounds appearance
Other		Food particles may be present

EMT Treatment

■ Provide oxygen.

- ■ At a minimum, provide low-flow oxygen at 4 to 6 L/min by nasal cannula.
- ■ Provide high-flow oxygen when the patient has significant bleeding, an altered mental status, or shortness of breath.

■ Position the patient.

- ■ Place the patient supine with the legs elevated.
- ■ If the patient is vomiting or nauseated, place in a lateral recumbent position (assuming the patient is breathing spontaneously).
- ■ Save vomitus if possible.

■ Consider the use of antishock trousers (MAST).

■ Ensure rapid provision of, or transport to, ALS services.

■ GALLBLADDER INFLAMMATION (CHOLECYSTITIS)

Acute cholecystitis occurs when a gallstone obstructs the duct leading from the gallbladder to the gastrointestinal tract. It is an uncommon cause for an EMT call, because most patients voluntarily go to their own physicians. Occasionally, however, the pain from cholecystitis may be misinterpreted by the patient as a heart attack. Unlike the pain from MI, the pain from cholecystitis is usually located in the right lower chest and right upper quadrant of the abdomen. It may be referred to, or radiate to, the right shoulder. There is no specific EMT treatment, although naturally, if there is any doubt about the patient having an MI, he/she should be treated as such.

■ ESOPHAGITIS

Esophagitis is inflammation of the esophagus. It is an uncommon cause for an EMT call, but on occasion the pain is interpreted by the patient as a heart attack. Unlike the MI, the pain from esophagitis is described as "burning" and can often be relieved by antacids. The pain is often described as being up and down the middle of the chest. Many patients will describe a history of esophageal reflux. The pain may be relieved by antacids. EMT treatment consists of keeping the patient in a sitting position. When any doubt exists about the presence of MI, treat for MI.

Miscellaneous Medical Conditions

■ ALLERGIC REACTIONS

Definition

Allergic reactions occur when the body's response to a foreign substance is not protective and defensive, but rather self-destructive. Foreign substances (antigens) can enter the body in several different ways:

- ■ *Injection*: drugs such as penicillin
- ■ *Ingestion*: foods such as shellfish or berries, or drugs such as penicillin
- ■ *Insect sting*: wasp, bee, yellow jacket, hornet (see Chapter 14)
- ■ *Inhalation*: pollens and other airborne allergens

Acute Scenario

The severity of an allergic reaction varies, ranging from mild symptoms of itching and burning to severe, full-blown anaphylactic shock (see Chapter 9), with generalized edema, respiratory distress, cardiovascular collapse, coma, and death occurring within minutes. It can be difficult to predict which patients with allergic reactions will progress to full-blown anaphylaxis. However, patients who experience progressively worsening allergic reactions to a substance may be at greater risk for anaphylaxis upon future exposures to the substance.

History: Subjective Reports

The patient with an allergic reaction may first be aware of a generalized warmth and itching, particularly of the hands and feet. Next, he/she may complain of a tightness in the throat or chest, with dyspnea and cough. This may be accompanied by nausea, vomiting, abdominal cramps, and diarrhea. The history of the present episode may reveal exposure to the foreign substance. The past medical history may include a known allergy, hypersensitivity, or asthma. Look for a medical ID tag. Ask the patient about the presentation and severity of previous reactions.

Examination: Objective Physical Findings

Like the symptoms, the signs of allergic reaction will vary with the severity of the reaction. Skin signs include raised red rash, hives, and swelling (edema) of the lips, tongue, eyelids, and hands. The location of the rash may be limited to a specific area (e.g., the arm if bitten by an insect), or it may be widespread (e.g., over the entire body if a medication is ingested). The systemic rash is commonly noted on the neck, face, scalp, chest, abdomen, and back. Respiratory signs include hoarseness, mild wheezing, and stridor. Gastrointestinal signs include vomiting and diarrhea. Cardiovascular signs include weak, rapid pulse and hypotension. The more severe respiratory and cardiovascular signs are associated with anaphylaxis (a severe form of allergic reaction).

EMT Treatment

■ Provide oxygen.

- ■ Provide low-flow oxygen.
- ■ If the symptoms progressively worsen, provide high-flow oxygen.

■ Identify the exposure substance if possible (e.g., penicillin, insect sting).

- ■ Prevent further exposure to the substance.
- ■ Remove the insect stinger if it remains embedded in the skin.

■ Treat severe allergic reactions as anaphylaxis.

- ■ Treat hypotension, if present, with elevation of lower extremities. Consider antishock trousers (MAST).
- ■ Ensure rapid provision of, or transport to, ALS services.

■ If you are trained and authorized to do so, assist the patient with prescribed medications, such as an anaphylaxis kit (epinephrine injection or antihistamine).

■ SEPSIS

Sepsis occurs when a local infection spreads throughout the body. Most commonly it originates with bacteria from the lung or urinary tract. These patients appear very ill. The most severely affected of them will be in shock, called septic shock (see Chapter 9). This usually occurs in elderly, debilitated, or alcoholic patients. Treatment consists of airway control, high-flow oxygen, supine positioning, and maintaining normal body temperature. Ensure rapid provision of, or transport to, ALS services.

■ DEHYDRATION

Dehydration is the excessive loss of body fluid. Volume depletion can originate from several sources, including

- Blood loss
- Protracted vomiting or diarrhea (particularly in children—see Chapter 16)
- Diabetic ketoacidosis (high blood glucose)
- Acute debilitation (as in an alcoholic who has been lying on the floor for several days)
- Sweating (as in classic heat stroke)
- Burns (see Chapter 11)
- Prolonged decrease in food and fluid intake

If the fluid loss is extreme, hypovolemic shock results (see Chapter 9).

■ KIDNEY (RENAL) DIALYSIS EMERGENCIES

Over 40,000 patients are undergoing dialysis in the United States. Many chronic renal failure patients have home dialysis units; most have had extensive training and many have helpers. The purpose of dialysis is to remove waste products that are normally removed by the kidneys and excreted in the urine. Hemodialysis patients undergo dialysis every 2 to 3 days. The usual "run" lasts for 5 to 6 hours, depending upon the size of the patient, the amount of kidney function remaining, and the type of dialysate used. In order to "hook up" to the dialysis machine, kidney patients have either an external arteriovenous shunt or an internal arteriovenous fistula. Another form of dialysis is referred to as peritoneal dialysis. In this type, dialysis fluid is instilled in the peritoneal space and drained later. This procedure is commonly performed at home and requires no special machine. The patient requires multiple dialysis treatments per day and/or week.

Kidney centers operate in most large communities and can provide valuable information over the phone.

Problems associated with dialysis generally fall into four categories:

- Shock
- Potassium imbalance
- Pulmonary edema
- Machine malfunctions

Shock

Shock may result from dialysis for a variety of reasons, including those listed here.

Extracellular Volume Depletion.   As a result of loss of saline during dialysis, the patient becomes lightheaded and woozy, but rarely unconscious. The patient will often recognize the problem and self-administer 50 ml of saline or more.

Hemorrhage.   There are two primary causes of cannula bleeding.

Intentional (Suicidal).   Dialysis patients have the highest suicide rate of patients with chronic disease. The patient will open the cannula and bleed out. If the cannula is pumping, clamp the open cannulas and apply direct pressure. If the bleeding cannot be controlled or the cannula cannot be clamped shut, apply a tourniquet to the limb above the cannula or shunt site.

Accidental.

Faulty connection.   A steady leak may be present. Re-establish the connection and apply pressure.

Arteritis.   There may be oozing around the arterial cannula. This usually occurs soon after placement of a new cannula. Applying direct pressure or clamping the cannula may worsen hemorrhage, since it increases the backpressure in the vessel.

Disconnection at Vein.   Arterial hemorrhage through the cannula and simultaneous venous leakage may occur. Immediately clamp the cannula. This may require a great amount of pressure because of the Teflon tube core. Disconnect the patient from the dialysis machine if a leak occurred during the dialysis run.

Cardiac (MI).   Dialysis patients have a high incidence of cardiovascular complications. If the patient experiences shock while on dialysis and has no apparent blood loss, then treat as for any other cardiogenic shock.

Duodenal Ulcer.   Dialysis patients have a high incidence of duodenal ulcers, which may bleed. If the patient is hypotensive with a history of tarry stools, treat for hypovolemic shock.

Subdural Hematoma.   Dialysis patients have a high incidence of spontaneous subdural hematoma because of anticoagulant therapy and usually *do not* give a history of head trauma. If the patient complains of severe headaches, especially while undergoing dialysis, stop dialysis and transport to the hospital.

Potassium Imbalance

Hypokalemia (low potassium in the blood) is found only while the patient is undergoing dialysis, or immediately following it. Usually, the patient is taking digoxin. Dialysis patients taking digoxin are much more likely to develop digitalis toxicity. Hypotension may be present. Arrhythmias and seizures may occur secondary to bradycardia.

Hyperkalemia (high serum potassium level) may occur prior to dialysis, and may cause arrhythmias. If alert, the patient will complain of profound weakness and difficulty with respiration (secondary to weakness). The patient may be unconscious and possibly even in cardiac arrest. The hyperkalemia must be treated with dialysis as soon as possible. Alert the hospital so that arrangements may be made.

Pulmonary Edema

Pulmonary edema is a common problem in dialysis patients, who usually gain 2 pounds of fluid per day. This fluid must be eliminated to keep weight and blood pressure normal and lungs clear. The examination is performed as in the pulmonary edema patient.

Machine Malfunctions

During a power outage, the patient may choose to stay connected to the machine and "wait it out." If the outage is short lived, no harm is done. If the outage is prolonged, the blood will cool and the patient may then be at risk from potassium-induced arrhythmias. Treat the patient by disconnecting him/her from the device, clamping the cannulas, and transporting to the hospital.

13 Poisoning and Overdose

General Principles

Definition

Overdose is the administration of or exposure to an excessive quantity of a potentially harmful chemical substance. An overdose may be intentional or accidental. Traditionally, this term has been used when referring to intentional administrations of excessive drug quantities. Overdoses have become the most common means of attempting and succeeding at suicide. For this reason, it is also important for the EMT to learn whether the overdose was intentional and whether the patient meant to cause harm or death to himself/herself. Such a determination assists the physician in determining the need for a psychosocial evaluation. In some states, law enforcement officers are authorized to order a detention (usually for 72 hours) of patients who are believed to be a threat to their own well-being pending psychosocial observation and evaluation.

A *poisoning* occurs with an exposure to a substance (poison) that, even in small quantities, causes damage or disturbance to a bodily structure or system. Although poisonings are typically accidental, intentional poisonings may occur. Intentional poisonings may be self-inflicted or result from an assault. Poisonings are the fifth most common cause of accidental death, following car accidents, falls, drownings, and burns. It is estimated that 5000 deaths per year occur as a result of accidental poisoning. As one would imagine, accidental poisonings occur most commonly in children.

There are several hundred poison control centers in the United States. Their personnel are available 24 hours a day with a detailed data base on toxic substances: drugs, chemicals, household products, and so on. The file for each substance contains information on chemical composition, toxic effects, and specific emergency medical treatment.

Routes of Entry

Poisons may enter the body through various routes of entry. These entry mechanisms would also apply to overdoses. The route of entry is typically dependent on the substance. Some substances have more than one possible route of entry.

197

Ingestion

- This is the most common route of entry in intentional overdose patients.
- Common substances of ingestion are nonprescription pain relievers (acetaminophen, aspirin), medications (antidepressants, sleeping aids), and household chemicals (bleach, rodenticides).

Inhalation

- While accidental inhalation is common, there is a rise in the practice of abuse through the inhalation of volatile chemicals.
- Common substances of inhalation include chlorine from a household chemical reaction, marijuana, crack cocaine, gasoline, cleaning solvents, and metallic paints ("huffing").
- The onset of symptoms when harmful substances are inhaled may be very rapid.

Injection

- Harmful substances may be injected either intentionally (IV drug use) or accidentally (insect sting).
- Common substances of injection include heroin, amphetamines, and bee venom.
- The onset of symptoms when substances are injected, particularly via the intravenous route, is very rapid.

Absorption

- Absorption of a substance typically is associated with an accidental poisoning.
- Common substances of absorption include nitrates, pesticides, and caustic or acidic chemicals.

Acute Scenario

An acute emergency generally develops for one of four reasons.

Unintended Effects (Adverse Effect)

- These effects are often from an overdose.
- The most common unintended effect is respiratory depression.

Withdrawal State

- The widthdrawal state is a mental and physical state caused by the termination or reduction of use of a substance that affects the mind through intoxication.
- The symptoms are usually specific to the substance.
- Withdrawal states commonly seen by the EMT are due to alcohol, stimulants (cocaine, methamphetamines), and narcotics (heroin, morphine).

Panic State

- The patient may develop anxiety symptoms that may or may not be directly related to the substance.

■ For example, after taking the first dose of a prescribed pain reliever such as Tylenol No. 3, the patient becomes nauseated and vomits. This increases pain and actually makes the patient feel worse than before. He/she becomes anxious and frightened, thinking this is an allergic reaction when it actually is a normal side effect of this drug; the result is a call to 911.

ALLERGIC REACTION

■ Allergic reactions to medications, foods, and environmental substances are relatively common.
■ The severity of the reaction is variable, as described in Chapters 9 and 12.

EMT Special Considerations

In the setting of an intentional overdose or the use of recreational drugs, the EMT will often be provided with information that is untrue, exaggerated, or incomplete. The EMT should not completely believe all information obtained in such cases. Above all, the examination and assessment should correlate with the information provided in the history-gathering process.

Ingested Poisons and Overdoses

■ GENERAL MANAGEMENT

History: Subjective Reports

The symptoms will depend upon the drug. The EMT needs to obtain a thorough past medical history. Of particular concern should be a history of suicidal tendencies, recent depression, and all medications accessible to the patient. In many patients, the past history, reports from family or friends, or the patient's story are the only significant clues of overdose or poisoning. If possible, a history of the present incident should be obtained, including the following information:

1. *What* was taken?
   a. Identify the name of the substance.
   b. Learn what the substance is used for (antihypertensive, metal parts cleaning fluid).
   c. The trade name, generic name, and/or brand name may all be useful bits of information.

2. *When* was it taken?
   a. What time was the substance ingested?
   b. Were other substances such as alcohol or other drugs also ingested?

3. *How much* was taken?
   a. When medications are ingested, determine how many pills were ingested and the dosage of the medication.
   b. If the ingested substance is a chemical, attempt to determine the volume ingested.

The EMT must be familiar with local street terms to interpret slang names for drugs. The drug abuser may use slang to identify the drugs ingested, such as "yellow jackets" when referring to pentobarbital.

Examination: Objective Physical Findings

The signs will depend upon the drug. The initial assessment, the focused history, and the physical examination must be thorough and must include estimation of respiratory, cardiovascular, and CNS status. Vital signs, including blood pressure, respiratory rate and depth, heart rate, and pupillary changes, may be the EMT's first indication of an accidental ingestion or overdose possibility. The survey should also include a search for unnoticed injury, such as compression injury (ischemia) to an extremity, as evidenced by a cold, swollen, cyanotic limb, and examination of extremities for needle marks.

Table 13–1 lists the characteristic presentations of drug overdose.

EMT Treatment

■ Assess the ABCDs.

   ■ If the patient is unconscious or lethargic, assure an open airway, administer high-flow oxygen, and assist ventilations as needed.

 Table 13-1   General Characteristics of Drug Overdoses

CLINICAL PRESENTATION	SUSPECTED DRUG TYPE
Lethargy, slurred speech, hypotension, hypothermia	Sedatives (barbiturates), tranquilizers
Pinpoint pupils (nonreactive), hypoventilation to respiratory arrest, stupor to coma, fresh needle marks	Opiates (narcotics)
Agitation, belligerence, diaphoresis, hypertension, hyperventilation, tachycardia, dilated pupils, chest pain	Stimulants (amphetamines), cocaine, crack
Hallucinations, dry/flushed skin, fever, dilated pupils, anxiety	Hallucinogens, atropines
Dystonic posture, profound hypotension, lethargy to coma, seizures	Phenothiazines
Cardiac arrhythmias, tachycardia, agitation, coma, seizures	Tricyclics, antidepressants
Hyperventilation, fever, vomiting	Salicylates, acetaminophen

■ If the patient is conscious and panicked, calm the patient in a reassuring manner.

■ Ingestion of poisons or overdoses creates an increased likelihood for vomiting. Be prepared with suctioning devices. Effective airway management and monitoring are crucial with overdose and poisoning patients.

■ If the patient is hypotensive, dizzy, or light headed, place in a supine position with legs elevated as necessary for hypotension.

■ If the patient is in cardiac arrest, immediately begin CPR. Ingestion of cocaine (rocks) can cause cardiac arrhythmias leading to sudden death. Apply an AED if available and you are authorized in its use.

Attempt to identify the substance or substances (multidrug overdoses are common) from the history or paraphernalia. Use special caution when handling the needles from an abuser of injectable drugs, in order to avoid exposure to blood-borne infectious diseases. Caution must also be exercised when handling even small amounts of hazardous chemicals (household pesticides, etc.) because absorption or inhalation exposure to the EMT could occur.

Call the local poison control center with the information on what was taken, how much, and when. In some communities, the EMT may be required to contact local medical control before or in place of contacting the poison control center.

If contact is made with the poison control center, the EMT may be given any of the following treatment instructions:

■ Dilute poison with water or milk.

■ Induce vomiting with syrup of ipecac (do not use fluid extract):
  – 2 tablespoons (30 ml) for adults
  – 1 tablespoon (15 ml) for children 1 to 12 years old
  – 1 to 2 teaspoons (5 to 10 ml) for infants

■ Follow the syrup of ipecac with 2 to 4 glasses of water (or 1 to 2 glasses of clear liquid). A gentle rocking motion (as in an ambulance on the way to the hospital) can help the ipecac work. Repeat after 30 minutes if no results.

■ *Do not give ipecac to these patients*:
  – Patients with an altered mental status
  – Patients who are having seizures or who have had seizures associated with this ingestion
  – Pregnant women or patients with an acute MI

■ *Do not give ipecac in cases of certain ingestions*:
  – Corrosives: acid, such as toilet bowl cleaner; alkali, such as lye, bleach, or drain cleaner; or any substance giving evidence of oral burns (warning labels usually state "May cause burns to skin or mucous membranes")
  – Petroleum products: gasoline, kerosene, lighter fluid, cleaning agents, furniture polish (warning labels usually state "Contains petroleum distillates")
  – Antiemetics: phenothiazine drugs, such as chlorpromazine (Thorazine), promethazine (phenergan), or prochlorperazine (Compazine)
  – Strychnine compound: some rat poisons
  – Cyclic antidepressants and cocaine

- Depending upon the policies of the receiving hospital, induced vomiting with ipecac may be withheld if transportation time to the hospital is short or if the time since ingestion has been prolonged. The use of ipecac is most beneficial when administered within 60 minutes of the time of ingestion. It is also useful for specific ingestions of substances not readily absorbed by charcoal (iron, lithium) and for sustained-release tablets.
- Administer activated charcoal, 2 tablespoons (30 ml) in a glass of water.
  - A commercially prepared sweet slurry of activated charcoal is available for use with children; the taste can be improved with sugar water.
  - Charcoal may be given after vomiting that was induced by ipecac but should never be used before the ipecac has worked, because the charcoal will inactivate the ipecac.
  - Do not delay transport while waiting to administer activated charcoal.
- Administer soothing agents such as milk or milk of magnesia.

Save vomitus (save initial vomitus separately) and take associated paraphernalia and drug or chemical containers to the hospital with the patient.

EMT Special Considerations

Consider conditions that may masquerade as a drug overdose, such as head trauma, meningitis, subarachnoid hemorrhage, hypoglycemia, poisonings, and brain tumor. In addition, patients who have both acute drug intoxication and head injury simultaneously present a special problem for assessment. Rapid transport after caring for the ABCDs is often the best care when ALS services are unavailable.

ALCOHOL ABUSE and OVERDOSE

Definition

Alcohol (ethanol), a CNS depressant drug, is the most abused drug in the United States. It is estimated that 10 million Americans are alcoholic (1 out of 20 people). Alcohol is associated with 50% of all arrests and 50% of all motor vehicle fatalities. Less than 5% of alcoholic persons are derelicts.

Acute Scenario

Alcoholic emergencies commonly seen by the EMT are of three types: acute intoxication, withdrawal seizures, and delirium tremens (DTs).

Acute intoxication is caused by ingestion of an excessive amount of alcohol. This results in high levels of alcohol in the blood, which may be exhibited by CNS effects that include:

- Muscular incoordination and balance disturbance (staggering and widened gait)
- Difficulty with speech
- Agitation with decreased inhibitions (swearing, abusive behavior)

- Decreased level of consciousness, including coma
- Respiratory depression and the inability to maintain airway control
- Increased pain threshold

Withdrawal seizures occur in the patient who has developed a physical dependence on alcohol and who has ceased intake of alcohol for at least a short period of time (12 to 48 hours).

Delirium tremens represents the most severe symptoms of the alcohol withdrawal syndrome. DTs can have a mortality rate as high as 15%.

History: Subjective Reports

The acutely intoxicated patient may have no complaints, but the patient's family or bystanders may relate a history of alcoholism. The family may also report changes in the patient's behavior, family life, and work performance. Withdrawal seizures usually occur 5 to 48 hours after the last drink. Withdrawal seizures are usually generalized, not partial, and cease after one or two seizures. DTs usually occurs 2 to 5 days after the last drink. Auditory or visual hallucinations are common.

Examination: Objective Physical Findings

The acutely intoxicated patient is generally aggressive and combative, but may be comatose, with hypoventilation and dilated pupils. Vomiting or vomiting of blood (see Gastrointestinal Bleeding in Chapter 12) can also occur. In the noncomatose patient, the EMT's exam may find coordination and balance difficulty, slurred speech, nausea and vomiting, and lethargy. It will be difficult for the EMT to accurately assess the intoxicated patient's level of consciousness or severity of injuries secondary to a traumatic event.

It is unlikely that the EMT will witness withdrawal seizures but, rather, will be called to the scene after the seizures. Because withdrawal seizures are part of an overall syndrome, the patient will likely exhibit signs and symptoms associated with the withdrawal syndrome in addition to those related to the seizure. The patient may have tremors, tachycardia, restlessness, sweating, weakness, nausea, and/or vomiting.

DTs presents with restlessness, tachycardia, disorientation, anxiety, delusions, tremors, fever, sleeplessness, hallucinations, and sweating. DTs can cause hypovolemic shock.

EMT Treatment

■ Protect the patient (and yourself) from injury.

■ If the patient is unconscious, assure an open airway, administer high-flow oxygen, and assist ventilations as necessary. Have suctioning equipment ready, because vomiting is common.

gen, ventilatory assistance, and rapid transport.

Whenever possible, transport the patient on his/her side to protect the airway should vomiting occur.

Delirium tremens is a medical emergency, and all patients suspected of having DTs must be transported to the hospital.

■ DRUG OVERDOSE AND POISONING (BY CATEGORIES)

Table 13–2 contains specific information and management regarding commonly seen major drug overdoses and poisonings listed by substance categories.

Substance Abuse and Recreational Drug Use

The EMT is frequently called to see a patient who is experiencing signs and symptoms consistent with substance abuse. At times, the EMT will gain information about substance abuse from friends, family, bystanders, or law enforcement officers. Without this information, the EMT must rely on the physical examination and assessment to determine if substance abuse may be the cause for a patient's presentation.

When the EMT is called to such patients, the substance involved is typically an opiate or derivative (heroin), a stimulant (cocaine, amphetamines), a hallucinogen (LSD, ecstasy), or a commonly used household product with CNS-depressant effects (metallic paints, hydrocarbon solvents, Halon fire extinguishers). In 1995, the Seattle–King County Health Department reported 130 heroin-related deaths in a population of 1.5 million. Of the 130 deaths, 100 involved the use of other drugs, typically cocaine and alcohol. While cocaine, heroin, and methamphetamines continue to be commonly used recreational drugs, the EMT will find in his/her community many new substances (often commonly found substances) being abused.

Table 13–3 lists some of the more commonly abused substances and recreational drugs. Refer to Table 13–2 for the management of other drug overdoses and poisonings.

EMT Special Considerations

When managing the potential overdose or substance abuse patient, the EMT must pay particular attention to safety. In addition to protecting the patient, the EMT must assure the safety of other emergency response personnel. If local policy allows, request law enforcement officers on all possible overdoses or substance abuse responses.

Table 13-2 Management of Drug Overdose and Poisoning

DRUG/SUBSTANCE	TRADE OR STREET NAME	SIGNS/SYMPTOMS	EMT MANAGEMENT	SPECIAL COMMENTS
Household Products				
Acids	Toilet bowl cleaners Rust removers Metal cleaners and polishes Tile and grout cleaners	Severe pain in mouth, stomach, chest (substernal)	NEVER INDUCE VOMITING Give patient Milk Milk of magnesia Egg whites (dilutes the acid)	Have patient sit up during transport
Alkalis	Automatic dishwasher detergent Drain cleaners Oven cleaners Washing soda Ammonia Bleach, floor cleaners	Severe pains in mouth, stomach, chest (substernal) Burns in mouth and esophagus Associated difficulty with swallowing	NEVER INDUCE VOMITING Attempt to dilute with fluids	Have patient sit up during transport Watch airway closely for edema causing restricted ventilation
Hydrocarbons	Petroleum products Gasoline Fuel oils Paint thinners Paint solvents Kerosene Lighter fluid Furniture polish	Most common symptoms are respiratory distress with coughing and choking Patient may develop pulmonary edema Abdominal pain may be present Convulsions (seizures) Patient may be comatose Monitor for arrhythmias	NEVER INDUCE VOMITING Treat with up to 100% oxygen depending on severity of overdose Control secretions with suction as required	Have patient sit up during transport, if possible

Table continued on following page

Table 13-2 (Continued)

DRUG/SUBSTANCE	TRADE OR STREET NAME	SIGNS/SYMPTOMS	EMT MANAGEMENT	SPECIAL COMMENTS
Cyanide	Laetrile overdose Contaminated fruit: seed crop fumigants Photo electroplating	Initial stage: Confusion Rapid respirations Later stage: Depressed respirations Vomiting Seizure Comatose	Some paramedic programs have cyanide antidote kits available. Support vital signs and respiration. If antidote is not available, transport patient to nearest medical facility having antidote.	
Pesticides	Warfarin base: Rat killer Strychnine base: Rodenticides Arsenic base: Insect sprays Ant and roach killers Liquid insect killers DDT pesticides Acetylcholinesterase Malathion	Warfarin type: Severe gastrointestinal symptoms Progressive lethargy/apathy Strychnine based: Acute illness Severe nausea/vomiting Respiratory distress Tonic stiffening Arsenic based: Acute gastrointestinal symptoms DDT: Severe gastroenteritis, ulcers	Warfarin poisoning: Patient must be seen at hospital for blood clotting problems Patients who are conscious with gag reflex can be given ipecac Support ventilation as required Tonic stiffening requires antiseizure medicines	Illicit drugs (e.g., heroin) are sometimes cut with strychnine Some pesticides contain anticholinergic agents

Perfumes/ deodorizers	Products containing perfumes and deodorizers are too numerous to list here	Produce severe gastroenteritis Respiratory problems from aerosol products may be present	Give oxygen as required Support vital signs	
Plants				
Poisonous plants	Glycosides: Foxglove Azalea Rhododendron Alkaloidal toxins: Hemlock Nightshade GI irritants: Philodendron Deiffenbachia Holly	Glycosides: Nausea/vomiting Hypotension May have bradycardia (heart rate <60/min) Alkaloidal toxins: Lethargy, which may progress to seizures and coma GI irritants: Severe nausea/vomiting Diarrhea Hypotension	Support with oxygen as required Support hypotension as with hypovolemia Use cardiac monitor, if available	Bring plant sample to hospital
Poisonous mushrooms	*Amanita muscaria*	10–30 minutes after ingestion: severe nausea/vomiting followed rapidly by seizures; death may occur	Support with oxygen as required Support hypotension as with hypovolemia Use cardiac monitor, if available	Bring plant sample to hospital
Hallucinogenic mushrooms	Psilocybin and psilocin	Severe mood disturbances Hyperventilation Nausea/vomiting Fever Reduced level of consciousness	Use ipecac if patient has gag reflex and is conscious Calm patient as necessary Support vital signs and ventilation as required	50–100 mushrooms can be fatal Onset 15–30 minutes after ingestion lasting up to 4–6 hours

Table continued on following page

Table 13-2 (*Continued*)

DRUG/SUBSTANCE	TRADE OR STREET NAME	SIGNS/SYMPTOMS	EMT MANAGEMENT	SPECIAL COMMENTS
Drugs				
Barbiturates (Long-Acting)				
Phenobarbital	Luminal (prescription); barbs, purple hearts (street)	Miotic pupils Respiratory depression to complete arrest Gradual onset of lethargy to coma Hypotension Hypothermia	Consult physician concerning ipecac, as drug may depress patient's gag reflex at the same time ipecac begins to work Support ventilations and blood pressure as per hypovolemia Check patient's gag reflex and level of consciousness frequently Use cardiac monitor, if available	Most abused drug next to Valium and alcohol May be used to reduce effect of amphetamines causing mixed overdose Usual dose: 15–30 mg three times per day
Barbiturates (Intermediate-Acting)				
Amobarbital	Amytal (prescription; blue ice, blue lady, turquoise blue birds (street)	Faster onset but shorter duration than phenobarbital	Same as phenobarbital	
Secobarbital	Seconal (prescription); red birds, red devils, downers, laybacks, reds (street)	Level of consciousness from agitated to comatose		

Pentobarbital	Nembutal (prescription); block busters, nemmies, nebbies (street)		Usual dose: 30 mg 3–4 times per day; 100 mg at bedtime
Pentobarbital/ amobarbital combination	Tuinal (prescription); Christmas tree, rainbows, tootsie (street)	Brain stem reflexes may be absent Pupils may be miotic Ankle clonus may be present (grasp leg at ankle, push foot back toward patient's nose, foot will jerk)	

Other Sedatives

Glutethimide	Doriden/CB, D	Rapid onset of coma (1 hour) Stupor or coma may alternate with alert or hyperactive behavior Pupils may be dilated/fixed Sudden apnea and hypotension may occur	Monitor vital signs and ventilation closely Avoid ipecac because coma may develop rapidly
Methaqualone	Quaalude (prescription); super/quads, soapers, roarers, ludes (street)	Sedative-hypnotic, action similar to that of short-acting barbiturates; coma and respiratory depression most common	Support ABCs as required
Methaqualone hydrochloride	Parest, Somnafac	Possible hallucinations	Abrupt withdrawal can cause serious side effects, including seizure, chills, general behavior change, anxiety
Methyprylon	Noludar	Pulmonary edema Diaphoresis Drowsiness, nausea, vomiting	If mixed with alcohol, drug can be fatal Usual dose: 400 mg at bedtime

Table continued on following page

Table 13-2 *(Continued)*

DRUG/SUBSTANCE	TRADE OR STREET NAME	SIGNS/SYMPTOMS	EMT MANAGEMENT	SPECIAL COMMENTS
Meprobamate	Miltown, Equanil, Mepriam, Saronil, Tranmep, Meprospan	Extreme drowsiness progressing to coma Possible hypotension Possible respiratory arrest	This drug is usually slow to produce severe effects; can use ipecac if given within 15–20 min after ingestion of drug Support ABCs as required	Large quantity of alcohol makes overdose possible with smaller dose Usual adult dose: 1200–1600 mg/day in divided doses
Ethchlorvynol	Placidyl	Onset of coma in 1 hour, which can be prolonged for days Seizures Depressed ventilation Absence of response to painful stimuli	Support vital signs and respiration Be prepared for seizure Avoid ipecac, as drug has rapid action in large quantities	Combination of Placidyl and amitriptyline can cause patient to be delirious Usual adult dose: 500–1000 mg
Diazepam	Valium	Unconsciousness from Valium, Ativan, and Tranxene is rapid (10–30 min) Unconsciousness from Librium, Dalmane, and Serax is slow (hours)	Do not use ipecac with Valium, Ativan, and Tranxene because of rapid action of drugs	Valium is the most widely prescribed and abused of all sedatives
Lorazepam Chlordiazepoxide Flurazepam Clorazepate Oxazepam	Ativan Librium Dalmane Tranxene Serax	Initially patient will be sleepy, confused; slurred speech with possible difficulty in controlling motor functions will progress to coma, respiratory depression, and/or respiratory arrest	Support vital signs and respiration as required	Alcohol is often used with these drugs; makes even small dose unpredictable Usual adult dose: 2–4 mg/day

Upiates and Derivatives				
Opium, Opium tincture, Laudanum, Morphine sulfate, Codeine, Diacetylmorphine, Hydromorphone, Oxycodone, Meperidine	Numbers in parentheses indicate potency equal to 10 mg of morphine sulfate: Paregoric (25 ml) Morphine Codeine (60–100 mg) Heroin (3 mg) Dilaudid (2 mg) Percodan (50 mg) Demerol (80–100 mg)	Pupils are miotic to pinpoint and are nonreactive Respiratory arrest is common; also shallow, slow respirations Patients are stuporous to comatose but are often arousable to painful stimuli; will return to unconsciousness when stimulus is relaxed Patients may have pulmonary edema and/or atrial fibrillation Look for fresh injection sites in arms, legs, between fingers and toes, as well as tattoos near large veins to hide needle marks	Support vital signs and ventilation as required Patient may be talking but not have gag reflex to protect airway Antidote is naloxone (Narcan), which is usually available from paramedics or most medical facilities These patients may have underlying communicable diseases from poor care of needles and poor living habits Treat pulmonary edema as required	Strychnine is often used to "cut" opiates; side effect is seizure and hypothermia Be alert; patients can be dangerous Do not relax vigilance in presence of patient or friends; stick to medical approach only Have police in attendance
Methadone	Dolophine (8 mg), Methadone, Amidon			Methadone often used in detoxification of heroin addicts; withdrawal symptoms are slower and less severe
Oxycodone and acetaminophen	Percocet			
Propoxyphene	Darvon	Pupils may not be pinpoint	Same as opiates	Can be refined and injected
Propoxyphene and acetaminophen	Darvocet, Darvocet-N	Can produce all other effects of opiates Darvocet-N may present with symptoms of hypoglycemia		
Etorphine hydrochloride	M99	Is 1000 times more potent than morphine, with sedative and respiratory effects	Same as opiates Diprenorphine hydrochloride (M50-50) counteracts ethorphine (antagonist as Narcan is to heroin)	Used only by veterinarians to immobilize large animals

Table continued on following page

Table 13-2 *(Continued)*

DRUG/SUBSTANCE	TRADE OR STREET NAME	SIGNS/SYMPTOMS	EMT MANAGEMENT	SPECIAL COMMENTS
Stimulants				
Amphetamine	Benzedrine (prescription); benz, bennies (street)	Agitation, flushing, perspiration, tachycardia, hypertension	Support vital signs and ventilation as required	Barbiturates often used to control "high"; therefore patient may have combined symptoms Usual doses: 5–60 mg/day
Dextroamphetamine	Dexedrine (prescription); dexies, copilots (street)	Patient may be hyperactive, with muscle twitching	Handle patient with caution — may have rapid mood changes	
Methamphetamine	Desoxyn, Methedrine, Obedrin-L (prescription); black beauties, ice (street)	Anxiety with visual hallucinations may occur Nausea, vomiting, abdominal cramps	May require restraints in best interest of patient	
Amphetamine and dextroamphetamine	Biphetamine	Hyperventilation Moderately dilated pupils	Ipecac should be considered if patient has active gag reflex and is conscious	
Methylphenidate	Ritalin (prescription); ritlins (street)	When severe, can lead to seizure and coma		Ritalin used for hyperactive children to reduce hyperactivty; often injected for street use, causing abscesses on skin and "cotton fever" from cotton ball fibers through which drug was strained for injection Usual dose 10–60 mg/day, divided 2–3 times per day

		Patient often combative		Combination of hallucinogen and phenothiazines may cause cardiovascular failure, shock, and death
Phenmetrazine Cocaine	Preludin (prescription); snow, coke (street), crack			
Hallucinogens, Psychedelics				
DMT (dimethyltryptamine), LSD, Mescaline, Peyote, Psilocybin		Pupils are large Patient is agitated, hot, flushed, delirious with hallucinations Toxic level of LSD usually lasts 12–24 hours	Protect patients from injury to EMT(s) and themselves Support vital signs and ventilation as required	
Phencyclidine	PCP, animal tranquilizer (prescription); angel dust, peace pill, angel fuzz, supergrass (with marijuana) (street)	Pupils may be midsize to large Combative behavior changing to depression Respiratory arrest Effect may last 2–4 days Hallucinations	Same as above This patient can be extremely dangerous; patients have been known to break their own limbs during restraint without acknowledging injury	PCP can be easily manufactured outside the lab in large quantity, with varied composition as a result Patient may react differently to same-size dose Used in many forms
Tetrahydrocannabinol	Marijuana, grass, pot, weed, Colombian gold, Thai sticks, etc. (street)	Anxiety, agitation Large pupils with "bloodshot" whites of eyes Appears drunk Hyperventilation secondary to surprising extra effect of "good" drug	Observation is usually sufficient Occasional hypotension when used in conjunction with alcohol Treat hyperventilation as usual	

Table continued on following page

Table 13-2 *(Continued)*

DRUG/SUBSTANCE	TRADE OR STREET NAME	SIGNS/SYMPTOMS	EMT MANAGEMENT	SPECIAL COMMENTS
Psychotropic agents				
Phenothiazines				
Chlorpromazine	Thorazine, Promapar, Chlor-PZ	Lethargy, which may progress to coma	Treat hypotension with elevated extremities	All phenothiazines lower the seizure threshold
Trifluoperazine	Stelazine	Orthostatic (postural) hypotension to profound hypotension	Support ventilation	
			Monitor cardiac arrhythmias if monitor is available	
Thioridazine	Mellaril	Pulmonary edema (Mellaril)	Be prepared for cardiac and/or respiratory arrest	
Prochlorperazine	Compazine	Cardiac arrhythmias	High-flow oxygen or bag mask assist	
		Dystonic reactions (swollen tongue, rigid jaw with face distorted)		
Haloperidol	Haldol	Limbs tonic, respiratory distress	These patients require immediate care to treat severe symptoms early	Patient can become extremely ill rapidly
Perphenazine	Trilafon	Dystonias, eyes locked, rigid face		
Antidepressants				
Tricyclics				
Amitriptyline	Elavil, Endep	Patients are often excited but can progress rapidly to coma	Treat same as phenothiazines	Patient can become extremely ill rapidly
Imipramine	Tofranil	Tachycardia and arrhythmias are very common	Cardiac arrhythmias with sudden death are the greatest danger	
Desipramine	Norpramin	Hypertension or hypotension		
Nortriptyline	Aventyl			

Doxepin Amitriptyline and perphenazine	Seizures May have symptoms of phenothiazines and tricyclics		
MAO inhibitors Tranylcypromine Isocarboxazid Nialamide Phenelzine	Same as tricyclics		Foods such as cheese and wine may cause symptoms of toxicity
Atropinics/ Anticholinergics			
Belladonna Atropine, belladonna	Classic atropine intoxication: delirious ("mad as a hatter"), flushed ("red as a beer"), dilated pupils ("blind as a bat"), absent perspiration ("dry as a bone")	Control hypotension as required Control hyperthermia as required	Jimson weed and nightshade contain belladonna
Antihistamines			
Diphenhydramine Benadryl	Sedative effect with low dosage	Same as anticholinergics	Commonly used by public as antinausea medicine
Dimenhydrinate Dramamine	Symptoms the same as anticholinergics in high dosage		
Mild Analgesics			
Salicylate Aspirin and others (over 400 preparations contain salicylate)	Initial symptoms: headache, nausea, hyperventilation Later symptoms: lethargy to coma Seizures Increased perspiration, hyperthermia	Use ipecac as soon as possible if patient is conscious; aspirin tends to form hard "ball" in stomach if not removed	

Table continued on following page

Table 13-2 *(Continued)*

DRUG/SUBSTANCE	TRADE OR STREET NAME	SIGNS/SYMPTOMS	EMT MANAGEMENT	SPECIAL COMMENTS
Acetaminophen	Tylenol, Datril, often combined with mild opiates	Same as salicylate Liver damage may occur in large-quantity overdoses	Use ipecac as soon as possible if patient is conscious Administer large quantities of fluid orally to cause excretion naturally	Overdose may be accidental because each patient's ability to metabolize this drug varies
Other Drugs Phenytoin	Dilantin	Slurred speech, hypotension Occasional dystonic posturing (see phenothiazine) Coma is rare except with massive overdose May develop atrioventricular block arrhythmia	Support vital signs and ventilation Put on cardiac monitor if available; be prepared to assist heart block with CPR should hypotension occur	
Lithium	Eskalith, Lithane	Muscle tremor, blackout spells, slurred speech, dizziness, blurred vision, dry mouth, fatigue, lethargy, confusion, stupor, coma; early signs of diarrhea, vomiting, dizziness	Support vital signs and ventilation	Lithium toxicity is closely related to serum lithium levels, and can occur at doses close to therapeutic levels Treats manic-depressive patients only

Iron

Ferrous gluconate	Fergon	Nausea, vomiting, diarrhea, stomach upset, weak/rapid pulse, decreased blood pressure	Induce vomiting with ipecac Hospital must pump stomach within first hour, because stomach may perforate from treatment
Ferrous sulfate	Feosol, Mol-Iron, others	Heavy dose can cause brisk bleeding in stomach/intestine and black tarry stools (from hemorrhage) Shock	
Ferrous fumarate	Feostat, others		

Alcohol Compounds

Ethanol	"Alcohol"	"Drunkenness"-like symptoms, coma and respiratory depression with large quantities Loss of gag reflex Dilated, slow-reacting pupils	Normally supportive May require aggressive airway management with children and young adults (often first-time users) Often used mixed with a variety of drugs
Methanol	Sterno	Usually takes 8–36 hours to take effect: headache, blurred vision, seizures, nausea, vomiting, abdominal cramps, to coma	Main treatment is performed by hospital Contact physician for ipecac in field As little as 2 teaspoons can be toxic; 2–8 oz can be fatal
Ethylene glycol	Antifreeze	Hyperventilation Coma occurs rapidly; may cause pulmonary edema seizures	Same as methanol As little as 100 ml may cause coma

Table 13-3 Commonly Abused Substances and Recreational Drugs

DRUG OR SUBSTANCE	COMMON NAMES	SIGNS/SYMPTOMS	EMT MANAGEMENT
Heroin (opiate, narcotic)	Horse, smack, black tar	Heroin use is commonly characterized by coma or a decreased level of consciousness, pinpoint pupils, respiratory depression or apnea, and a history or evidence of drug abuse. Since heroin is usually injected, track marks may be evident (new or old).	After quickly assessing the ABCDs, the EMT must focus on securing the airway, providing high-flow oxygen or assisting ventilations if needed, and providing CPR if the patient is in cardiac arrest. Request ALS services. Attention to EMT safety is crucial since the heroin overdose patient may suddenly awaken and be unaware of his/her surroundings.
Cocaine (stimulant)	Coke, blow, snow, rock, crack	The patient's presentation may vary. Cocaine use is commonly characterized by irritability, euphoria, agitation, tachycardia, and hypertension. The patient may progress to having seizures, cerebral hemorrhage, hyperthermia, chest pain, acute MI, ventricular arrhythmias, pulmonary edema, coma, and cardiac arrest. Cocaine may be inhaled (snorting), injected (shooting up), smoked as crack (freebase), or applied to the mucous membranes.	After assessing the ABCDs, the EMT should treat the signs and symptoms identified in the focused history and physical exam. Provide high-flow oxygen and minimize exertion and further agitation. Treat seizures, chest pain, and other symptoms as with any other patient. The patient should be evaluated in an emergency room. Attention to EMT safety is crucial since the cocaine patient may become paranoid and violent.

Heroin & cocaine mixture	Speedball	This mixture of heroin and cocaine is usually injected. Signs and symptoms of both drugs may be present.	Treat as with heroin or cocaine abuse or overdose.
Methamphetamine (other amphetamines include dexedrine, Ritalin, ephedrine)	Crank, speed, ice	The signs and symptoms of amphetamine-type drugs are similar to those of cocaine. These drugs may be injected, ingested, snorted, or smoked depending on the type of drug. Amphetamines are commonly used in diet pills (dexedrine), in decongestants (ephedrine), and for attention deficit disorder in children (ritalin). Long-term use may lead to paranoid syndromes.	The treatment for amphetamine-type drug abuse or overdose is similar to that of cocaine.
Phencyclidine	PCP, angel dust, krystal	PCP abuse or overdose may present with loss of pain perception, lethargy, euphoria, hallucinations, violent or bizarre behavior, disinhibition, hyperthermia, tachycardia, seizures, or coma. PCP is often added to marijuana and LSD. It may be injected or ingested but is usually added to another substance to be smoked.	The PCP overdose patient can be extremely hazardous to the EMT. Ensure EMS provider safety first. Assess and treat ABCDs. Treat signs and symptoms as with other patients. If possible, restrain patient with soft restraints during treatment and transport.

Table continued on following page

Table 13-3 [Continued]

Drug or Substance	Common Names	Signs/Symptoms	EMT Management
LSD, MDMA (hallucinogen type)	Acid, ecstasy, Adam	The patient using hallucinogen-type drugs may experience mood changes (euphoria or depression), anxiety, visual disturbances, and hallucinations. Chronic users may experience "flashbacks." Severe intoxication may result in seizures, hyperthermia, hypertension, and cardiac arrhythmias.	Assess and treat ABCDs. Provide oxygen. The most effective treatment provided by the EMT will be gentle reassurance in a calming manner.
Rohypnol (flunitrazepam)	Roachies, roofies, rophies, rope	This relatively new drug has been referred to as a "date rape" drug. It is related to drugs such as diazepam (Valium) and alprazolam (Xanax). Although the drug is not manufactured in the United States, it is available in other countries, including Mexico. This rapidly acting drug (within 30 minutes) has sedative and amnestic effects. The patient may simply appear to be intoxicated. The effects may last for hours. Although commonly ingested, it may also be snorted, smoked, and used intravenously. Alcohol significantly enhances the intoxicating effects.	The treatment is similar to that of any drug overdose with sedative or depressant properties. Of utmost importance is the protection of the airway. Respiratory status may be depressed. Provide high-flow oxygen and assist ventilations if necessary. Transport patient to the hospital for evaluation and observation.

Substance	Description	Treatment
GHB (gamma-hydroxybutyrate)	Liquid ecstasy, liquid X, liquid E	Originally produced as an anesthetic, the sale of this drug was banned by the FDA in 1990. GHB is reported to have caused seizures, unconsciousness, and respiratory failure. Other effects include vomiting, bradycardia, and bradypnea. At least one death has been linked to the accidental ingestion of GHB. The effects of the drug are noted within 15–30 minutes. The effects may last for up to 4 hours if ingested alone. Alcohol significantly enhances the symptoms of GHB. Although it can be produced as a white powder, it is commonly used as a clear liquid mixed in another drink.	Patients are treated symptomatically. The primary focus must be on airway control and ventilations. Provide high-flow oxygen and assist ventilations if necessary. Transport patient to the hospital for evaluation and observation.
Commonly abused household chemicals (hydrocarbon solvents, paints, and aerosols)	Paint thinner, paint stripper, gasoline, varnish, kerosene, metallic paints, Halon fire extinguisher	The effects of hydrocarbons vary depending on the type of chemical, degree and route of exposure, and complications from the exposure. The patient may experience generalized CNS depression, seizures, cardiac arrhythmias, and irritation to the mucous membranes and respiratory system. GI upset leading to vomiting may result in aspiration pneumonia. Inhalation has a higher order of toxicity than does ingestion. The placing of solvent vapors or metallic paints in a plastic bag and then inhaling the vapors while placing the bag over the mouth and nose has become a popular fad among young people. This process, called "huffing," has been demonstrated to be lethal.	Safely remove the patient from the toxic environment. Assess and treat ABCDs. Provide high-flow oxygen and ventilate if needed. Treat other focused history and physical exam findings as with other patients. Use caution when providing advanced drug therapy with catecholamines (epinephrine, nonselective beta agonists) because this may increase the likelihood of arrhythmias. Request ALS services and transport.

Because CNS effects are commonly associated with abused substances, the EMT must be prepared for sudden changes in behavior, including sudden awakening, violent behavior, mood swings, and paranoid reactions.

Inhaled Poisons

■ Carbon Monoxide

Definition

Carbon monoxide (CO) is a colorless, odorless, tasteless gas produced by the incomplete combustion of organic materials, such as wood, gasoline, natural gas, and coal. It is produced and found in harmful concentrations in poorly ventilated areas, such as a closed garage with a running automobile engine, or when using briquettes for cooking in a closed space. It can also be produced in heating systems, wood stoves, or camp stoves in trailers. Moderately elevated CO levels may develop in persons in accidents on busy freeways in underpasses or tunnels. House fires and industrial fires are common sources of CO poisoning, especially for firefighters if they have inadequate respiratory protection. Even smoking in a closed room can cause mild elevations of CO. According to the Consumer Products Safety Commission, nearly 200 people per year die as a result of accidental CO poisoning.

Acute Scenario

Carbon monoxide has an affinity for the hemoglobin in the red blood cell, displacing oxygen. When the lungs do not pick up oxygen for delivery to the bloodstream, a low blood oxygen level (hypoxemia) results. The end result is decreased oxygen availability to the tissues.

History: Subjective Reports

Although suicide attempts are usually obvious, other cases of CO poisoning may not be obvious. For the most part, CO poisoning is not perceived by the patient as a problem, because one of the results of hypoxemia is a generalized feeling of well-being. The degree of symptoms is related to the length and concentration of exposure.

- *Mild exposure*: Symptoms include lightheadedness, mild headache, nausea, and dimness of vision. Some patients may have symptom relief with removal to fresh air and provision of oxygen.
- *Moderate exposure*: Symptoms include dizziness, blurred vision, weakness, and severe headache.
- *Severe exposure*: Symptoms include headache, confusion, apathy, and lethargy. The potential for long-term effects is significant in pregnant women, children, and the elderly.

The history of the present episode may reveal clues to the source of the CO poisoning. The EMT should be especially suspicious of CO upon finding an outbreak of symptoms in several people all in the same place at the same time, such as a house or a schoolroom. Other common scenarios leading to exposure include:

- The use of portable generators and/or charcoal briquette stoves during power outages, particularly when cool temperatures exist.
- The use of charcoal cooking devices by those unaware of the potential hazards (recent immigrants).

Examination: Objective Physical Findings

The degree of objective signs also depends upon the length and concentration of exposure. Low exposure produces irritability and impaired judgment. High exposures produce tachycardia, seizures, coma, and cardiovascular collapse. The classic sign of "cherry-red" mucous membranes and skin is rarely seen.

EMT Treatment

The EMT should be protected against any potentially toxic environment with breathing apparatus. Once safe access to the environment is gained and rescue operations are complete, begin ventilation of the area as necessary.

Terminate exposure of the patient to the toxic environment as soon as possible. Provide the patient with an oxygen mask during rescue, if possible.

Provide high-flow oxygen.

Support ventilations as needed.

Complete the focused history and physical exam. Obtain a history of underlying illnesses that may be affected by the CO exposure (heart disease, chronic respiratory disease, pregnancy).

When CO exposure results from smoke (e.g., firefighting), consider the possibility of exposure to other toxic gases, including cyanide.

All CO poisoning patients should be evaluated at a hospital emergency department. Hyperbaric chambers, when available, are used to treat serious CO poisonings.

■ Smoke Inhalation

Definition

Smoke inhalation results from exposure to fire without adequate respiratory protection. House or industrial fires produce a number of toxic combustion products, especially from plastics such as polyvinyl chloride (PVC).

Acute Scenario

The results of smoke inhalation can be life threatening and include:

- Edema of the upper airway
- Bronchospasm
- Pulmonary edema
- CO poisoning
- Cyanide poisoning

The smoke inhalation victim is at risk of developing these serious conditions as late as 5 to 8 hours after the exposure, even if the initial symptoms are minimal or absent.

History: Subjective Reports

Dyspnea may be the only complaint and may range in severity from mild to severe. The patient may also complain of a sore throat, burning sensation of the nasal passages and oropharynx, or headache. All patients with a history of significant exposure to smoke, especially if in an enclosed space or with an altered mental status, need hospital evaluation.

Examination: Objective Physical Findings

The victim of smoke inhalation may have hoarseness, raspy voice, cough, wheezing, black sputum, facial burns, or singed facial hairs. Any of these signs indicates the need for hospital evaluation.

EMT Treatment

■ Safely remove the patient from the smoky environment, using respiratory protection if needed.

■ Provide high-flow oxygen (humidified oxygen if available). Assist ventilations if needed.

■ If rales are present, place in a sitting or semireclining position.

If facial burns, hoarseness, an altered mental status, or stridor is present, request ALS services and provide rapid transport to the hospital.

■ TOXIC GAS EXPOSURE: CL_2, H_2S, CN, CS, AND OC

Chlorine Gas (Cl_2)

Chlorine is an irritant, poisonous gas. Inhalation of the toxic gas can occur as a result of transportation accidents, industrial accidents, leaks at swimming pools, or household mixing of bleach (sodium hypochlorite) with acid, usually in a misguided effort at cleaning a toilet bowl. Chlorine becomes a strong acid itself when it dissolves into the moisture of a person's mucous membranes, resulting in burning sensations of the eyes, nose, and throat. Other symptoms include chest tightness, headache, and nausea. Physical findings include cough, wheezing, rales, hoarseness, cyanosis, seizures, shock, and coma.

Treatment consists of safely terminating the exposure. Protection within a toxic environment can include makeshift masks of wet cloths. If there are several victims, those with signs of pulmonary edema have highest priority. Second priority goes to those with other forms of respiratory distress, who are treated simply with oxygen (humidified oxygen if available). Lowest priority patients are those who require only irrigation of the eyes. External decontamination of patients with significant exposure (chlorine cloud) may also be necessary as a protective measure for EMS and hospital personnel. While the effects of chlorine inhalation exposure are normally short term, there has been at least one report of newly developed chronic asthma persisting years after the chlorine exposure.

Hydrogen Sulfide (H_2S)

Hydrogen sulfide is a highly toxic, flammable, colorless gas. It is also a mucous membrane irritant. Inhalation of H_2S can occur as a result of occupational or industrial exposure to sewer gas, such as that found in septic tanks, in crude oil drilling sites where high sulfur levels exist, or in petroleum refineries. The gas is notable for its smell of "rotten eggs." Victims of H_2S exposure may complain of burning sensations of the eyes, nose, and throat; chest tightness; headache; nausea; and skin irritation. Physical findings include vomiting, confusion, seizures, rapid respirations, and sudden respiratory arrest. Substantial exposures may result in immediate cardiovascular collapse.

Treatment consists of safely terminating exposure and providing high-flow oxygen. Assist ventilation as required. Irrigate eyes and flush the skin as needed. Thorough external decontamination may be necessary as a protective measure for EMS and hospital personnel with significant exposures.

Tear Gas or Chemical Mace (CN and CS)

Inhalation of the toxic gases chloracetophenone (CN) and chloro-benzylidenemalononitrile (CS) can occur as a result of exposure to tear gas or chemical mace. These agents were the first chemical mace agents used by the police and the military for crowd control or personal protection. More recently, chemical mace has become available to the public for personal protection. Increasingly, these products are being used by criminals as well.

CN is a mucous membrane and respiratory tract irritant as well as a powerful skin sensitizer. Exposure to high concentrations can cause pulmonary edema, and victims may complain of burning sensations and dyspnea in addition to skin irritation. Physical findings include tearing, salivation, cough, and rales.

Like CN, CS is a mucous membrane and respiratory tract irritant as well as an extremely powerful skin sensitizer. Exposure to CS may result in complaints of headache, nausea, vomiting, eye and nose irritation, burning sensation of the skin, excess salivation and coughing. Burns to the skin may also occur.

Treatment consists of safely terminating exposure, providing high-flow oxygen for respiratory distress, and providing appropriate decontamination. Victims should face into the wind and remove contaminated clothing. Irrigate the eyes as needed, caution victims not to rub their eyes, and wash the face and hands of the patient. Notify the emergency department in advance, and wash down the victim in a shower facility outside the emergency department, if possible. Decontaminate the ambulance after transport to remove traces of CN or CS, if present.

Oleoresin Capsicum (OC)

The *Capsicum* plant, a chili pepper, produces the main ingredient in this now-popular form of chemical protection device. Commonly referred to as "pepper spray," OC has a characteristic peppery odor. Police and others are now frequently carrying OC for personal protection. Although not as toxic as CS or CN, pepper spray can be highly effective. OC spray is also a mucous membrane irritant and skin sensitizer that causes burning and tearing of the eyes, spasmodic closing of the eyelids, and pain on exposure to skin. Once safe removal from the exposure is accomplished, treatment includes high-flow oxygen for respiratory distress, irrigation of the eyes and skin, and decontamination for severe exposures. Remove any contaminated clothing. Decontamination prior to transport may be necessary as a protective measure for EMS and hospital personnel.

Chemical forms of personal protection devices using combinations of CS, CN, and OC are now available. Exposures to these combined forms are likely to be seen by EMTs. Fortunately, the treatment is essentially the same:

■ Assure the safety of all emergency services personnel. Wear appropriate protective equipment.

■ Provide high-flow oxygen for respiratory distress.

■ Remove contaminated clothing.

■ Irrigate the eyes thoroughly.

■ If possible and appropriate, decontaminate all exposed skin surfaces.

■ Provide advance notice to the receiving hospital (if transporting) and decontaminate per hospital procedures.

■ Decontaminate the EMS transport vehicle once the transport is complete.

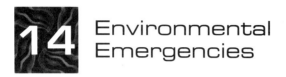

Environmental Emergencies

Water

■ DROWNING AND NEAR-DROWNING

Definition

Drowning is the fourth leading cause of accidental death. *Drowning* is death due to submersion. *Near-drowning* is submersion under water that does not result in death.

A predictable sequence of events can occur in drowning. First, large amounts of water are often swallowed. Next, small amounts of water in the hypopharynx and larynx (upper airway and voice box) cause coughing and laryngospasm, closing off the trachea (windpipe). If the victim is rescued at this point, there will be little or no water in the lungs. The laryngospasm makes further breathing attempts useless, whether the victim is under water or at the surface. (It also makes rescue attempts at this stage difficult.) Lack of breathing results in hypoxia and unconsciousness. Prolonged hypoxia inevitably leads to cardiac arrest.

Eventually, anoxia causes muscular relaxation. The relaxation of the larynx allows water to enter the lungs. When a large volume of fresh water enters the lungs, it is rapidly taken up into the bloodstream, causing an increase in blood volume and an electrolyte imbalance. In addition to asphyxia, these physiologic changes can result in ventricular fibrillation. By comparison, a large volume of aspirated salt water draws fluid out of the bloodstream, resulting in increased pulmonary edema.

The differences that can occur in fresh water as opposed to salt water do not affect the EMT's treatment of the near-drowning patient. The treatment priorities are still the basic ABCDs. What does make a difference in the treatment rationale is a history of near-drowning in cold water. Near-drowning victims have recovered completely after up to 40 minutes of complete submersion in cold water. Survival after cold water submersion is attributed to the mammalian diving reflex. This reflex slows metabolism, decreases the body's oxygen needs, and shunts oxygenated blood from the periphery to the heart and brain. The maximum water temperature considered as "cold water" in submersion cases is unknown, although most sources indicate the temperature must be below 50°F. Because of the diving reflex concept, all cold water submersion victims (particularly children) should receive aggressive resuscitation efforts. This belief led to the creation of the common expression (when referring to the cold water submersion victim), "the patient isn't dead until he is warm and dead."

Acute Scenario

The near-drowning victim has been deprived of oxygen, causing hypoxia. It is the hypoxia that causes the initial physiologic changes to the near-drowning victim. The aspirated water (if any) is unlikely to produce major physiologic effects in the time the EMT may be caring for the patient. However, the effects of aspiration and fresh versus salt water effects will have an impact on the long-term care of the resuscitated near-drowning victim.

History: Subjective Reports

The patient most likely will be unable to give any history of the incident. Bystanders are often not completely reliable for estimating the time of submersion, although that estimate should be solicited, if possible. Family or friends may relate other aspects of the incident, such as a dive into shallow water, alcohol or drug intoxication, or pertinent past medical history. Significant history for the near-drowning patient includes

- All symptoms stated by the conscious near-drowning victim
- An estimate of the time of submersion and the temperature of the water (cold versus normal temperature)
- The possibility of trauma resulting from a diving, skiing, or boating accident
- Symptoms or events prior to the submersion indicating the submersion may have been caused by an illness (hypoglycemia, syncope), trauma (assault, boating accident), or an intentional act (suicide attempt)
- A history or known use of alcohol or recreational drugs
- Past medical history, including medications and allergies

This information as well as the type of water (fresh vs. salt) will be valuable to the ALS responders and the receiving hospital.

Examination: Objective Physical Findings

Assess the ABCDs, but do not waste time attempting to remove water from the lungs. Examine the patient for trauma. Assume that all submersions resulting from diving, skiing, or boating accidents may have caused a cervical spine injury. Check the patient for evidence of hypothermia. Give all patients a thorough physical exam after resuscitative measures have begun.

EMT Treatment

The treatment priorities for the near-drowning patient include rapid removal of the patient from the water, management of the ABCDs, resuscitation, provision of or transport to ALS services, and EMT safety. The patient will not be well served if the rescuers become additional victims.

■ If the patient is still in the water, the EMT must ensure that attempts to rescue the victim do not create additional victims.

- Keep in mind the "throw, tow, row, then go" rule. If possible, throw a flotation device, tow with a rope or pole, or use a boat.
- If these attempts fail, swim to the victim only if you are trained to do so. Do this only if it can be done safely.

■ Once the patient is reached (in or out of the water), maintain manual cervical immobilization. If a cervical spine injury is suspected, place the patient on a backboard and apply a cervical collar as soon as time permits.

■ Control the airway.

- Open the airway, avoiding hyperextension if cervical spine injury is suspected.
- Do not attempt to remove water from the lungs. Such attempts are likely to cause vomiting and do little good for the patient.
- Assume all near-drowning patients will vomit during the resuscitation. Have suctioning equipment ready for use.

■ Provide oxygen and assist ventilations as necessary.

- If the patient remains in the water and you are trained to do so, begin ventilations in the water. Do this only if it can be done safely.
- Once out of the water, provide positive pressure ventilation with 100% oxygen.
- If the patient is conscious and has adequate ventilations, provide high-flow oxygen.

■ Initiate CPR as necessary.

- Apply an AED to the patient if you are trained and authorized to do so.
- Follow standard defibrillation protocols or appropriate defibrillation protocols for hypothermic cardiac arrest patients.

■ Treat immersion hypothermia, if present. Most near-drowning victims will have some degree of hypothermia. All near-drowning victims are at risk for hypothermia.

- If mild to moderate hypothermia exists, remove all wet clothing, insulate the patient, and rewarm the core before the extremities (heated oxygen or hot packs to chest, groin, and neck).
- If severe hypothermia exists, handle the patient gently, remove all wet clothing, and insulate the patient. Provide rapid transport.
- CPR should not be abandoned in a victim of immersion hypothermia until the victim has been rewarmed.

Transport all victims of near-drowning to the hospital, even if they are conscious and alert.

■ DIVING (SCUBA)

Scuba (*self-contained underwater breathing apparatus*) diving is becoming increasingly popular, and untrained or inexperienced divers encounter three types of problems: descent, bottom, and ascent. When these problems cause medical conditions directly resulting from the changes in pressure, the results are often referred to as "barotrauma." Examples include a pneumothorax and ruptured eardrum.

Descent Problems

A diver with existing blockage of nasal or sinus passages (such as that resulting from a head cold or ear infection) has an inability to equalize the internal pressure with the increasing external environmental pressure at depth. This may result in rupture of the eardrum (tympanic membrane). The diver may experience intense pain in the ear or nasal sinuses, causing him/her to ascend rapidly. If the eardrum ruptures, sudden loss of balance will result. Nausea, vomiting, and disorientation may also occur as the cold water contacts the ruptured eardrum. Treatment by the EMT consists of transport to the hospital and treatment for ascent problems if present.

Bottom Problems

Underwater unconsciousness can occur for a variety of reasons, including carbon monoxide poisoning from an improperly filled tank, and nitrogen narcosis. *Nitrogen narcosis* is due to the effect of nitrogen on the CNS and results initially in mild to moderate intoxication. This sense of euphoria has been called "rapture of the deep." The diver who loses consciousness underwater may drown. Carbon monoxide poisoning should be suspected in the diver complaining of nausea and headache and who has an altered mental status.

Ascent Problems

Definition

Ascent that is too rapid can cause either barotrauma to the lungs or decompression sickness. *Barotrauma to the lungs* occurs when rapid ascent causes the increasing pressure of air in the lungs (relative to the external environmental pressure) to rupture alveoli. Air then leaks into the chest, possibly creating a pneumothorax, or into the blood vessels, causing an air embolism. An *air embolism* is an air bubble that can block the flow of blood wherever it lodges.

Decompression sickness (the bends) occurs when rapid ascent causes nitrogen gas, which had been dissolved in the blood under pressure, to suddenly form bubbles in the blood vessels as the external environmental pressure decreases on ascent. This mechanism is very similar to the sudden formation of CO_2 bubbles when a bottle of carbonated beverage is opened. To avoid the bends, Scuba divers are trained to ascend slowly and to wait for intervals at various depths.

Acute Scenario

Barotrauma to the lungs can result in respiratory distress from pneumothorax or neurologic disorder from an air embolism lodged in the brain. The bends results when nitrogen bubbles (nitrogen emboli), which can block circulation, deposit in the muscles or joints. The formation of nitrogen bubbles in the joints and muscles causes the pain symptoms.

History: Subjective Reports

Barotrauma to the lungs, as in a pneumothorax, is manifested by the sudden onset of shortness of breath (dyspnea) and chest pain. An air embolism can present with disorder of the CNS, such as visual disturbances, dizziness, or sensory loss.

Decompression sickness, as in the bends, is usually manifested by pain in the muscles and joints. The diver may also complain of a headache and muscle cramps and of being tired. The onset may be delayed up to 48 hours and is occasionally seen in the diver who goes on an airline flight within 12 hours of a dive. Another form of decompression sickness occurs when the nitrogen embolism affects the pulmonary vasculature. Symptoms include chest aching, coughing, and dyspnea. These symptoms are often referred to as the "chokes."

The EMT must obtain as much information about the recent dives as possible. Questions asked to obtain dive information include

1. When was the last dive? How many dives were made this day?
2. What was the depth?
3. Did the diver ascend quickly?
4. Did the diver make decompression stops during the ascent?
5. When did the symptoms begin?
6. What were the initial symptoms? How did the diver look immediately following the dive?

Examination: Objective Physical Findings

Barotrauma to the lungs may produce the signs of a pneumothorax: cough with bloody sputum (hemoptysis) and decreased breath sounds unilaterally. The exam may also reveal subcutaneous air and an altered mental status. A tension pneumothorax may develop, with signs of hypotension, tachycardia, and tachypnea. Tracheal shift away from the affected side is a late sign of tension pneumothorax and is rarely seen.

Air embolism may present with CNS disorder, such as confusion, difficulty in speaking, motor loss, loss of consciousness, or seizures. Any unconscious diver seen by the EMT should be assumed to have experienced the effects of gas embolism.

The bends may be manifested by mottled skin, evolving rash, or muscular cramps. When the "chokes" are seen, the patient may also have cardiac involvement leading to cyanosis and shock. The patient may experience paraplegia and other peripheral neurologic conditions.

EMT Treatment

Management of barotrauma to the lungs and decompression sickness may require immediate use of hyperbaric oxygen in a decompression chamber. Until arrangements for hyperbaric decompression can be made, the patient should be treated based on the signs and symptoms.

■ Assess the ABCDs.

- Position the patient supine with the feet and legs elevated so that they are higher than the head.
- Ensure that the airway is open and clear.
- Provide ventilations if necessary.
- Provide high-flow oxygen.
- If needed, begin CPR. Implement defibrillation protocols if trained and authorized to do so.

■ Conduct a focused physical examination.

- Note any additional injuries found.
- Assess the lung sounds for the possibility of a pneumothorax. Monitor for the progression to a tension pneumothorax.
- Conduct a neurologic survey. Neurologic signs should be recorded and changes monitored on a neurologic check sheet (see Appendix 7).

■ Prepare the patient for rapid transport.

- Ensure rapid provision of, or transport to, ALS services.
- Contact medical control to determine if the patient needs to be transported directly to a facility with a hyperbaric chamber (preferably a hospital with a chamber).

■ The EMT or medical control may wish to contact the Divers Alert Network at 919-684-8111.

Heat and Cold

■ HEAT SYNCOPE

Heat syncope (fainting) is a transient state of unconsciousness, occurring in a hot environment, from which the victim has recovered.

Heat syncope is classified as orthostatic syncope, which means that it is caused by venous pooling. The victim will usually have been standing motionless for a prolonged period, often as a spectator at an event. Upon fainting, the body becomes horizontal and the victim wakes up. The patient usually has no complaints and no physical findings unless injured while falling. Treatment consists of removing the patient from the hot environment. Because heat syncope is merely a mild form of heat exhaustion, the patient's condition may progress to the more typical heat exhaustion if the exposure to the hot environment continues.

■ HEAT CRAMPS

Heat cramps occur in the individual exercising in a hot environment, commonly while replacing sweat losses with only water and not salt. The patient complains of the sudden onset of muscular pain, which may range from mild tingling to severe pain in the extremities or abdomen. Muscle cramps will be evident. Treatment consists of rest, removal to a cool environment, electrolyte and water replacement, and transport to a hospital if evidence of heat exhaustion is present or if symptoms do not resolve rapidly.

■ HEAT EXHAUSTION

Definition

Heat exhaustion is a common heat illness. It occurs as a result of excessive water and/or salt loss, usually with strenuous exercise, although it may occur in the elderly or inactive person. The victim may be in mild hypovolemic shock if significant amounts of fluid have been lost through perspiration. Heat exhaustion occurs when the rate of heat loss (through vasodilation of the skin vessels and evaporation of sweat) is less than the rate of heat gain (through exercise, external heat sources, and/or simple metabolism).

Acute Scenario

In heat exhaustion, the victim experiences symptoms that usually provide sufficient warning of heat loss mechanism failure, but fortunately before the body temperature rises dangerously. (In heat stroke, in contrast, the body temperature rises dangerously before collapse occurs.) Heat exhaustion may begin with something as simple as heat syncope or heat cramps.

History: Subjective Reports

The heat exhaustion victim complains of weakness, dizziness, headache, and nausea. Muscular cramping, including abdominal pain, may also be present. The symptoms may begin gradually and often follow exercise. The setting may be outdoors and recreational, or indoors and occupational. The EMT must therefore obtain information regarding the following factors:

1. What activity or work was being done by the patient?
   a. Was the patient doing heavy manual labor?
   b. Was the patient standing for prolonged periods in a hot environment?

2. How long was the activity or work being done?
   a. Had the patient just begun work?
   b. Is the environment new to the patient? Has he/she had time to become acclimatized to the hot environment?

3. What are the environmental conditions of the area where the work or activity was being performed?
   a. How hot is the environment (temperature)?
   b. Does the environment have high humidity?

4. How much and what type of clothing was being worn by the patient?
   a. Was the patient dressed with many layers of clothing?
   b. Was the patient wearing impervious or specialized protective clothing (e.g., rubber suit)?

5. What were the frequency of rest breaks and the degree of rehydration?
   a. Had the patient taken rest breaks frequently?
   b. Had the patient been regularly drinking fluids (other than plain water) during the work or activity?

6. What is the patient's recent and past medical history?
   a. Does the patient have any recent illness or activity that may have added to his/her fluid losses (excessive alcohol consumption, respiratory or GI infection)?
   b. Is the patient taking any medications that may cause him/her to lose additional fluid (diuretics such as furosemide [Lasix], decongestants such as pseudoephedrine [Sudafed])?
   c. Has the patient been using recreational stimulant drugs (e.g., cocaine, methamphetamines)?

Examination: Objective Physical Findings

The primary sign in heat exhaustion is skin that is of subnormal temperature. It will generally feel cold and clammy to the touch, and its color will be pale or gray. When significant fluid loss has occurred and mild hypovolemia is present, signs can include a rapid, weak pulse and postural hypotension. When significant sodium loss has occurred, the patient may have seizures. If the heat exhaustion is allowed to progress, the patient may become disoriented, although unconsciousness is rare.

EMT Treatment

■ Remove the patient from the hot environment and/or strenuous activity.

■ Position the patient flat with the lower legs elevated.

- ■ Monitor the airway closely because vomiting may occur.
- ■ If the patient remains nauseated and/or is vomiting, place the patient in a lateral recumbent position.

■ Provide oxygen.

- ■ Provide low-flow oxygen.
- ■ If the patient has an altered mental status or is exhibiting signs of shock, provide high-flow oxygen.

■ Provide rehydration.

- ■ If the patient is conscious and able to drink, provide electrolyte-containing fluids (e.g., sports drinks).
- ■ Avoid large quantities of drinks containing excessive sugar or caffeine.
- ■ *Do not provide salt tablets to the heat exhaustion patient.*
- ■ If the patient is unable to drink due to excessive vomiting or an altered mental status, request ALS services (if available).

■ Although heat exhaustion rarely progresses to heat stroke once treatment is initiated for the patient, the EMT must monitor for signs of heat stroke (particularly an altered mental status).

■ Transport the patient to a hospital.

■ HEAT STROKE

Definition

Heat stroke occurs when heat loss mechanisms fail or are overburdened. The body temperature subsequently rises to dangerously high levels. It is the least common heat illness, and the most deadly.

There are two common types of heat stroke: classic and exertional (see Table 14–1). In *classic heat stroke*, the heat loss mechanisms fail as a result of the victim's becoming too dehydrated to continue to sweat. This often occurs in the elderly, especially in those with chronic diseases, during heat waves. Obesity, skin disorders, and certain drugs, such as diuretics, can also be factors. In *exertional heat stroke*, the heat loss mechanisms in the body fail to keep up with the heat produced by strenuous exercise in a hot and humid environment. High humidity reduces the effectiveness of sweating for evaporative heat loss because the rate of evaporation is decreased. Even a trained and acclimatized young adult can overexercise directly into

Table 14-1   Characteristics of Types of Heat Exposure Emergencies

CHARACTERISTICS	HEAT EXHAUSTION	CLASSIC HEAT STROKE	EXERTIONAL HEAT STROKE
History			
Collapse	Sudden	May be gradual	Sudden
Exertion	May precede	Not present	Present
Mental status	Usually clear, may be confused	Disorientation, convulsions, coma	Disorientation, convulsions, coma
Skin			
Temperature	Normal or cool	Hot	Hot
Color	Pale	Red	Red
Moist/dry	Moist	Dry	Usually dry
Vital signs			
Pulse	Rapid, weak	Rapid, weak	Rapid, full
Blood pressure	May be low	Low	May be low

heat stroke, which is the second leading cause of death in athletes (after trauma deaths). Excessive heat generation can also occur with certain drugs, such as an overdose of thyroid hormone.

Acute Scenario

The onset of classic heat stroke can be gradual, and these patients are often discovered at home by family or friends, generally in an advanced stage of heat illness. The victim of exertional heat stroke can collapse suddenly and rapidly become comatose. Body temperatures above 41°C (105°F) are not long tolerated and must be lowered rapidly. Heat stroke has a very high mortality rate.

History: Subjective Reports

The heat stroke patient may complain of the same symptoms as the heat exhaustion patient (headache, weakness, dizziness, visual disturbances, and confusion). The patient may state that he/she feels extremely hot. The history obtained by the EMT should be identical to that obtained for the heat exhaustion patient discussed previously in this chapter.

Examination: Objective Physical Findings

For the most part, all heat stroke patients have the same signs. Disorientation, seizures, or coma may be present. The primary sign in heat stroke is skin that is hot to the touch. It is usually also red (in Caucasians) and dry, although in about one third of exertional heat stroke victims, the skin is moist. In either case, sweating is decreased. The body temperature will be elevated. The pulse will be rapid, as will the respirations. Patients with classic heat stroke, with dehydration and vasodilation, may have a weak pulse and a low blood pressure. Exertional heat stroke patients may have a full pulse and a normal blood pressure.

EMT Treatment

■ Cool rapidly.

- ■ Immediately move the patient to a cooler environment.
- ■ Cooling may be accomplished by immersion in a tub of cool water, if feasible.
- ■ Another method involves placing cold packs at the neck, armpits, and groin, and covering the patient with wet towels or sheets.
- ■ The patient's temperature must be monitored to avoid hypothermia and shivering.

■ Provide high-flow oxygen.

■ Be prepared for possible seizures.

■ Ensure rapid provision of, or transport to, ALS services.

■ Frostbite

Definition

Frostbite occurs when localized cooling causes tissue damage. When the water within and between cells freezes, the sharp edges of the ice crystals damage the cells. Cellular damage also occurs as a result of ischemia caused by blood vessel injury or constriction. Freezing can occur when the heat supply to an affected part is less than the heat loss.

Frostbite can be categorized like burns. *Frostnip* (first-degree frostbite) is shallow, initial frostbite, often of the face, fingertips, or toes. *Superficial frostbite* (second-degree frostbite) involves the surface and subcutaneous tissue. *Deep frostbite* (third-degree frostbite), additionally involves underlying muscle and bone, generally of the hands or feet.

Acute Scenario

Frostbite requires rapid rewarming to avoid permanent loss of function or even tissue death and amputation of the affected body parts.

Refreezing after rewarming will cause additional tissue damage. Frostnip, however, may be warmed at a slower rate.

History: Subjective Reports

The patient with frostnip is generally not aware of it. The area may be painless, and the onset is gradual. On rewarming, the area has a tingling sensation. The patient with superficial frostbite complains of numbness. On rewarming, the area stings initially and then throbs or aches. The patient with deep frostbite may complain of numbness, and on rewarming experiences extreme pain.

Examination: Objective Physical Findings

Frostnip appears white, turning red on rewarming. Superficial frostbite appears white and waxy. The superficial tissue is firm, but the underlying tissue is soft. On rewarming, the area becomes mottled blue and swollen initially, and then blisters appear.

Deep frostbite appears pale or yellow. The skin is cold and hard. On rewarming, the area becomes purple or black initially, and then blisters form.

In addition to the frostbite, the patient may be at risk for hypothermia. Other generalized signs of hypothermia may also be noted in the examination.

EMT Treatment

In the case of *frostnip*, hold the skin area against a warm part of the body, such as the armpit. The area may also be held against a warm object.

In the case of *superficial frostbite*, rewarm the area with body heat. Remove any wet clothing near the frostbitten area, such as socks. Apply gauze between fingers and toes if possible. Apply a dressing to protect the area (especially blisters), and transport with the extremity elevated.

In the case of *deep frostbite*, keep frozen and transport to the hospital unless transport time is over 1 hour. Keep the injured area dry and protected during transport.

If transport time to the hospital is expected to be several hours, or if the area has previously been partially thawed, provide rapid rewarming in a warm water bath. The water should be kept carefully between 38°C and 40°C (100°F and 105°F) for 20 to 30 minutes, or until the area stays red after removal from the water and feeling returns. Dress and protect blisters. Place gauze between fingers or toes, and transport with extremity elevated. Avoid refreezing. The process of rewarming is likely to be extremely painful for the patient.

■ Assess the patient for hypothermia and treat accordingly.

■ HYPOTHERMIA

Definition

Hypothermia, or generalized body cooling, is the term used for what was previously called "exposure." It occurs when the temperature of the core of the body (the internal organs of the trunk) is below 35°C (95°F).

Acute hypothermia occurs when a person has been immersed in cold water and becomes very quickly cooled. It is also called immersion hypothermia and can occur in water as warm as 21°C (70°F). Thin persons, especially children, are particularly at risk for rapid heat loss from cold water immersion.

Subacute hypothermia occurs when a person is exposed to a cold environment, usually outdoors, without adequate preparation (insulation, shelter, food, and so on). Hikers and hunters can die in outside temperatures of 30°F to 50°F, especially if unexpected rain and wind develop, which is why this is often called the "killer of the unprepared."

Chronic hypothermia occurs when elderly persons, or persons with chronic diseases, are exposed to cold over an extended period, usually indoors in poorly heated homes. Alcoholics also can develop chronic hypothermia because of decreased sensitivity to the cold, as well as vasodilation induced by alcohol, which increases generalized cooling.

Acute Scenario

Mild to moderate hypothermia exists at a core body temperature of 30°C to 35°C (85°F to 95°F). At lower temperatures (>85°F) severe hypothermia exists. The victim of hypothermia has lost the ability to maintain body temperature without medical intervention.

History: Subjective Reports

The victim of hypothermia is generally aware of feeling cold only when the body temperature remains above approximately 35°C (95°F). Below that temperature, although the victim may be aware of uncontrollable shivering and problems with numbness and difficulty using the fingers, the strongest feeling is that of apathy. The hypothermia victim does not care anymore. The patient with moderate hypothermia will experience gradual degeneration of his/her mental status.

Some severely hypothermic patients exhibit "paradoxical undressing": removal of clothes because of a sensation of heat, possibly because of failure of peripheral vasoconstriction at very low body temperatures.

The onset of hypothermia varies with its origin: minutes in acute immersion hypothermia, hours in subacute hypothermia, and days in chronic hypothermia. Of particular importance to the EMT will be information regarding additional risk factors for hypothermia. Risk factors include

- Age—neonates, children, elderly persons
- Chronic disease—cardiovascular disease, diabetes, hypothyroidism, anemia.
- Recent or current use of intoxicating and depressant substances—alcohol, antidepressants
- Current state of immobility—bed bound, unable to move as a result of an acute injury
- Current illness or condition—malnutrition, dehydration, exhaustion
- Inadequate protection from the environment—lack of heat in a cold home, inadequate clothing for the environment

Examination: Objective Physical Findings

The physical and mental signs and symptoms of hypothermia are related to the patient's core body temperature (Table 14–2).

Table 14-2   Physical Findings in the Hypothermia Patient

Core Temperature	Signs of Hypothermia	Mental State
>35°C (95°F)	Shivering	Withdrawn, discouraged
32–35°C (90–95°F)	Difficulty speaking ↓ Motor ability	Confused, indecisive, apathetic
30–32°C (85–90°F)	↓ Shivering Blue skin Stiff muscles	Poor judgment, lethargic
27–30°C (80–85°F) (SEVERE)	Ice-cold skin Rigid muscles ↓ Pulse ↓ Respirations	Irrational
<27°C (81°F)	Pupils dilated/nonreactive Blood pressure unobtainable Pulse difficult to palpate Respirations as low as 2–3/min Pulmonary edema	Unresponsive, coma

EMT Treatment

FOR MILD TO MODERATE HYPOTHERMIA

■ Prevent further heat loss.

- ■ Remove the patient from the cold environment.
- ■ Replace wet clothing with dry clothing.
- ■ Add insulation to the patient.

■ *Rewarm the core* before the extremities by insulating the arms and legs separately, not next to the body.

■ Rewarm with external heat (during transport).

- ■ Provide heated (42°C to 46°C), humidified air or oxygen, if available.
- ■ Apply heat packs to the neck, armpits, and groin.
- ■ Apply an electric blanket to the trunk, if available.

■ Provide carbohydrates, if the patient is able to swallow—sugar, candy, and so on.

■ Carefully examine for other injuries.

FOR SEVERE HYPOTHERMIA

■ Prevent further heat loss.

- ■ Remove the patient from the cold environment.
- ■ Replace wet clothing with dry clothing.
- ■ Add insulation to the patient. Cover all parts, including the head.

■ Handle the patient gently.

- ■ Ventricular fibrillation is easily induced in the severely hypothermic patient.
- ■ *Do not use oropharyngeal airways.*

■ Provide oxygen (preferably heated to 42°C to 46°C). Assist ventilations as needed.

■ Start and continue CPR if the patient is unconscious and pulseless.

- ■ Follow defibrillation protocols for hypothermic patients.
- ■ *No victim of hypothermia is considered dead until after rewarming.*

■ Position with head lower than the body.

■ Ensure rapid provision of, or transport to, ALS services. Provide rapid transport to a hospital.

EMT Special Considerations

If the transport time to the hospital is less than 15 minutes, do not attempt to rewarm the patient unless warm moist oxygen is available. In rescue situations, particularly cold water immersion, when there may be many victims, the most severely hypothermic patients will be the quietest. Do not be distracted by those complaining most bitterly about being cold.

The most likely victims of hypothermia seen by the EMT will be the neonate and the elderly fall victim. Even if the environment does not appear cold to the EMT, these victims may become hypothermic. Assume all neonates and elderly patients who have been immobile for a prolonged period of time in a cold environment have some degree of hypothermia.

Bites and Stings

■ ANIMAL BITES

Animal bites from wild animals, particularly skunks, bats, raccoons, and foxes, pose a special risk of rabies. In some communities, over 10% of bats have rabies. In addition, a bite by a pet or domestic animal, *especially* if the bite is unprovoked or the animal is acting in a strange manner, may suggest rabies. Bites from mice, rats, gerbils, hamsters, squirrels, guinea pigs, or rabbits pose essentially no risk of rabies to humans.

People bitten by animals are often anxious and fearful. They need to be reassured that most bites are not serious. Obtain a careful history of the incident. Wash the wound extremely well, cover with a sterile dressing, and transport. All wild animal bites must be evaluated by a physician.

The EMT's responsibility is patient care. Police or animal control officers may be needed to identify or capture the animal.

■ SNAKEBITES

Definition

Two types of snakes are poisonous in the United States: pit vipers (rattlesnakes, cottonmouths, water moccasins, and copperheads) and coral snakes. Not all bites from poisonous snakes, however, result in venom deposited in the body (*envenomation*). Less than 20% of all snake bites in the United States result in envenomation.

Acute Scenario

Pit viper venom is primarily toxic to the cardiovascular system. Coral snake venom is toxic to the nervous system.

History: Subjective Reports

All victims of snakebite are extremely anxious and fearful. Some may faint; others may be nauseated or vomit. All snakebites hurt. These are not specific signs of envenomation.

It is often difficult to identify a snake in the field, and any unidentified snake is assumed to be poisonous. The information provided in Table 14–3 can help in the identification of snakes.

Examination: Objective Physical Findings

The EMT needs to be able to identify the signs and symptoms of envenomation in order to guide treatment (see Table 14–4).

EMT Treatment

■ Approach the victim cautiously. Ask, "Where is the snake? Are you *sure* it is gone/dead?"

■ Calm and reassure the victim. Keep the victim still.

■ Quickly rinse the bite area with mild antiseptic. *Do not apply ice to the bite.*

■ Assess the ABCDs and treat accordingly. Provide high-flow oxygen to the symptomatic patient.

■ Remove rings, bracelets, and any other objects that may cause constriction once swelling begins.

■ If the bite is on an extremity, immobilize using a loose splint. Place the extremity below the level of the heart.

■ There is considerable controversy over the use of constricting bands or pressure dressings for snakebites. The following is one available option. Follow your community's protocol.

  ■ Apply constricting bands above and below the bite site to reduce venous and lymphatic flow. These should be placed 2 to 3 inches on either side of the wound, and the bands should be tight enough to restrict venous return but not reduce arterial flow. Check for an arterial pulse below the bands.
  ■ Constricting bands are of little benefit if applied more than 30 minutes after the bite.
  ■ Because of the rapid absorption of the coral snake's venom, a constricting band will be of no use.

■ Monitor vital signs. Treat for shock and assist ventilations as needed.

Table 14-3 Identification of Snakes

CHARACTERISTICS	PIT VIPER	CORAL SNAKE	NONPOISONOUS SNAKE
Head	"Pits" between the eyes and nostrils, look like extra nostrils	—	—
	Large fangs	Small fangs	No fangs
	Triangular, broad flat head, wider than neck	Black nose	—
	—	—	—
Eyes	Vertical pupils	Round pupils	—
Body	Thick	Small: 10–18 inches	—
	—	Colored bands: red on yellow	If colored bands: red on black, not red on yellow
Bite mark	Two puncture wounds: 0.5 inch apart	Tiny puncture or scratch-like wounds	Teeth marks, no fang marks
		Bites on small part, such as fingers	
Speed	Quick strike	Slow, chewing action	
Found where	Copperhead, cottonmouth: Texas to the Carolinas	South: Florida, Arizona, Texas	All states
	Rattler: all states, except Alaska, Hawaii, Maine	—	

Table 14–4   Symptoms and Signs of Envenomation

REACTION	PIT VIPER	CORAL SNAKE
	Symptoms	
Immediate/local	Severe burning pain at site of the bite	Minimal pain
Delayed/systemic	Weakness	Weakness
	Faintness	Numbness at the site or at
	Numbness at the site	the lips, tongue, or scalp
		Visual disturbances
		Difficulty speaking
	Signs	
Immediate/local	Swelling	Minimal swelling
	Discoloration	Slight bruising
Delayed/systemic	Hemorrhagic blisters	Bizarre behavior
	Adrenaline response (rapid pulse, sweating)	Paralysis of the eyelids and respiratory muscles
	Cardiovascular collapse	CNS depression
	Seizures	Seizures
	Coma	Coma

■ Identify or bring the snake, if dead.

  ■ The EMT's responsibility is patient care. Those handling the snake should use caution because accidental envenomation may still occur for some time after the snake is dead.

  ■ Police or animal control officers may be needed to identify or capture live snakes.

  ■ Notify the hospital of the snake identification, if possible.

■ Transport the patient rapidly to a hospital.

■ There is considerable controversy regarding the use of incisions for snakebite treatment. Incision and drainage may be indicated by local protocol for poisonous snakebites when transport times are prolonged. It should only be done if

  ■ Ordered by the medical control physician

  ■ Signs and symptoms of envenomation occur

  ■ The bite occurred less than 30 minutes earlier

  ■ The bite is on an extremity

The technique is performed by making a longitudinal incision, 0.5 inch long and 0.25 inch deep directly over the fang mark, extending toward the suspected venom deposit point. Mechanical suction from a commercially available snakebite kit is then applied. The most commonly recommended device is a Sawyer Extractor. If the suction device is ineffective or not available, *suction by mouth can be used as a last resort*. Any swallowed venom will be neutralized by stomach acid, although it is best not to swallow it and to rinse out the mouth. This procedure is considered to be a last resort used only when transport time will be considerably prolonged.

EMT Special Considerations

Do not pack the area in ice. The cooling effect can cause additional tissue damage, which can produce a greater problem than that caused by the injection of venom.

■ INSECT STINGS AND SPIDER BITES

Insect Stings from Hymenoptera (Bees, Wasps, Hornets, and Ants)

The class of insects known as Hymenoptera includes bees, wasps, hornets, yellow jackets, and ants. These insects inject venom. Although it would require a great number of bee stings to inject sufficient venom to produce lethal effects, it may only take one sting to produce an anaphylactic reaction. Approximately 5% of the population are allergic to Hymenoptera venom. Stings cause twice as many deaths each year as snakebites. Anaphylactic shock and hypersensitivity reactions are discussed in greater detail in Chapters 9 and 12. The identification of the offender may be difficult, because the insect has often disappeared.

Local symptoms of Hymenoptera sting include a painful, itching wheal. Systemic symptoms include anxiety and may include signs of allergic reaction. Local signs include a white, firm, elevated wheal, surrounded by redness and rapid swelling. Systemic signs may be seen if an allergic reaction occurs (Chapter 12). Signs of respiratory distress and cardiovascular collapse may result if the allergic reaction progresses to anaphylactic shock (Chapter 9).

Treatment is limited to removing the stinger, if it is still attached, and monitoring for any progression to signs of hypersensitivity reaction or anaphylaxis. Transport if any sign of systemic allergic reaction occurs, if the victim has multiple stings or was stung around the eye, or if the patient has a history of allergic reactions to stings. Application of cold to the site may be comforting. *Do not apply cold (ice or ice packs) directly to the skin*. Commercially available "sting relief" treatments may provide additional pain relief. Treat for shock if the signs and symptoms of the reaction continue to worsen.

Spider Bites

Black Widow Spider

The black widow spider (*Latrodectus* species), generally found in warmer climates, is a glossy black spider about 1 inch in size. It may be distinguished by a red-yellow or orange marking (often in the shape of an hourglass) on the abdomen. It often inhabits pit toilets. The venom injected by its bite is toxic to the CNS.

The bite may be barely noticeable initially, but can cause a dull pain that rapidly spreads to result in headache, chest tightness, and dyspnea. Symptoms may not be noted for 30 minutes or longer. Signs of systemic reaction include muscular cramps in the bitten extremity that then spread to the abdomen, chest, and back. Paralysis, seizures, cardiovascular collapse, or respiratory arrest may occur. The patient's presentation may be mistaken for an MI or abdominal distress.

Treatment is aimed at reducing the absorption of toxin from the site of injection and supporting basic life functions. As with snake-bite, treatment includes the following steps:

■ Immediately cleanse the site with antiseptic, alcohol, or soap and water.

■ Immobilize the extremity by splinting.

■ Assess the ABCDs and provide appropriate care. Provide high-flow oxygen. Assist ventilations as necessary.

■ Monitor the vital signs, and treat for shock as necessary.

■ Identify the insect if possible, and transport with the patient. Take precautions to avoid envenomation of responding emergency service personnel.

■ Hospital treatment may include administration of antivenin.

Brown Recluse Spider

The brown recluse spider (*Loxosceles* species) is usually found in the southeast and midwest but may be found in other parts of the United States. The spider is pale yellow or dusty brown, and about 0.5 inch in size. It may be distinguished by a brown violin-shaped design on its back. It likes dark corners.

The bite of the brown recluse spider produces severe local effects. The bite causes tenderness and a red, swollen area within a few minutes. Over the next few hours, the area eventually blisters. An ulcer may appear and remain for days or months. When systemic effects occur, they include weakness, fever, chills, nausea, and shock. Treatment is limited to rapid transportation to the hospital. As with all spider bites, cleanse the bite area with antiseptic, alcohol, or soap and water. Ice may be applied (indirectly to the skin) for pain relief. No approved antivenin is currently available.

Scorpion Stings

Scorpions are primarily found in the arid desert areas of the south-western portion of the country. Most scorpions are relatively harmless, although their stings may produce local pain and swelling. The only truly dangerous scorpion is the bark scorpion (*Centruroides exilicauda*), found mostly in Arizona and New Mexico. The bark scorpion (sometimes referred to as the Arizona sculptured scorpion) injects a venom that is toxic to the CNS. Young children are particularly affected by the systemic effects of the bark scorpion. Symptoms include local pain at the site and a pins-and-needles sensation. Signs include local swelling and discoloration, which can progress to muscular contractions, increased salivation, abnormal eye movements, restlessness, tachycardia, seizures, cardiovascular collapse, and respiratory arrest. Adults may also exhibit hypertension and tachypnea.

Treatment for most scorpion stings is limited to removing the patient from the environment, cleansing the site, applying ice, and monitoring for additional symptoms. Treatment steps for bark scorpion stings include the following:

■ Remove the patient and responders from the possibility of additional scorpion stings.

■ Cleanse the site of the sting with antiseptic, alcohol, or soap and water if possible.

■ Immobilize the extremity with a loose splint. Minimize activity of the patient. Project a reassuring attitude in order to calm the patient.

■ Assess and treat the ABCDs as required.

   ■ Assist ventilations as needed.
   ■ Provide high-flow oxygen for patients exhibiting systemic signs.

■ Monitor vital signs and treat for shock as needed.

■ Hospital treatment may include administration of anti-venin. Contact with a regional poison control center may be necessary for information regarding antivenin.

■ MARINE ORGANISM INJURIES

Stings

Stings can result from jellyfish, Portuguese man-of-war, anemone, or coral. The stinging cells (nematocysts) stick to the skin and release venom into the skin when ruptured. The stings can be lethal if the quantity is great enough or if systemic allergic reaction occurs. Occasionally, severe stings on the chest can cause cramping of the chest muscles, drowning a swimmer. The patient normally complains of an immediate stinging and burning pain. The sting area may become red and edematous, and may begin to itch. Systemic signs and symptoms may occur, including weakness, nausea, headache, abdominal pain, tachycardia, and chest pain. The patient may progressively worsen to the point of experiencing seizures, paralysis, coma, and cardiac arrhythmias. Deaths have been reported from the sting of the Portuguese man-of-war.

Treatment consists of several steps to be done in order.

■ Assess and treat the ABCDs.

  ■ Assure control of the airway.
  ■ Provide high-flow oxygen. Assist ventilations if needed.
  ■ Monitor the pulse frequently because cardiac arrhythmias may occur.

■ Treat other conditions such as seizures or coma.

■ Avoid breaking the nematocysts. Wash the sting areas using sea or salt water. Do not use fresh water. The EMT must protect himself/herself from stings. Use double gloves or heavier weight gloves.

■ Except in the case of jellyfish stings, soak the sting areas with alcohol or vinegar. These substances may cause jellyfish nematocysts to discharge.

■ Apply a solution of baking soda (sodium bicarbonate) to neutralize the acid venom.

■ Apply a dry powder to make the nematocysts stick together. Talcum powder, flour, or baking powder are adequate, but meat tenderizer contains an enzyme (papain) that can also inactivate venom.

■ Scrape the nematocysts off with a knife and wash again in salt water.

■ For severe cases, a boxed jellyfish antivenin may be useful for pain relief and systemic effects. Contact with a regional poison control center may be necessary to obtain information regarding the antivenin.

Punctures

Punctures can result from stepping on spiny animals such as sting rays, sea urchins, or salt-water catfish. Systemic allergic reactions are rare. Look for broken-off pieces of spine in the wounds. Place the injured part in hot water for at least 30 minutes to inactivate the venom. Avoid burning a numbed foot by placing both feet in the hot water, if feasible. Once removed from the hot water, examine the foot again for pieces of spine. Elevate the extremity and transport the patient.

Poisons

Rarely, poisoning can be caused by the eating of a marine organism usually containing a toxin such as tetrodotoxin (puffer fish), scombroid (mackerel, tuna, bonita, mahi mahi), or ciguatera (barracuda, red snapper, grouper), or by eating contaminated shellfish ("red tide") such as mussels and clams. The signs and symptoms are slightly variable; however, each of the previously mentioned poisonings leads to gastroenteritis. The onset of symptoms varies from minutes to a few hours. Severe cases may result in respiratory failure in the case of shellfish poisoning and anaphylactic signs with scombroid poisoning.

Treat as for any poison. Assess and treat the ABCDs. Assure airway control and provide high-flow oxygen. Signs of laryngeal edema (hoarseness or stridor) indicate the need for rapid provision of, or transport to, ALS services. A thorough history will be valuable to the hospital and poison control center in deciding upon additional treatment.

Man-Made Hazards

■ RADIATION EXPOSURE (IONIZING)

Definition

Radioactive material releases ionizing radiation. This can be in the form of alpha particles, beta particles, gamma rays, x-rays, or neutron radiation. Radiation sources include isotopes used in hospitals or industry for research or treatment, radioactive wastes from research or nuclear power plants, radiation leaks from nuclear power plants, and materials used in the production of nuclear weapons. Trucks or other vehicles transporting radioactive materials are always clearly marked with purple and yellow signs and are heavily protected. The possibility of leakage of radiation material from a well-packed container is slight, although real. Microwaves, radio waves, and magnetic fields are nonionizing forms of radiation and therefore are not discussed in this chapter.

Accidents involving radioactive materials generally occur where radiation experts are present to direct safety procedures, and often any needed decontamination of the environment and the patient(s) will be done before the EMT arrives. (These are called "clean" accidents.) If not, the risk from exposure is estimated by measuring the radiation with a Geiger counter, which registers units of roentgens (R). Local protocol will determine how the EMT dispatcher obtains advice in the case of the "dirty" accident.

In the case of a radiation accident, the patient or patients must be considered as "contaminated." Without proper decontamination, radioactive materials in the environment or on the patient(s) may contaminate other persons. This case poses many more difficulties for the EMT than the case of a person who is simply irradiated (exposed to excessive radiation but not contaminated).

Acute Scenario

Ionizing radiation causes changes in the ways in which all the body cells function. Some effects are immediate (hours to days), and some effects are delayed (years). Exposure is cumulative over one's lifetime. Biologic effects include hair loss, cataracts, sterility, birth defects, bone necrosis, and cancer. There is no known treatment providing recovery from the long-term effects.

Several factors will influence the outcome of exposure to ionizing radiation. They are the type and strength of the radiation, the duration of exposure, the distance from the source, and the protective shielding in place. Time, distance and shielding, must be kept in mind by the EMT in order to minimize exposure during a response to a radiation accident.

History: Subjective Reports

Ionizing radiation cannot be heard, seen, or felt. The patient will likely have some information regarding the exposure. Of particular importance to the EMT should be information regarding the patient's exposure, including time, distance, and shielding. Symptoms of acute radiation sickness occur in stages. The symptoms are directly related to the dose of radiation received. Initially, the symptoms include nausea and anorexia. The effects of severe exposures may quickly worsen. When obtaining the history, the EMT should ask, if possible

1. How long were you exposed to the radioactive material? What was the material?
2. What was the distance from you to the material?
3. Was there any shielding between you and the material? What type?
4. How are you feeling now? When did the symptoms begin?

Examination: Objective Physical Findings

Patients exposed to ionizing radiation can be divided into two groups: those posing no risk to the EMT and those posing some risk. The first group consists of persons exposed to a source of radiation that has subsequently been shielded (noncontaminated patient), and persons who have inhaled, come in contact with, or swallowed radioactive material (contaminated patient). Patients exposed to a source of radiation do not become radioactive themselves. However, clothing and skin may become contaminated with radioactive particles or liquids if a fire or explosion has occurred. This second group of contaminated patients poses some risk to the EMT.

Patients exposed to radiation may not have external signs of injury. Therefore, external injuries associated with accidents during

Table 14-5   Signs and Symptoms of Radiation Exposure

Roentgens	Effects of Short-Term Whole-Body Radiation Exposure
20–100	Blood cell changes
200–400	Nausea, vomiting, hair loss
	Marked reduction in white blood cells, leading to some deaths from infections
300–600	Diarrhea, destruction of bone marrow, sterility, 50% chance of death within 30 days
1000–2000	Severe diarrhea, death likely within 2 weeks
Over 2000	CNS damage, death within hours

transportation are generally the result of the vehicle accident and are not due to exposure to radioactive materials. At the scene of a transportation accident, do not allow the presence of radioactive materials in the involved vehicle (such as low-level wastes) to delay initiation of examination of the accident victim. The EMT must, however, assure the safety of all emergency services personnel.

The acute radiation sickness patient may exhibit signs of vomiting, abdominal cramps, and diarrhea (see Table 14–5). Severe exposures can lead to an altered mental status, signs of shock, coma, and death. Chronic, systemic disease and complications of high-dose radiation exposure will not be seen in the time the EMT is with the acutely exposed patient.

EMT Treatment

Approach the patient only after a qualified person has determined that the risk of contamination is low or absent.

- If the source of radiation (e.g., the radiation accident scene) remains, do not approach the scene unless protective measures have been taken.
- Request assistance from a qualified radiation safety officer, if available on scene. Many facilities using radiation are required to have a designated radiation safety officer. The assistance of this person should be requested.
- Contact may also be made with the Radiation Emergency Assistance Center and Training Site (REAC/TS) operated for the U.S. Department of Energy at Oak Ridge, Tennessee, (423) 481-1000.
- If the patient and scene are not contaminated and the patient was merely overexposed to radiation, approach the patient using normal procedures.

Take precautions to minimize self-exposure if the patient or the area is suspected of being contaminated. Protection is based upon decreasing the time of exposure, increasing the distance from the source, and increasing the protective shielding.

- Park response vehicles away and upwind.
- Rescue, if needed, should be well planned. It should be quick; victims may have to be moved without regard for injuries. If extrication is required for a person trapped near a radiation source, the work should be divided so that no one rescuer receives excessive radiation exposure.
- Appropriate protective clothing, including hoods, respirators, masks, lead aprons, gowns, gloves, and shoe covers, should be worn.
- Avoid dust and smoke by staying upwind whenever possible.

Decontamination may be necessary before beginning emergency medical care.

- Decontaminate patients exposed to particle-emitting radioactive substances.
- If possible, remove the patient from the contaminated area.
- Remove the patient's clothing. Bag the clothing to prevent further contamination.
- Wash the patient with soap and water. The waste water must now be treated as contaminated also.
- Wrap the patient in clean blankets or other disposable clothing (e.g., Tyvek suit).

Move the patient to the final transport vehicle.

- Minimize the number of personnel and vehicles that may become contaminated by the patient.
- Place plastic covering on the floor, bench seats, and stretcher of the transport vehicle to minimize accidental contamination.
- Do not transport other contaminated materials, including the bagged clothing.
- Provide advanced notice to the hospital. Follow the hospital's directions for handling contaminated patients.

Medical care consists of the treating the ABCDs.

- Flush wounds well with saline solution at the scene.
- If the patient is merely externally contaminated or is noncontaminated, treat the patient's symptoms as with any other patient.
- If the patient has ingested radioactive material, contact medical control regarding the induction of vomiting using syrup of ipecac.

Once the transport is complete, decontaminate the vehicle as directed by a qualified radiation safety officer. EMTs may need to shower before returning to service.

■ Electricity

Injuries caused by *electricity* can occur from downed power lines, malfunctioning home appliances, construction and maintenance work, or improper use (as when a child chews through an electric wire). Similar injuries are seen when a person is struck by *lightning*. The sudden surge of electricity through the body can cause extensive burns, cardiac or respiratory arrest, or fractures. Examination must be particularly thorough and must include a search for entrance and exit wounds, signs of spinal fracture or shoulder dislocation, and neurologic signs such as motor or sensory loss.

The first priority is to approach the victim safely.

- Ask, "Is the power still on?" Be *sure* it is shut off before proceeding.
- Advise victims trapped in cars by downed power lines to stay put until electric company experts arrive.
- Once it is safe to do so, remove the patient from the hazardous area.

The next priority is the assessment and treatment of the ABCDs.

■ Assume that the unconscious patient has a spinal injury and use the jaw thrust, if necessary.

■ Victims of electrical shock are likely to have respiratory arrest or impairment. Assist ventilations if needed. Provide high-flow oxygen if spontaneous respirations are adequate.

■ Assess the pulse and blood pressure. Shock may occur as a result of injuries or cardiac dysfunction.

■ If the patient is pulseless, immediately begin CPR.

■ Attach a defibrillator to the patient following defibrillation protocols if a defibrillator is available and you are authorized to use it. The risk for lethal cardiac arrhythmias is high.

■ Treat for shock.

■ Perform a focused physical examination and treat accordingly.

- Treat burn wounds.
- Splint fractures.
- Transport on a backboard using cervical spine precautions.

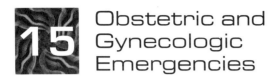

Obstetric and Gynecologic Emergencies

Emergency Childbirth

■ GENERAL ASSESSMENT AND UNCOMPLICATED DELIVERY

Definitions

Delivery prior to arrival at a hospital may occur despite the most careful plans. Most deliveries in the out-of-hospital setting occur without complications. With this in mind, the EMT's primary responsibility is to assist the mother in the delivery and assess the newborn baby. The mother will deliver the baby, not the EMT (or MD). The EMT should provide assistance and much-needed reassurance to the mother. Although emergency childbirth is a challenge, it can also be wonderfully gratifying for an EMT to assist a prospective mother in the delivery of her child.

A *primigravida* is a woman having her first pregnancy. A *multipara* is a woman who has had two or more previous deliveries. The *fetus* is the developing baby while in the uterus. *Labor* refers to rhythmic contractions. *Bloody show* is the mucus plug expelled at the start of labor. *Breaking water* is the gush (or occasionally slow trickle) of watery fluid from the vagina when the amniotic sac ruptures. *Presentation* refers to the part of the baby that comes out first.

Acute Scenario

Delivery can become unexpectedly abrupt. Transportation difficulties, such as a storm or transport vehicle breakdown, may also cause unplanned out-of-hospital birth. Regardless of these factors, the well-trained EMT must be prepared to assist in a sudden delivery.

History: Subjective Reports

When seeing the pregnant patient for any reason, the EMT should be concerned with three specific issues:

- Is delivery potentially imminent?
- Is the pregnancy considered to be high risk?
- Are there other medical or traumatic conditions that may adversely affect the mother, baby, or delivery?

Imminent Delivery

To determine whether there is time for transportation to a hospital (the delivery is not imminent?), ask these questions:

1. Is this the first baby? For the primigravida, the stages of labor are generally prolonged. For the multiparous patient, the stages of labor are more rapid. The multiparous patient is often the best judge of imminent delivery. This mother knows when delivery is close based on her past experiences.

2. How advanced are the pregnancy and labor? To obtain this information, ask the woman
   a. "What is your due date?" The prediction of the due date is often very accurate when regular prenatal care has been a part of the pregnancy. When the pregnancy is close to or past the due date, the likelihood of precipitous delivery is obviously greater.
   b. "How frequent are the contractions?" Contractions that are less than 2 minutes apart are a sign that delivery is imminent.
   c. "Has your water broken (rupture of the amniotic sac)?" Although the rupture of the bag of water is not necessarily a sign of imminent delivery, it most often indicates that the woman is in the final stages of labor.

3. Is there a sensation of rectal fullness? If the woman feels as though she has to move her bowels, this is another sign of imminent delivery. This sensation results from the fetal head pressing against the rectum through the vagina.

High-Risk Pregnancy

The EMT should then attempt to determine if the pregnancy is considered to be high risk. This may have to be accomplished while preparing for a delivery if the initial history suggests imminent delivery. High-risk pregnancies are indicated by the physician's suspicion that complications of delivery or fetal development may be likely. These deliveries may require ALS and special transport destinations for the neonate. In making the assessment, ask the patient:

1. "Does your doctor consider this a high-risk pregnancy?" "Have any of your previous pregnancies been high risk?" "Did you have any complications with your previous pregnancies and deliveries?" The pregnancy may be considered high risk for many reasons. Common reasons include difficulties with past pregnancies and/or deliveries, a history of premature labor, identified fetal abnormalities, pre-eclampsia, chronic disease (hypertension, seizures, or cardiac disease), and recreational drug use or substance abuse.

2. "Are you a diabetic?" Diabetic mothers often give birth to larger babies. These babies are also at a higher risk for hypoglycemia after birth.

3. "Do you smoke?" Maternal smoking typically results in a lower birth weight baby. There is believed to be a higher risk for spontaneous abortion and stillbirth when mothers smoke during pregnancy.

4. "Have you used any recreational drugs or alcohol during this pregnancy?" Babies born to mothers who drink alcohol during pregnancy may develop fetal alcohol syndrome. Such babies may be born with a variety of abnormalities. Increased rates of miscarriage, preterm delivery, and abruptio placentae have been associated with the use of cocaine during pregnancy. The use of narcotics, including heroin, during pregnancy can cause drug dependence for the baby. The risks of the baby experiencing respiratory depression or prolonged apnea are significantly increased.

History of Chronic Disease or Trauma

The EMT must obtain a past medical history as is done with all other patients. A history of chronic disease or recent trauma may create new complications for the mother, baby, or delivery process. Ask the patient questions regarding medications being taken, past medical history (diabetes, hypertension, seizures, cardiac problems, and lung disease), allergies, and recent trauma. Even minor traumatic events may precipitate labor.

Examination: Objective Physical Findings

If the answer to any of the history questions indicates that delivery may be imminent, then the EMT needs to examine the woman for crowning (Fig. 15–1A). *Crowning* is the bulging out of the presenting part (usually the fetal head) at the vaginal opening. Often crowning is evidenced only by the bulging at the vaginal opening, without actual visualization of the head. When the history suggests the possibility of increased risks, the EMT must pay particular attention to:

- The mother's vital signs (especially blood pressure)
- The respiratory rate and ventilations
- Signs of vaginal bleeding and/or shock
- Indications of a concurrent medical illness exacerbation
- A history or exam findings suggesting traumatic injury.

EMT Treatment

In some instances, it is obvious that delivery will occur promptly, and arrangements should be made for delivery at the scene. When there is some doubt, local protocol may call for contacting the hospital for advice.

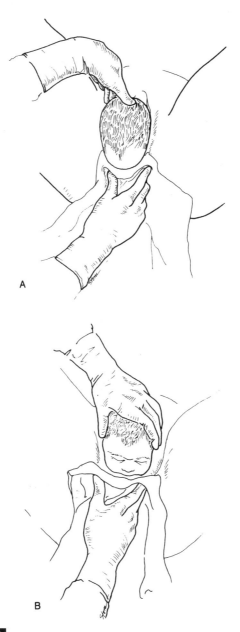

Figure 15-1

Delivery. *A*, Initial presentation. *B*, Emergence of the head. *Illustration continued on following page*

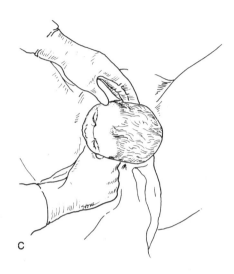

C

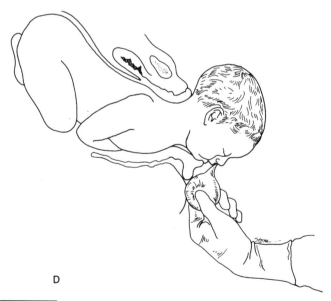

D

Figure 15-1

Continued   *C*, Checking for the cord around the neck; 90-degree rotation. *D*, Initial suctioning of nostrils.

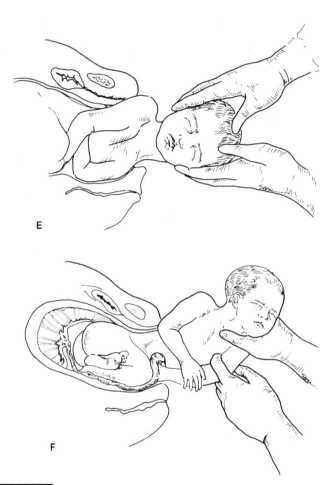

Continued   *E*, Emergence of the shoulder with gentle downward traction. *F*, Gentle upward traction to free both shoulders.

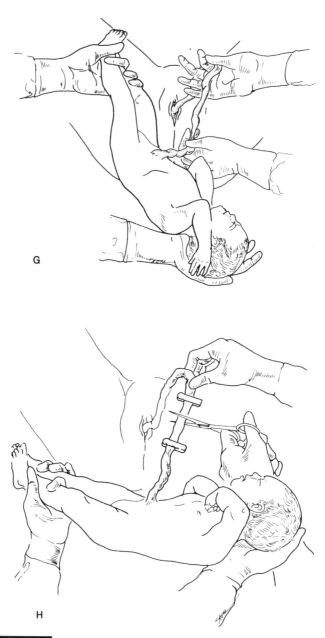

Figure 15–1

Continued   G, Preparing to clamp the cord. *H*, Clamping and cutting the cord. Note that the infant's head is lower than the feet.

Preparation for Delivery

In preparation for delivery at the scene, the EMT must

Reassure the woman. An unplanned delivery causes anxiety in addition to the normal strain of childbirth. Tell the primigravida that rectal pressure is normal and does not indicate that she needs to move her bowels. One person (a family member or EMT) should stay at the woman's head for the duration, to provide reassurance and hold her hand. An emesis basin should be present. Coaching the woman about her breathing involves giving these instructions:

- Pant through the mouth during contractions.
- Avoid bearing down or pushing until told to do so.
- Rest between contractions.

Prepare the environment for delivery. Position the woman on her back or side with a clean sheet beneath her buttocks. The woman should be positioned so that her knees are bent and can be spread apart. For sterile supplies, open the obstetrics (OB) kit first, then wash hands well before putting on gloves. If there is time, sterile drapes can be placed under the buttocks, between the legs, across the abdomen, and over each thigh. Open the OB kit and ensure that all necessary supplies are present. Ensure that towels for drying the baby are nearby. Additionally, ensure that all resuscitation equipment is nearby and ready for use. At a minimum, this equipment must include an infant bag-valve mask with a neonate-sized mask, oxygen, suctioning equipment, blankets, and heating devices. The emergency responders should also don appropriate protective equipment (gloves, gowns, eye protection).

Delivery

Assist with birth of the head. Place the palm of your hand over the head of the baby and exert very gentle pressure to prevent an explosive delivery. This reduces the chance of tearing of the area around the vagina and/or losing control of the baby. This is also accomplished by having the mother bear down to push only after the baby's head is presenting. Avoid placing fingers over the fontanel, which are the soft spots on the midline near the front and near the back of the head. Release pressure when the contraction ends and reapply when it starts again. Although the pressure is released, the EMT's hands must remain near the head to provide continued support from beneath as the baby emerges (Fig. 15–1*B*).

Look and feel for the cord around the neck (Fig. 15–1*C*). If the umbilical cord is wrapped around the neck, gently loosen it and slip it over the head carefully. Have the mother stop pushing and pant until the cord is released from around the neck. If it is too tight to be easily slipped over the head, the cord should be clamped at two sites 2 inches apart and cut between the clamps. Extreme caution must be used when using instruments near the baby to avoid accidental injury.

When the face is visible, look for and puncture the amniotic sac if it ■ is present. Remove the sac from the baby's face. At this time, the EMT may also look for signs of (or the absence of) meconium. *Suction with the bulb syringe* (compress, insert, release) two to three times (Fig. 15–1*D*). In suctioning the mouth, insert the syringe about 1 to 1.5 inches; in suctioning each side of the nose, insert the syringe about 0.5 inch. Suction the mouth first and then the nostrils.

Assist with birth of the shoulders. Support the baby with both hands ■ (Fig. 15–1*E*). Guiding the head downward can assist with delivery of the upper shoulder. Guiding the head upward can assist delivery of the lower shoulder (Fig. 15–1*F*).

Position the baby on the table, bed, or floor between the mother's ■ legs at the level of the vagina or lower, with the baby's head slightly lower than its body. Wipe the baby's face and *repeat bulb syringe suction* of the mouth and nostrils. Quickly dry the baby. Wrap the baby well in blankets or towels. The baby should be breathing at this point. If not, gently rub the baby's back or snap your finger against the soles of the feet. Evaluation of the newborn infant's condition at this point and at 5 minutes after birth may include calculation of the APGAR score (see Appendix F). *Feet that are initially blue are not abnormal.*

Clamp and cut the umbilical cord. Wait for the pulsations to cease ■ first and then clamp about halfway between the baby and the mother (Fig. 15–1*G*). Try to leave at least 6 inches of cord attached to the baby, and have 2 to 3 inches between the clamps. Cut with sterile scissors, if available (Fig. 15–1*H*). Local protocol may call for the addition of umbilical tape tied on the baby's end of the cord, about 0.5 inch from the clamp toward the baby. Apply umbilical tape very slowly and carefully.

Wait for the placenta to deliver. This usually occurs 15 to 20 minutes ■ after the birth of the baby. Evaluate the mother's condition during this time, and immediately transport if there is heavy bleeding (postpartum hemorrhage). If the baby is doing well, it can be put to the mother's breast during this period, and this will aid in contraction of the uterus. It is not necessary to delay transport simply because the placenta has not yet delivered. When the placenta is delivered, wrap it in a plastic bag and take it to the hospital for examination. After the placenta is delivered, massage the abdomen above the uterus (mid to lower midabdomen) using firm rubbing in a circular motion.

■ *Record* the time of birth and any calculated APGAR scores.

Prepare for transportation to the hospital with clean linen, a sanitary napkin over the vaginal opening, and direct pressure on any lacerations to stop bleeding. As soon as possible, direct someone to turn on the heater to the transport vehicle. Nearly all babies born in the out-of-hospital setting experience some degree of hypothermia. The vehicle should be too warm for the EMT in order to be appropriate for the baby.

■ PROLONGED DELIVERY

Prolonged delivery is defined as labor lasting more than 20 minutes after contractions have become 2 to 3 minutes apart. The fetus may be too big to deliver vaginally, although there are other causes. Appropriate management is transport to the hospital.

Complications of Delivery

■ PROLAPSED UMBILICAL CORD

The term "prolapsed cord" refers to the situation that exists when the umbilical cord comes out of the birth canal before the fetus (Fig. 15–2). It can occur at the same time as the breaking of the waters (rupture of the membranes) and usually occurs early in labor, so that delivery is not imminent. The danger in a prolapsed cord is that the cord can be compressed between the fetal head and the sides of the birth canal. The result of this compression is that the flow of oxygenated blood to the fetus can be diminished or totally blocked.

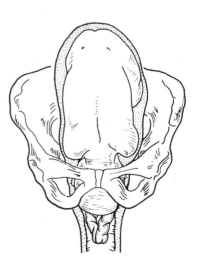

Figure 15-2

Prolapsed umbilical cord.

If the cord is visibly coming out of the vagina before the fetus, the EMT treatment is aimed at keeping the fetal head out of the birth canal and away from the cord.

■ Immediately have the mother stop pushing. Have her pant through the contractions as much as possible.

■ Place the mother in a position that will allow the weight of the baby to be taken off the prolapsed cord.

  ■ Place the mother on her left side. Elevate her hips and legs so that they are higher than her shoulders.

  ■ An alternate position is the knee-chest position. Place the mother on her hands and knees with the knees up to the chest. The mother's head should be down and the buttocks should be up.

■ Using a gloved hand, feel the prolapsed cord. If no pulsations are felt in the cord, insert two fingers into the vagina to relieve pressure on the cord. Maintain this position until the patient is transferred to the hospital.

■ This (along with complicated breech delivery) is the only instance in which it may be necessary to insert a hand into the woman's vagina.

■ Provide high-flow oxygen to the mother.

■ Transport rapidly to the hospital.

■ Keep the cord moist en route to the hospital by wrapping it in a moistened, sterile towel from the OB kit.

■ Notify the receiving hospital of the prolapsed cord while en route.

■ BREECH PRESENTATIONS

There are two types of breech presentation, the buttocks presentation and the limb presentation (Fig. 15–3). With the *buttocks presentation*, delivery is usually slow, allowing time for transport to the hospital. When delivery is too rapid to allow time for transport, a special problem may occur. After the buttocks and trunk have been delivered, the head may be delayed in the birth canal. The pressure of the fetal head in the birth canal against the umbilical cord can diminish or totally block the flow of oxygenated blood to the fetus. At the same time, once the chest has been delivered, the baby will attempt to breathe spontaneously. However, the face is still in the birth canal, and thus the airway is blocked.

If delivery of the head does not occur within 3 minutes after delivery of the trunk, the procedure given here is followed:

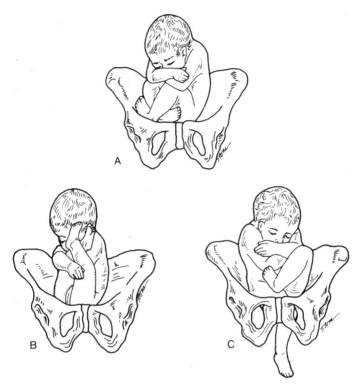

Figure 15-3

Breech presentations. *A*, Complete. *B*, Frank. *C*, Incomplete (single footing).

■ Continue to support the baby's legs and trunk.

■ Immediately have the mother stop pushing. Have her pant through the contractions as much as possible.

■ Provide high-flow oxygen to the mother.

■ Using a gloved hand, the EMT should place two fingers into the vagina, forming a "V" with the fingers on either side of the baby's nose. The vaginal wall should be pushed away from the baby's face until the head emerges spontaneously, which it will usually do. *Do not pull on the baby at any time.* If possible, the cord should pass through the opening created by the fingers. This (along with prolapsed cord) is the only instance in which it may be necessary to insert fingers into the mother's vagina.

If the head is not delivered within 2 to 3 minutes, rapid transport to the hospital is indicated. Continue to maintain the open airway using the fingers to move the vaginal wall away from the baby's nose. En route, notify the hospital.

With the *limb presentation*, delivery in the field is not possible. Rapid transport to the hospital is indicated. Provide high-flow oxygen to the mother. Position the mother as with prolapsed cord. Elevate the mother's hips and legs higher than her shoulders. Alternatively, the mother may be placed in the knee-chest position. In this position, the mother is on her hands and knees with the knees up to the chest. The head is down and the buttocks are up. Notify the receiving hospital in advance.

■ MULTIPLE BIRTHS

In general, the birth of two or more infants is handled in the same fashion as delivery of a single infant. Usually, the patient is aware of carrying twins (or other multiple babies), although the EMT should suspect multiple birth if the mother's abdomen is unusually large after the birth of the (first) baby.

Twins are usually small and may be premature. Therefore, they deserve special handling, as described under premature births.

■ PREMATURE BIRTHS

A baby is considered premature if it is born before the 37th week of gestation. The premature baby usually is small, weighing less than 5.5 pounds (<2.5 kg). Babies weighing as little as 1 pound have been known to survive. Premature infants have major problems with heat loss and respiratory distress.

A premature infant looks smaller, thinner, and redder than the normal baby, with a disproportionately larger head. Its skin may seem particularly thin and shiny, and creases on the soles of the feet may be absent. EMT treatment is as follows:

Keep the infant warm, to about 32°C (90°F), in an infant carrier, if ■ available.

- ■ Protection against heat loss can be improvised by wrapping the baby well, first in a blanket, then in aluminum foil. Avoid burning a premature infant's tender skin by direct contact with hot objects.
- ■ An alternative, if an infant carrier is unavailable, is to use an empty drawer (as in a drawer from a chest of drawers). Place blankets in the drawer for padding and insulation. Wrap the baby in a clean, dry, well-insulating blanket. Place the baby in a reflective blanket (e.g., rescue blanket). Place chemical heat packs in the drawer between the insulating blanket and the reflective blanket. *Do not allow the heat packs to contact the baby's skin.*
- ■ Wrap the baby so that only the face is visible.

■ Assure an open airway. Keep the air passages clear, especially the nostrils, by suctioning with the bulb syringe. When positioning the infant supine for transport, ensure that the large occiput does not create flexion of the neck, thereby occluding the airway.

■ Administer humidified oxygen, if available, at 2 to 3 L/min into a tent improvised from a sterile towel or aluminum foil. If this is unavailable, simply provide blow-by oxygen to the area near the baby's nose.

■ The significantly premature infant most likely will be unable to adequately breathe spontaneously. Assist ventilations using an infant bag-valve mask if there are any signs of respiratory distress or hypoxia (cyanosis, bradycardia, or decreased respiratory rate or volume, or the baby becomes progressively quiet).

■ Be especially careful with the umbilical cord. Observe it closely for bleeding from the cut, and apply an additional clamp or tie if indicated.

■ Avoid contamination. A surgical mask (on the EMT) can prevent the transmission of infection.

■ The premature infant typically requires care in a neonatal intensive care unit (NICU). Contact local medical control or follow protocols for transport to the appropriate hospital for the premature infant.

Note: Premature infants born at 20 weeks of gestation or less rarely survive.

■ MECONIUM-STAINED NEWBORN

Meconium is the first bowel discharge of the newborn infant. When meconium is released by the fetus while still in the uterus, it can create problems. The meconium-stained newborn is at risk for respiratory complications, and the mortality rate can be as high as seven times normal. Particularly ominous is dark green or black, thick fluid appearing on rupture of the amniotic sac (breaking of water) early in labor.

EMT treatment involves special care of the newborn's air passages (suctioning with the bulb syringe). When meconium is observed during the delivery, the EMT must suction the mouth and nostrils as soon as possible but prior to delivery. It may be necessary to have the mother stop pushing during a contraction to allow adequate suctioning before proceeding with the delivery. Once the delivery has occurred, suctioning must be performed immediately and before applying any stimulus to induce spontaneous respirations. Many infants will have meconium present in the airways even when diligent airway suctioning was accomplished.

The EMT should request ALS responders (if available) any time meconium staining is noted. The infant must be rapidly transported to the hospital if meconium aspiration is suspected or if respiratory distress with meconium staining is present. Contact local medical control to determine the appropriate transport destination for this type of infant. When possible, the infant with a high risk of meconium aspiration and/or respiratory distress with meconium staining should be transported to a hospital with a NICU.

■ STILLBIRTH AND ABANDONMENT

Most newborns are healthy and start breathing within 30 seconds of birth. Some do not and require infant resuscitation (CPR). The stillbirth is a fetus that has been dead for some time in the uterus before birth. The stillborn baby is easily recognized by a foul odor, skin covered with blisters, extremely wrinkled skin, and a soft head. CPR is not indicated for a stillbirth. If there is any doubt, opt in favor of the patient; assume that some possibility for life exists, and attempt resuscitation.

Increasingly, the EMT is encountering neonates that have been abandoned or neglected for the first few minutes or hours of life. Often the neonate is found in a trash can or dumpster, or is left in a conspicuous location for others to find. These are difficult situations to manage. The EMT may have little or no information regarding the time of birth. When family members are present, the EMT may be provided with inaccurate information in an attempt to protect the mother. Regardless of the situation, the EMT must quickly decide whether to attempt resuscitation. In making the decision, the EMT should keep in mind that cyanosis, cool skin, respiratory arrest, and cardiac arrest can occur rapidly in the neonate. Therefore, these conditions do not provide the EMT with good indications of the length of time since respiratory or cardiac arrest occurred. Again, when any doubt exists, begin attempts at resuscitation.

■ POSTPARTUM HEMORRHAGE

Excessive bleeding after delivery is called postpartum hemorrhage. It may result from internal or external bleeding and is defined as bleeding resulting in more than four to five soaked sanitary pads in the 30 minutes following delivery. Internal bleeding may be caused by retained placenta, ruptured uterus, or uterine inversion. External bleeding usually results from tears of the perineal area. Blood loss can be severe enough to cause shock.

EMT treatment involves adding sanitary napkins as needed. Place the pad over the vaginal opening. Do not insert dressings into the vagina. Save soaked pads in a plastic bag so that blood loss can be estimated by hospital personnel. Place the mother supine and elevate her legs. Encourage the baby to suck at the mother's breast, which will aid in contraction of the uterus. Massage the lower abdomen by firmly rubbing in a circular motion (uterine massage). When signs of shock are present, treat as usual with high-flow oxygen. Request ALS services if available. Consider antishock trousers (MAST), and provide rapid transport.

■ UTERINE INVERSION

Uterine inversion is a rare complication following delivery in which the uterus turns inside out. It can occur either spontaneously or as a result of pulling on the umbilical cord. It is a very serious condition, and shock may occur rapidly. Wrap the inverted uterus in moistened sterile towels and transport the patient rapidly to the hospital. Treat the patient for shock. Place the patient supine with the legs elevated. Provide high-flow oxygen.

■ PULMONARY EMBOLISM

Pulmonary embolism is a very rare complication of childbirth. It can be caused by amniotic fluid escaping into the woman's circulatory system and lodging in a blood vessel in the lungs. An amniotic fluid embolism is usually associated with a difficult labor. Symptoms, signs, and treatment are as described in Chapter 12.

Complications of Pregnancy

■ TOXEMIA OF PREGNANCY (ECLAMPSIA)

Definition

The exact *cause* of toxemia of pregnancy is unknown. It is more common in the first pregnancy and often appears at about the 24th week. *Pre-eclampsia* is characterized by hypertension and edema. The advanced stage, *eclampsia*, is marked by seizures.

Acute Scenario

Eclampsia seizures have a high mortality rate. Although toxemia of pregnancy occurs in only a small percentage of all pregnancies, it is the third most common cause of mortality in pregnant women. Fetal mortality is also high as a result of the increased risk of premature delivery.

History: Subjective Reports

The pregnant woman with toxemia generally complains of headache, visual disturbances, or epigastric pain. She may notice recent swelling of the face, fingers, or legs. In less severe cases, the pre-eclampsia patient may have been diagnosed by her physician as having hypertension.

Examination: Objective Physical Findings

Signs of mild toxemia of pregnancy (pre-eclampsia) include high blood pressure and swelling (edema) evident in the face, hands, or feet. Severe toxemia of pregnancy is characterized by seizures, mental confusion, and/or other significant neurologic abnormalities. The pregnant patient's blood pressure is generally considered high when it is greater than 140/90 mm Hg in the third trimester. Any pregnant patient, beyond the 20th week, presenting with new-onset seizures, severe headache, an altered mental status, blurred vision, hypertension, or seizures should be assumed to have toxemia of pregnancy.

EMT Treatment

■ Provide high-flow oxygen.

■ Reduce external stimuli that could precipitate a seizure. Keep the lights dim before and during transport. Keep noise to a minimum; avoid using the siren unless absolutely necessary. Minimize the activity of or work done by the patient.

■ Position the patient lying down or, preferably, on her side. Keep the head slightly elevated.

■ If available, request ALS services and provide rapid but gentle transport to the hospital.

■ ECTOPIC PREGNANCY

An ectopic pregnancy occurs when the fertilized egg implants outside the uterus—for example, in the fallopian tube. Early in the first trimester it can rupture, causing internal bleeding. Shock may result. The woman will complain of acute abdominal pain of sudden onset. She may also relate an incident of dizziness or syncope. Assume that any woman of child-bearing age who presents with acute, unilateral lower abdominal pain has an ectopic pregnancy until it can be proven otherwise. Attempt to determine if the patient may be pregnant. Questioning may include

1. "Is there any possibility you may be pregnant?"
2. If the answer is no, ask
   a. "Why do you believe you are not pregnant?" If the patient is not sexually active or has had a hysterectomy, the possibility cannot exist.
   b. "When was your last menstrual cycle?" If more than 28 days ago, then ask, "Is it normal for you to have long cycles?"
   c. Keep in mind that birth control devices are not 100% effective.

Physical findings may include slight or no vaginal bleeding and signs of shock. When postural signs or other signs of shock are found, treat as usual for shock: give high-flow oxygen, use supine positioning with the legs elevated, and consider antishock trousers (MAST). Ensure rapid provision of, or transport to, ALS services.

■ First Trimester Vaginal Bleeding

Definition

The medical term "abortion" refers to the termination of a pregnancy within the first 20 weeks. It may be spontaneous or induced. The term "miscarriage" is the word most nonmedical people use for spontaneous abortion. Induced abortions can be done safely in a medical setting by qualified medical professionals.

Acute Scenario

When an abortion is incomplete and some portion of the placenta remains, uterine bleeding can be profuse. In addition, self-induced or criminal abortion can result in perforation of the uterus, causing massive hemorrhage. Complications may also result following both spontaneous and induced abortions.

History: Subjective Reports

The patient may complain of abdominal pain, often similar to menstrual cramps. The pain often occurs at 6 to 8 weeks of the pregnancy. Dizziness and weakness may also be present if bleeding is also occurring. The patient's history regarding the possibility of pregnancy must be assessed if the woman did not know she was pregnant.

Examination: Objective Physical Findings

Vaginal bleeding may be minimal or profuse. Tissue may be passed. The patient may exhibit signs of compensated shock: tachycardia; pale, sweaty skin; and orthostatic syncope.

EMT Treatment

After caring for the patient's ABCDs, conduct a focused physical examination. Vital signs should include postural blood pressure and heart rate.

Save any tissue passed or protruding from the vaginal opening.

Observe closely for signs or symptoms of shock. Treat for shock if necessary.

The priority of transport is determined by the clinical condition: routine if vital signs are stable; rapid if shock is present.

■ THIRD TRIMESTER VAGINAL BLEEDING

Definition

There are several causes of third trimester vaginal bleeding. *Placenta previa* occurs when the placenta is abnormally located over the opening of the uterus into the birth canal (cervix) (Fig. 15−4). When the cervix dilates early in delivery, the blood vessels in the placenta tear and bleed. *Abruptio placentae* is premature separation of the placenta from the wall of the uterus (Fig. 15−5). *Uterine rupture* can occur in a woman who has previously undergone delivery of a baby by cesarean section (surgery).

Acute Scenario

Vaginal bleeding in the third trimester can be minimal or can be severe enough to be a life-threatening emergency for both the mother and the fetus.

History: Subjective Reports

Although placenta previa is initially painless, abruptio placentae presents with abdominal pain. A history of multiple pregnancies, chronic

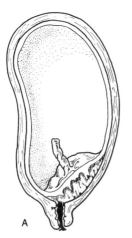
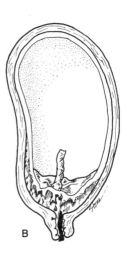

Figure 15−4

Placenta previa. *A*, Partial. *B*, Complete.

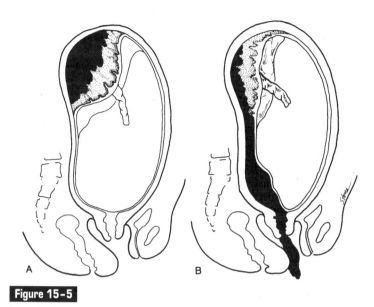

Figure 15-5

Abruptio placentae. *A,* Concealed. *B,* Apparent.

hypertension, or trauma to the uterus places the patient at higher risk for abruptio placentae. The ruptured uterus presents as "tearing" pain in a specific area, with abdominal tenderness, and the uterine contractions of childbirth may stop.

Examination: Objective Physical Findings

Vaginal bleeding may be minimal or massive. In some cases of abruptio placentae the bleeding may be concealed, hidden inside the uterus. When blood loss is significant (external or internal), signs of shock will be present.

EMT Treatment

▓ Provide high-flow oxygen.

▓ Place sanitary napkins over the vaginal opening as needed. Save soaked pads in a plastic bag so that blood loss can be estimated by hospital personnel.

▓ Position the woman on her side. Elevate the legs if necessary to treat for shock.

Request ALS services. Notify the hospital and provide rapid transport, especially when signs of shock are present.

Trauma

■ Trauma in Pregnancy

Although the treatment of the pregnant trauma patient is essentially the same as that of any other traumatically injured patient, physiologic changes to the patient and the inclusion of a second patient (i.e., the fetus) must also be recognized by the EMT. Most commonly, trauma to the pregnant woman occurs as a result of motor vehicle accidents, falls, and assault. The most important rule in caring for the traumatically injured pregnant patient is, "Providing optimal care for the mother will improve the baby's chances of survival."

In the early stages of pregnancy, the fetus is protected by the pelvis. As the pregnancy advances, the uterus (and hence the abdomen) becomes more prominent and, therefore, more susceptible to injury. In the third trimester, the mother's total blood volume has increased, her heart rate is increased, and her blood pressure is slightly lower (although usually normal at term). The uterus begins to push upward on the GI system and the diaphragm. The respiratory rate may subsequently increase, although the depth of ventilations may be decreased. The weight of the uterus on the inferior vena cava readily causes hypotension in the mother when she is in the supine position. Because digestion is slowed during the latter stages of pregnancy, the stomach can contain food for hours.

Because of the increased blood volume, the mother may lose a significant amount of blood before signs and symptoms of shock appear. Unfortunately, the placenta may have inadequate blood flow before shock becomes evident. Additionally, direct injury to the baby may occur, particularly with lap safety belts, high-speed deceleration, or even blunt trauma to the baby's head. Injury to the placenta (abruptio placentae) may also occur. This places both the mother and baby at significant risk of death.

In addition to standard trauma care, treatment for the traumatically injured pregnant patient should include the following steps:

■ Rapidly assess and package the woman.

■ Place the mother in the left lateral recumbent position (if cervical spine injury is not suspected). When the patient is secured to a spinal immobilization device, the device should be elevated on one side (preferably the left) to displace the weight of the uterus off of the inferior vena cava.

■ Provide oxygen regardless of the patient's condition. High-flow oxygen is indicated if the patient has any signs of shock, or complains of abdominal or pelvic pain.

■ Ensure rapid provision of, or transport to, ALS services.

■ Avoid unnecessary delays in transport.

■ Contact local medical control to determine the appropriate transport destination for the pregnant patient who does not have major trauma. The facility should have the capability to provide fetal monitoring and emergency obstetric care.

■ SEXUAL ASSAULT

"Rape" and "sexual assault" are legal terms, not medical terms. Medical personnel should use the term "history of sexual assault." The victim's treatment should be similar to treatment for any other victim of violent assault. This particular type of violence produces both physical and emotional trauma. The victim who relates a history of sexual assault thus needs both physiologic and psychological care.

■ Conduct yourself in a soothing and calming professional manner. Do not display personal curiosity, and do not moralize.

■ Control obvious bleeding, and treat other injuries in the standard fashion. Do not examine the genital area, unless considerable bleeding is obvious.

■ Inform the victim of the need for medical care for treatable injury, infection, or pregnancy. Advise the patient not to wash, urinate, or defecate until seen by a physician, in order to preserve evidence. The victim has the right to ignore this advice.

■ If the victim refuses transport to the hospital, provide the local rape crisis/counseling center telephone number. Try not to leave a victim alone; encourage contact with a friend who can come and help. If that is not possible, call the local rape center and then put the victim on the line.

■ Because sexual assault and rape are crimes, most states require reporting to the police by EMS personnel.

■ Record all details carefully. Use the victim's own words, in quotes, in the report. The EMT may be called to testify in a future court proceeding regarding the incident. An accurate and complete incident report form will be in the best interests of the EMT and the patient.

Pediatric Emergencies

Many of the specific emergencies that can occur in childhood are the same as emergencies that occur to adults. The difference is that children are not just small adults. The assessment and examination of the young child can prove to be difficult for even the best of EMTs. In the infant and toddler, communication skills are not yet developed. In these cases the EMT must rely on the parents, older siblings, or other caregivers to provide a medical history. Even as the child becomes older, communication may be difficult because the child may be reluctant to speak to a stranger. The examination may need to be delayed or, in some cases, waived due to the child's resistance to the EMT's physical closeness. Younger children also have physiologic differences that may be noted in the examination. Normally healthy children invariably respond to stress with an adrenaline response. Tachycardia, tachypnea, cool and pale skin (especially peripherally), decreased appetite, and lethargy are commonly seen in the ill child.

For discussion of other causes of injury or illness that can be seen in children, see the information on airway obstruction and choking in Chapter 8, burns in Chapter 11, asthma and abdominal pain in Chapter 12, and poisoning in Chapter 13. Examination of the child is covered in Chapter 2. Other types of specific emergencies that occur primarily in childhood are the subject of this chapter.

Respiratory Distress

■ CROUP

Definition

Croup is a viral infection that often follows a cold or other upper respiratory illness. The common age of occurrence is 6 months to 3 years. Although it can occur anytime, outbreaks of croup are common in the late fall and winter.

Acute Scenario

Acute attacks often occur at night. Swelling of the tissues around the larynx, just below the epiglottis, can restrict the flow of air and cause respiratory distress.

History: Subjective Reports

The patient may not be old enough or willing to provide any history, but the parents may relate the history of recent respiratory illness.

278

The common elements of the story related by the parent are the child appeared normal acting throughout the day, had slight respiratory infection symptoms recently, and awoke during the night with respiratory distress.

Examination: Objective Physical Findings

The three most notable signs are high-pitched stridor or a wheezing sound on inspiration, a barking cough (called "seal bark"), and hoarseness. A low-grade fever may be present. Signs of respiratory distress may include the use of flaring nostrils, intercostal muscles, and supraclavicular retractions during inspiration. Signs of decreased oxygen may include restlessness, agitation, lethargy, and tachycardia.

EMT Treatment

Provide cool, humidified (if available) oxygen. Both the humidification and the coolness are beneficial. Often the child may feel somewhat better when taken outside in the cool, damp night air.

Place in the position of comfort, which normally is sitting.

Gentle handling includes avoiding looking in the mouth. Croup can be difficult to distinguish from epiglottitis.

When respiratory distress of any severity is reported, the child should be transported to the hospital for evaluation.

EPIGLOTTITIS

Definition

Epiglottitis is a bacterial infection seen in all ages but most commonly seen in children 2 to 7 years old. There is usually a history of recent upper respiratory illness.

Acute Scenario

Epiglottitis is a life-threatening emergency because the swollen epiglottis can cover the larynx, causing total obstruction of the airway.

History: Subjective Reports

The patient will complain of pain on swallowing and a sore throat. The patient (or the parents) will usually relate a history of sudden onset of the acute symptoms.

Examination: Objective Physical Findings

The patient with epiglottitis is usually frightened and prefers to remain still. The position of comfort is upright and leaning forward with the chin thrust out. Drooling will be evident. Stridor, dyspnea, and tachycardia will be present. Intercostal and supraclavicular retractions may be seen when respiratory distress is present. Lung sounds may be diminished as the child chooses to breathe shallowly in order to minimize movement. Other signs may include a high fever, cough, and hoarseness. The most important observation by the EMT will be that the child appears profoundly ill and anxious.

EMT Treatment

■ Allow the child to remain in a position of comfort. Sitting up with the jaw forward is the preferred position.

■ Provide high-flow oxygen (humidified if available). If the child does not tolerate a mask due to anxiety, hold the mask near the child's face.

■ Avoid any stimulation of the mouth or throat. *Do not use airways. Do not use suction. Do not inspect the mouth or palpate the neck.*

■ Ensure rapid provision of, or transport to, ALS services. Transport to an appropriate pediatric hospital if at all possible. Rapid but gentle transport is critical.

■ The EMT must use infection control measures.

■ Foreign Body Obstruction

Definition

The vast majority of deaths occurring from foreign body airway obstruction occur in young children. Most of these occur in infants.

Acute Scenario

The introduction into the upper airways of foreign objects that are subsequently aspirated can result in airway obstruction. Obstruction of the trachea causes the inability to breathe. Obstruction of one bronchus or the lower airways generally will not totally impede breathing but may produce marked respiratory distress.

History: Subjective Reports

When complete airway obstruction is present, the child will be unable to speak, cough, or cry. Parents, siblings, or other caregivers may relate a history of sudden onset of respiratory distress. The child may have been heard coughing or gagging near the time of initial onset. Possibly the most important information obtained from those with the child relates to the activity of the child prior to the onset of respiratory distress. Often the child was eating or had recently finished eating, or the child may have been playing with small toys or objects. Upper airway obstruction may also be caused by serious infections such as epiglottitis. A history consistent with epiglottitis may be present.

Examination: Objective Physical Findings

The most important finding in the initial assessment is the inability to breathe. The child may be conscious or unconscious. Initial observations may also reveal cyanosis. In the partially obstructed airway or the lower airway obstruction, the child may have unilateral wheezing or the absence of lung sounds unilaterally. The sudden onset of severe respiratory distress, apnea, and unconsciousness in a child should be assumed to be foreign body airway obstruction until proven otherwise.

EMT Treatment

If the child or infant is unable to audibly cough or speak, or is unable to breathe, assume the child has a completely obstructed airway.

- Attempt ventilations. If unsuccessful, reposition the airway and reattempt ventilations. If ventilations remain unsuccessful, perform obstructed airway maneuvers.
- For the child, use the Heimlich maneuver (abdominal thrusts) as described in Chapter 8.
- For the infant, use back blows and chest thrusts as described in Chapter 8.

If the child or infant is able to audibly cough or speak, or is able to breathe spontaneously, assess the child or infant for a partially obstructed airway.

Any partially obstructed airway can, in a child or infant, quickly progress to a completely obstructed airway. Monitor the patient's respiratory status continuously.

If the airway is cleared or remains partially obstructed, provide high-flow oxygen or ventilations as necessary.

Ensure rapid but gentle provision of, or transport to, ALS services.

The child with a history consistent with epiglottis who now has an obstructed airway must be immediately transported to the nearest facility capable of advanced airway management.

Miscellaneous Pediatric Emergencies

■ SUDDEN INFANT DEATH SYNDROME (SIDS)

SIDS is defined as the sudden and unexpected death of an apparently healthy infant, which remains unexplained after a scene investigation, review of the infant's medical history, and complete postmortem studies. SIDS is the leading cause of death in infants between 1 month and 1 year old. The peak incidence of SIDS is between 2 and 4 months of age. An estimated 6000 to 7000 deaths occur each year in the United States, which is roughly two to three SIDS deaths per 1000 live births. The cause is unknown, and no early warning signs have yet been identified.

The infants usually die during sleep in their cribs at night (SIDS is often called "crib death"). Because much time may elapse before the infant's death is discovered, postmortem changes may be noted by the EMT. These include blood-tinged mucus near the nostrils or on the bedding, pooling of blood on the body's underside (anterior surface if the baby was prone), and white skin areas on the nose or face when the baby was found prone.

Risk factors for SIDS have been identified; however, they are non-specific because they are often associated with other causes of infant death. These factors include

- Male sex
- African-American or Native American ancestry
- A recent mild respiratory infection
- Prematurity
- Young mother with many children
- Lower socioeconomic status
- Drug use or cigarette smoking by the mother during pregnancy
- Smoke exposure of the baby
- Prone sleep position

EMT treatment for SIDS will vary depending on the appearance of the baby and local protocols. In general, CPR should be initiated in the absence of signs that the baby is obviously dead (rigor mortis, livor mortis). The EMT may choose to begin resuscitation attempts when the family apparently is unable to accept the infant's obvious death. Such measures may make the family feel that every effort was made to save their baby. However, the EMT should be honest with the family and avoid providing misleading hope. Transport will largely depend on local policies. In some communities, the infant may be pronounced dead at the scene and must remain at the scene pending a death investigation. In other communities, efforts may not be ceased on cardiac arrest victims and transport must occur.

Although the first priority is the infant, SIDS is a family disaster, and the parents will be panicked and grief stricken. Some parents will have intense guilt feelings. Keep the family informed, as much as is possible, with accurate and truthful information. Provide reassurance that everything possible was done for the baby. Dealing with the death of a child is an extremely difficult task for EMTs. The EMT must maintain a professional yet caring attitude. The reactions of family members will vary greatly. Hospital personnel may want to initiate special counseling for the parents, once SIDS has been diagnosed.

SIDS foundations across the country are promoting SIDS risk reduction education. Risk reduction includes

- Placing healthy babies on their backs or side to sleep
- Placing babies on a firm mattress or other firm surface; avoiding bedding such as fluffy blankets, comforters, or sheepskin under the baby, and waterbeds.
- Keeping babies warm but not too warm; the room temperature should feel comfortable to you
- Pregnant women getting early prenatal care and not using alcohol or drugs (unless prescribed by a doctor)
- Preventing exposure of the baby to smoke

■ FEBRILE SEIZURES

Definition

Fever can be seen in a variety of common childhood illnesses. It is defined as an abnormally high body temperature. Causes of fever in children include infection (viral or bacterial) or exposure to a particularly hot environment (classic heat stroke). About 5% of children with fever develop seizures. Febrile seizures typically occur in children between the ages of 6 months and 6 years. The seizure is typically generalized and lasts less than 15 minutes (typically less than 10 minutes).

Acute Scenario

Febrile seizures generally are not life threatening, although the panicked family may think they are. Febrile seizures are generally limited to a single event (one seizure per episode). Many children who experience a febrile seizure will experience another childhood seizure associated with a subsequent fever. Multiple seizures suggest some other cause. Generally, febrile seizures are believed to occur as a result of a rapid rate of temperature rise rather than elevation of the temperature to a specific point.

History: Subjective Reports

The child will generally be too young or disoriented to relate complaints, but the family may be able to give details about the character of the seizure. Febrile seizures are usually generalized, with symmetrical tonic-clonic motor activity, whereas the finding of focal motor activity may indicate a more serious condition, such as meningitis. A history of a recent fever or symptoms of an illness (e.g., ear infection, respiratory infection) should be related by the family or caregiver. The EMT should also ask the family whether the child has had a seizure associated with a fever in the past.

Examination: Objective Physical Findings

By the time the EMT arrives, the seizure will usually have stopped, and the only physical findings on examination may be the postictal state and warm, red skin. A stiff neck may be suggestive of meningitis or encephalitis. Often the child or infant will be lethargic. After completing the tremendous physical work associated with a seizure, the child should be expected to be tired and tachycardic. Bradycardia in a child is often a sign of hypoxia. If the child's temperature is taken, it will be slightly elevated or normal. At this point, the temperature does not provide much information.

EMT Treatment

■ The standard approach to seizures involves the following measures:

- Protect the child from injury. Place the child on a large, flat surface to avoid accidental falls. Avoid hard surfaces that may cause injury to the head.
- Provide high-flow oxygen, and suction as necessary.
- Position the patient on his/her side when the postictal phase begins.

■ If skin temperature is particularly hot, remove the clothing to aid natural cooling. Sponging with lukewarm water may be indicated in cases of heat stroke. *Do not use alcohol or ice water.*

■ Have the parents consult with their pediatrician about the use of antipyretic (antifever) medications such as acetaminophen. If the EMT is authorized to provide acetaminophen, assist the parents in providing the child with a dose of 15 mg/kg. Often, parents know exactly how much to give from past experiences with fever and past instructions from their pediatrician.

■ Transport the child if heat stroke, meningitis, or some cause other than a simple infection may have triggered this seizure. Otherwise, the parents may choose to transport if the child is now awake, breathing normally, did not appear to aspirate during the seizure, and is not bradycardic. The EMT must follow local protocols regarding transport.

■ MENINGITIS (BACTERIAL)

Meningitis is defined as an inflammation of the meninges that surround the brain and spinal cord. There are many causes of meningitis, both viral and bacterial. Meningitis may occur at any age. The incidence for children is highest in the first 2 years of life. Although meningitis caused by bacteria is typically more severe, it is nearly impossible for one to differentiate between viral and bacterial meningitis in the field. The symptoms may be very similar.

Initially the signs and symptoms may include fever, headache, stiff neck, and vomiting. The signs and symptoms can become severe in a relatively short time (within 24 hours). The child may progress to being lethargic, irritable, confused, or comatose. Seizures may occur. The disease may continue to progress to a septic state, leading to shock. Meningitis caused by meningococcus often results in the finding of petechiae (small, pinpoint, purplish-red spots) or purpura (small areas of purplish, mottled-looking skin). Although viral causes of meningitis may also result in petechiae or purpura, the EMT should assume the cause of the meningitis is meningococcus bacteria when a rash is noted until proved otherwise.

EMT actions and treatment include the following:

■ Use infection control precautions.

   ■ When bacterial meningitis is suspected (particularly if petechiae, purpura, or a rash is noted), respiratory protection and/or a face mask should be worn by those having close contact with the child.
   ■ Minimize the number of personnel and amount of equipment having close contact with the child.
   ■ After transport, decontaminate equipment and the transport vehicle.
   ■ EMS personnel should follow local exposure reporting procedures. The personnel should follow up to determine if prophylactic treatment is necessary.

■ Provide high-flow oxygen. If needed, assist ventilations.

■ Treat for shock.

   ■ Place the child supine or lateral recumbent with the legs elevated.
   ■ Maintain normal body temperature. Avoid overheating and possibly causing a febrile seizure.

■ Ensure rapid provision of, or transport to, ALS services.

■ Notify the receiving hospital of the potential infectious state of the child. When one is available without additional delay, transport the child or infant to a pediatric hospital.

■ DEHYDRATION AND HYPOVOLEMIA

Volume depletion in infants and children may result from dehydration due to fever, vomiting, diarrhea, a decreased fluid intake, and/or blood loss due to trauma. Relatively small amounts of fluid loss can be catastrophic, since there is proportionately less fluid reserve in children than in adults. Although signs of acute blood loss may be obvious, signs of dehydration may be subtle. They include lethargy, dryness of the lips and oral mucosa, tachycardia, decreased frequency of urination, prolonged capillary refill time, tachypnea, and a depressed fontanel (in infants).

Mild dehydration is often treated at home with oral fluids. These fluids usually contain balanced solutions of sugars and electrolytes. EMT treatment includes providing high-flow oxygen (humidified if available), anticipating vomiting, and placing the child supine or lateral recumbent with the legs elevated. Ensure rapid provision of, or transport to, ALS services. Continue treatment for shock as required. If possible without delays, transport to a pediatric hospital.

Trauma

■ Accidental Injury

Trauma continues to be the leading cause of death in children. Injuries to a child may occur for a wide variety of reasons. As a result of their curiosity (and later, in adolescence, their feeling of invincibility), children often experience accidental trauma. Unfortunately, intentional trauma (e.g., assaults) continues to become more frequent in children. Trauma may be either blunt or penetrating. The most common causes of trauma in children are falls and motor vehicle accidents. The subtle differences in physiology and communication abilities of children, and the relative inexperience of most prehospital providers with pediatric patients, can make the task of caring for the pediatric trauma patient a difficult one.

The EMT must always be mindful of the effective compensatory mechanisms of children, the typical progression of shock symptoms in the child, and the most common causes of traumatic death in children. Head injuries are responsible for most pediatric trauma cases and pediatric trauma deaths. The effective management of the child's airway and attentive effort to improve oxygenation can significantly reduce mortality in the pediatric head-injured patient. When traumatic injury leads to shock, the child has extremely efficient compensatory mechanisms. As a result, the early signs of shock in the pediatric shock patient will nearly always include tachycardia (which may progress), increased capillary refill time, restlessness, cool skin beginning at the periphery, and tachypnea. Hypotension and a decreased level of consciousness are nearly always late signs of shock in the pediatric patient.

EMT treatment of the traumatically injured pediatric patient is similar to that of the adult, with emphasis placed on areas where physiologic differences exist. Treatment includes the following steps:

■ Rapidly assess the ABCDs.

   ■ Maintain cervical immobilization when cervical spine injury is suspected or when a mechanism for such an injury exists.

- Ensure that the airway is open and clear of foreign bodies or fluids. Ensure that the large occiput of the young child does not cause neck flexion when the child is supine.

- Assess the ventilations. If inadequate or absent, provide positive pressure ventilation using 100% oxygen.

- Hyperventilate the child with a suspected head injury or a decreased level of consciousness. Do not provide excessive volumes or rapid, forceful ventilations in the child or infant. This will increase gastric distention.

- When spontaneous respirations are adequate, provide high-flow oxygen.

- Assess the pulse and capillary refill. Absent peripheral pulses or increased capillary refill time in the pediatric trauma patient may indicate moderate shock. Control any major bleeding with direct pressure.

- Assess the level of consciousness. In the very young child, the EMT should assess the behavior and actions of the child.

- Obtain a complete set of vital signs.

If necessary because of complications found in the ABCDs or as a result of obvious major trauma, perform a rapid extrication of the patient. Protect the cervical spine as much as possible.

Place the child supine on a spinal immobilization device.

- Ensure that the neck is not flexed and/or the airway compromised by the large occiput of the child's head. If necessary, place a towel or blanket under the child or infant's shoulders.

- Treat for shock by elevating the foot of the board if necessary.

Remove all clothing to perform a rapid trauma exam.

- Cover the child with blankets to maintain body temperature. Children can lose body heat very quickly.

- Place in the back of a transport vehicle if possible.

When a properly sized cervical collar is not available for the child, use a rolled towel or small blanket. The rolled towel or blanket is placed behind the child's neck with the two ends crossing at the chest just below the anterior neck.

Quickly prepare the child by packaging securely and readying for transport.

Ensure rapid provision of, or transport to, ALS services. Quickly transport the child to an appropriate hospital for pediatric trauma patients (if possible).

■ CHILD ABUSE (BATTERED CHILD)

Definition

Child abuse is considered to be a social problem that affects all socioeconomic groups. There are four types of abuse: physical, emotional, sexual, and neglect. It is not a rare problem; as many as 10% of all children under age 5 seen in hospital emergency departments are battered children. Ninety per cent of these children may be abused by their parents; 10% are abused by others, such as babysitters or friends of the family.

Acute Cause

Child abuse incidence can progress from minor injury to increasingly severe injury. The battering parent is likely to abuse the child again unless some intervention occurs. One in every 500 battered children dies; about 35% may be permanently damaged. When child abuse is suspected, it is important to protect the child from further abuse and to assist the family in seeking treatment.

History: Subjective Reports

When child abuse is suspected, the EMT has two patients: the physically (and/or emotionally) injured child *and* the emotionally disordered parent.

THE CHILD.   Get down on the same level as the child by kneeling or sitting down. The child may be too young or too fearful to voice complaints, so adopt a reassuring and comforting manner. Do not ask detailed questions about what happened, especially if the suspected abuser is still in the same room. The history should remain focused on assessing the child's injuries first, followed by his/her emotional well-being. If abuse is suspected, the history must not dwell on the exact cause of the injury or illness. This may cause anger or anxiety in the nearby parent, which will ultimately affect the child.

THE PARENT(S).   Do not question the parent in front of the child. Do use supportive interview techniques. Although a history of multiple "accidents" in the past is suggestive of child abuse, do not contradict the history given by the parent (or by the child, for that matter). That history may seem odd; the parent(s) may be vague or evasive, and they may have waited an excessive amount of time before calling for emergency help.

Examination: Objective Physical Findings

THE CHILD.   The child may not be crying despite an obvious injury and may be withdrawn and fearful. Carefully explain the need for examination before touching the child. If the severity of the injury permits, allow time for friendly conversation with the child before proceeding to the physical exam. Trauma that may seem bizarre, especially if the history does not match the injury, is suggestive of battering. Unexplained burns, especially cigarette burns, are suggestive of abuse. "Glove-like" or "sock-like" scald injuries or patterned burns (such as iron-shaped burns) are also suggestive. Unexplained fractures are suggestive. Multiple injuries at different stages of healing, such as old and new bruises, are particularly suggestive.

THE PARENT(S).   The parent's (or parents') behavior may seem odd. They may seem detached or unconcerned and may make little attempt to comfort the child. Occasionally, the parents may show signs of substance abuse or be openly hostile or uncooperative.

EMT Treatment

Attempt to transport the child to the hospital, even if the injuries seem trivial, if battering is suspected. *Do not give the parents the option of transporting the child by themselves.* In most communities, local law enforcement officers will come to the scene to assist in encouraging the parents to permit EMS transport.

Maintain a calm, professional, nonjudgmental manner toward the parents. They may be asking for help in a fashion that is difficult to recognize.

Continue to maintain focus on the care of the child. Treat all injuries and illnesses as with any other child.

When making plans for transport, be aware that the child may react negatively to the idea of separation from the parents, even if only for the trip to hospital.

The EMT can be most helpful if he/she makes precise observations and includes detailed notations of indications of child abuse, neglect, or molestation. These notes must be objective, accurate, and specific. The observations of the EMT may enable child welfare authorities to take appropriate action.

If the parents refuse to allow transport, do not argue over the child. If local law enforcement officers are unable to assist, contact local medical control before leaving the scene. Use a telephone rather than the radio, if possible.

The EMT must learn and observe state and local laws on reporting cases of suspected child abuse. Most states require the reporting of suspected child abuse to child welfare agencies.

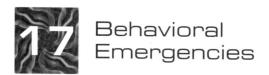

17 Behavioral Emergencies

General Principles

A behavioral emergency is the sudden appearance of unusual, disordered, or socially inappropriate behavior. "Unusual" refers to behavior or lifestyle that is not normal or "usual" *for the person in question.* "Disordered" behavior lacks pattern or purpose. Behavior is "inappropriate" when it does not match the setting (the time or place) or the particular cultural or age group.

Behavioral emergencies can vary in severity. A *life-threatening emergency* exists when an individual is dangerous to self or others. This can occur when the person is out of control, assaultive, acutely suicidal, or acutely homicidal. In addition, patients can present with a behavioral emergency that is related to an acute life-threatening medical emergency. This can occur in the context of substance abuse or some other medical condition. The way in which the EMT handles such a patient can convert a life-threatening situation into a non–life-threatening one, or vice versa.

■ IDENTIFICATION OF A LIFE-THREATENING EMERGENCY

To identify a life-threatening behavioral emergency, the EMT needs to observe the person's appearance and behavior, listen to the person, and assess the physical (medical) status. Appearance and behavior observations include the person's posture, facial expressions, speech, motor activity, and mannerisms. Listening includes being aware of sensitive topics that increase the person's agitation; focusing on the person's ability to distinguish what is real from what is not; and noting an erratic mood, poor impulse control, or questionable judgment. Assessment of medical status must be particularly thorough if there is reason to suspect a medical emergency and if the patient is irrational or uncooperative.

■ MANAGEMENT OF A LIFE-THREATENING EMERGENCY

Management of a life-threatening behavioral emergency includes

- ■ Treatment of any medical condition
- ■ Psychological management
- ■ Controlling the environment
- ■ Physical restraint when necessary

290

Medical treatment starts with the assessment of the patient for a medical cause of the behavioral disorder, such as hypoxemia or drug overdose, as discussed later.

Psychological management starts with establishing rapport by active listening—reflecting feelings by paraphrasing, acknowledging, and validating those feelings (fear, sadness, or anger). Clarify misperceptions of external reality, without contradicting the person's internal reality. Set limits by labeling inappropriate behavior, and ask the person to cooperate.

Controlling the environment involves using trusted family or friends when possible but removing them from the immediate environment when they are contributing to the crisis by further agitating the person. Removing the person from a hostile or frightening environment may also be helpful. Police may be required to help with managing the environment, especially when crowd control may be a problem. The overall goal of controlling the environment is to enable the person to feel safe. The EMT must keep a safe distance, not crowding or cornering the person. Additionally, the EMT must control the environment by ensuring the safety of EMS responders. This includes observing for nearby potential weapons (knife, bat, gun, etc.), attempting to remove potential weapons from the area or removing the patient from the area, and always ensuring an escape path for EMS responders should the patient become violent.

Physical restraint is the treatment of last resort. Local laws and policies may dictate specific actions, but the person who is out of control is generally acknowledged to be in danger. Special training can allow EMTs and others to use a minimum of force in restraint. The basic principles are adequate personnel, good coordination (team leader), securing the extremities one at a time, using padded leather restraints, and especially careful observation to avoid aspiration if the patient vomits while restrained. Additional precautions regarding restraint are noted in the Psychosis and Violence section of this chapter.

Most behavioral emergencies are *non–life threatening*. However, as mentioned earlier, the actions of the EMT can convert a non–life-threatening situation into a life-threatening one. Therefore, the EMT needs to be continually aware of the signs of dangerousness while assessing the person's mental status.

Assessment

Assessment proceeds as usual. Obtain a chief complaint; obtain a history of the present illness, past medical (and psychiatric) history, and medications; and record the symptoms and signs. Use the person's own words (in quotes) to describe thought content and mood. Objective findings include such descriptions as the following.

APPEARANCE

- *Posture*, such as appearing sleepy or weak
- *Facial expression*, such as an angry or sad expression

- *Actions*, such as being curled up in a room corner or holding a gun to his/her head
- *Motor activity*, such as experiencing tremor activity of one arm
- *Mannerisms*, such as frequently brushing imaginary insects off his/her body.

SPEECH

- *Rate*, such as talking very fast or with slurred speech
- *Volume*, such as weak or very loud
- *Quantity*, such as not wanting to talk or seeming unable to stop talking

THOUGHT FLOW

- Logical sequence
- Rambling thoughts
- Repetition of thoughts or questions.

AFFECT (APPARENT MOOD)

- Sad
- Angry
- Depressed
- Ambivalent

PERCEPTION

- Illusions
- Hallucinations

REASONING

- Orientation
- Attention span
- Memory
- Judgment
- Coherent expression

Medical Causes

Medical causes of behavioral emergencies are similar to the range of causes of coma listed in Chapter 5, which are either structural or metabolic. Structural causes include head injury, brain tumor, and CVA. Metabolic causes include low blood sugar (hypoglycemia), oxygen deficit (hypoxemia), toxic state from substance abuse (drug or alcohol), and fever or infection (such as meningitis). In any of these conditions a life-threatening state may exist that is primarily medical, not behavioral. The behavioral disorder may indeed be only a transitional state, preceding the onset of unconsciousness and death. However, the delirious patient may be out of control and dangerous to others, which also creates a life-threatening emergency.

Some findings in the patient assessment are typical of medical causes of behavioral emergencies. The history may reveal hallucinations (visual or auditory), headache, recent illness, past history of a chronic illness, past history of substance abuse, or problems with memory or orientation. Objective physical findings may include a decreased level of consciousness, an empty facial expression, slurred speech, fever, stiff neck, severe hypertension, or motor deficits. These, or any other signs of an acute medical condition, indicate that medical treatment takes the first priority. Treat life-threatening emergencies as is medically appropriate.

When the condition is not life threatening, treatment is supportive: provide reassurance and transport to the hospital. Special reassurance is required for *senile dementia*, which is marked by decreased reasoning power and memory loss in the elderly. Unlike *delirium* (the acute confusional state described earlier), dementia is slow and insidious in onset.

Situational Anxiety

■ Reactions to Injury or Illness

Fear and anxiety are common reactions to acute illness or injury. Patients are often fearful about pain and the possibility of future disability or death. The feeling of helplessness, or loss of personal control, naturally causes anxiety. Some fearful patients will react with denial and some will react with anger, occasionally directed at the EMT. In some patients, the reaction to injury or illness is "regression" to child-like behavior, such as demanding or whining. The EMT treatment (beyond whatever is medically necessary) is supportive: provide reassurance and transport. Give a realistic appraisal of the situation in order to help patients cope. Do not confront the patient with denial, but be concerned and supportive.

■ Grief and Reactions to Death

Both sudden death and anticipated death cause great emotional reactions in people. By virtue of their profession, EMTs frequently encounter death. It is difficult for families to cope with sudden death, particularly suicide or the death of a child. Anticipated death, as in the patient with a known terminal disease, presents the EMT with both family reactions and the emotional reactions of the patient.

The person expecting to die may go through a number of phases: denial, anger, bargaining, depression, and acceptance. Family reactions are very similar. The EMT may encounter individuals in any of these phases. Family members are not as frequently exposed to death as is the EMT; therefore, their initial response to sudden death may be one of disbelief and dismay. Some people, particularly in some cultural groups, become wildly hysterical. In cases of suicide, family members may be overcome with feelings of guilt and self-blame. As family members realize what has happened, emotions of depression or anger may become evident. Anger may be directed at the EMT. Realistic coping comes later. Some individuals react quickly; others react slowly over weeks.

The EMT may also react emotionally in this type of emotionally charged situation. To provide efficient care, the EMT must control these feelings. At the same time, sensitivity as a human being needs to be maintained. The EMT must not become immune to his/her own deep-felt emotions as well as to the grief and emotion experienced by others. Unfortunately, the nature of the job requires the EMT to continue to perform his/her duties. Often, family members function better when they see someone, such as an EMS professional, taking charge of the situation. In cases of death following a long-term chronic illness, the family members have been in the position of being the care providers for so long they are now exhausted. They need someone to allow them to relinquish their care provider roles for a while.

The EMT can play a comforting role in situations of grief by expressing empathy. Empathy involves responding on a feeling level, using active listening skills to paraphrase, acknowledge, and validate others' feelings. This giving of "emotional permission" for venting of intense feelings is very important. In addition, try to be realistic in the use of language about death, particularly with children. Do not confront the fear of death in patients or family, but instead acknowledge those feelings of denial and fear in a straightforward, empathetic manner.

Although the exposure to death and dying may become a common thing for the EMT, he/she must keep in mind that this exposure is relatively uncommon for most people. The EMT may be looked to as the expert. The family may ask, "So what comes next? What do you need me to do?" It is important to explain the anticipated procedures and actions that will occur as a result of this death. This may include explaining why a coroner, medical examiner, or police officer is coming to the scene; what resuscitation measures were taken, if any; and how to contact local support groups (such as a SIDS foundation, etc.) if they so desire. Above all, the EMT must demonstrate concern for all those involved. The victim's body must be handled with dignity and respect. If the victim was moved from the bed to the floor during resuscitation attempts, ask the family if they would like you to move him/her back into his/her bed (assuming no police or medical investigation is anticipated). The EMS responders should ensure that any equipment, supplies, or trash are removed from the area (e.g., in a bedroom) so that the family does not need to do this later. Then, observe the family for medical changes. Older family members may experience angina or shortness of breath. Younger members may experience anxiety or hyperventilation. Above all, do not leave the family alone soon after the death. Someone (a police officer, EMT, chaplain, etc.) should attempt to remain with the family long enough to ensure transport of the victim's body and to observe family members for potential medical conditions.

■ DISASTERS AND MASS CASUALTY INCIDENTS

Strongly emotional reactions occur in natural disasters (earthquake, storm, flood) or man-made disasters (explosion, crash, fire, building collapse). The EMT will be faced with both physical injuries and psychological distress. People may be suddenly isolated from their families and other supports, as well as possibly losing the security of their homes.

Most people react with initial numbness, followed by anxiety ranging from nervousness to blind panic. A few people (a minority) stay "numb" for prolonged periods. Many may resist transport from the scene because of concern about their homes or other family members. It may turn out that only a small minority of individuals involved in a mass casualty incident remain calm. In this context, the EMT or other rescuer may also be overwhelmed.

The EMT needs to concentrate on the tasks at hand: safety and control of the scene, and triage, treatment, and transportation according to established protocol. When individuals are resistant to transport from the scene, balance the need for transport with other needs. Children, especially, do better if reunited with family before transport. When people are confused, agitated, and uncooperative, set limits on their behavior. Assign nervous people specific tasks to accomplish. Isolate the panicky individual by physically removing him/her from the scene and assigning a calm individual to remain with the panicky one to avoid the spread of panic.

Psychiatric Causes

■ ACUTE ANXIETY

Everyone experiences anxiety as a response to stress. When the level of anxiety is such that it interferes with the ability to function, then it becomes a psychiatric disorder. The term "acute anxiety" is used here to cover a wide variety of disorders:

■ *Anxiety neurosis* describes the patient who is nervous, fearful, and hyperalert, with various physical symptoms such as a rapid pulse; pale, cool, clammy skin; dry mouth; and nausea.

■ *Panic attack* occurs unpredictably and usually lasts only minutes. The patient has feelings of terror and fear of losing control or "going crazy," with physical symptoms such as faintness, sweating, and shaking.

■ *Phobic disorder* is the irrational fear of a specific object, situation, or activity.

■ *Hyperventilation syndrome* is marked by numbness and tingling in the fingers, toes, and lips; dizziness; diffuse chest pain; contractions of the fingers (carpopedal spasm); and, of course, rapid breathing.

■ *Conversion reaction* occurs when the reaction to stress is converted into physical symptoms such as blindness, paralysis, or sensory loss.

■ *Pseudo-coma* is a type of conversion reaction, often recognized by fluttering eyelids, especially when they are touched lightly.

- *Hysterical seizures* are another type of conversion reaction, appearing as bizarre thrashing motions.

In general, acute anxiety is a "diagnosis of exclusion," which is to say that it is considered only when other possible causes of the behavior, whether medical or psychiatric, have been reasonably ruled out. For example, it is important to consider alternative causes of hyperventilation, such as CHF, before treating the condition as acute anxiety (see Chapter 3).

EMT treatment of acute anxiety is generally supportive: provide reassurance and transport. Separate family members from the patient if they are contributing to increased agitation (but let them stay if the patient becomes more agitated at the suggestion that they leave the room). Provide realistic information, and identify or label the disorder if it is certain. Explain what will happen, and involve the patient in decisions, if possible. Set limits on behavior, when necessary.

Hyperventilation syndrome can usually be treated by reassurance. Sometimes the use of a paper bag or a rebreather mask can be helpful. *Use extreme caution when employing this method.* Continued hyperventilation is preferable to the EMT causing increased hypoxia. Local policy and procedures may govern the use of noxious stimulants in suspected pseudo-coma; ammonia inhalants in particular may be contraindicated in hypertensive patients. Patients with hysterical seizures can be controlled by wrapping their forearms together. This is done by holding the arms together overlapping, so that the fingers of the hand are at the elbows of the other arm, and wrapping both forearms together with elastic gauze, such as Kerlix. Regardless of what method of treatment is used for acute anxiety, the EMT must ensure that medical conditions have been ruled out and that no further harm is done to the nonviolent patient.

■ DEPRESSION AND SUICIDE

Definition

Everyone experiences sad or depressed feelings as a response to the frustrations and disappointments that are an inevitable part of daily life. When these depressed feelings are persistent and oppressive, they constitute a psychiatric disorder. Suicidal behavior can range from an active threat (such as the person standing on a ledge) to a minor overdose. Suicide is the ninth leading cause of death.

Acute Scenario

The person with a major depressive illness is at risk of suicide. All suicidal patients are treated as being in life-threatening emergencies for two reasons: first, suicide "gestures" can be unintentionally fatal; and second, intense suicidal feelings are generally short lived. Thus, if the EMT can intervene and prevent suicidal behavior, the patient can benefit.

History: Subjective Reports

The depressed patient will report feeling "blue" and despairing. He/she commonly feels hopeless, helpless, and worthless. A major depressive illness is marked by symptoms lasting over 2 weeks, such as these:

- Disorders of sleep or eating
- Lack of interest in usual activities
- Overwhelming fatigue
- Guilt feelings
- Difficulty concentrating
- Persistent thoughts of death or suicide

All depressed patients should be asked about suicidal ideas and behaviors. Suicide gestures are generally cries for help, although death can accidentally occur. A suicide attempt may be ambivalent or serious. Table 17–1 gives a profile of suicidal patients.

To evaluate the seriousness of suicidal thoughts or behavior, ask the patient specific questions and consider the following:

1. "Were you trying to kill yourself?" "Did you want to die?"
2. "Have you tried harming or killing yourself before?" "How many times?" "How did you try to do it then?" Attempt to discreetly obtain this information from a family member or friend also.
3. Has the patient experienced a recent loss such as a death, divorce, or job loss.
4. Were the patient's plans vague or specific. The suicide attempt that was obviously well planned is a serious gesture.
5. Did the patient have the means available to accomplish his/her plan (highly lethal method, such as a gun or jumping)?
6. Does the patient have a family history of suicidal behavior?
7. Does the patient have a chronic or terminal medical illness?

Examination: Objective Findings

The patient may appear very sad, may be crying, and may appear despairing and hopeless (flat affect). Scars may be present from previous suicide gestures or attempts. The patient may also be very angry that the attempt failed. Violent behavior should be anticipated rather than merely considered.

EMT Treatment

The first concern is the safety of all present. The out-of-control person with a weapon, even if seemingly only threatening suicide, pre-

Table 17-1 Characteristics of Suicidal Individuals

Types	Age	Sex (M:F)	Method	Setting
Suicide gesture (death accidental)	15–35	1:3	Overdose (minor) Wrist lacerations	In the presence of others Impulsive act Overly manipulative Lovers' quarrel History of gestures
Ambivalent suicide attempt (mixed motivations)	35–45	1:1	Overdose (serious) Wrist lacerations	Help is available Ambivalent wish to die Wants relief from suffering, not necessarily death Usually not an impulsive act
Serious suicide attempt (survival accidental)	35–45	2:1	Hanging Gunshot wound Drowning	Isolated setting Expressed wish to die Discovery and survival accidental
Completed suicide	45+	Male more common	Gunshot wound Jumping	Isolated setting History of serious attempts Recent loss of loved one, status, or health

sents a danger to all in the immediate vicinity. Disarming the person and the situation is a police responsibility, not the EMT's.

Once the threatening situation has been diffused, restraint of the potentially violent patient should be accomplished to protect the patient and the EMS personnel. The EMT should ensure that the police have secured all weapons (pocket knives, cigarette lighters, matches, and needles) the patient may have on his/her person.

Life-threatening medical emergencies are treated in the standard fashion, starting with the ABCDs.

Treatment of the depressed patient is supportive. It may be helpful to have only one EMT talk to the patient privately. When one EMT is successfully communicating with the patient, all others should refrain from interfering in any way.

Ask all depressed patients about suicidal ideas and behaviors. Do not leave these patients alone.

Be definite in the plan of action. Indicate that the patient is expected to go to the hospital by phrases such as "let's go to the ambulance now," rather than asking for the patient to agree.

When the acutely depressed or suicidal patient adamantly refuses transport, local laws may apply. Most states have an involuntary treatment act that allows hospitalization against the person's will if he/she is at risk for suicide or self-harm. States differ regarding who is empowered to carry out these laws—it may be local police, physicians, or specially trained mental health professionals. Physical restraint and transport by the EMT may be indicated (or prohibited). Understand and obey local policy.

■ Psychosis and Violence

Definition

The term "psychosis" covers a wide range of psychiatric disorders, all of which commonly involve a loss of contact with reality. The psychotic patient has difficulty with the activities of daily living, distorted thoughts and perceptions, and confusion between subjective ideas (internal reality) and what is objective (external reality). The psychotic patient is fearful, mistrustful, and sometimes angry. Psychotic disorders range from the harmless recluse who acts and dresses bizarrely to the violently wild and out-of-control person who thinks everyone is trying to kill him/her.

Acute Scenario

The psychotic patient can be dangerous to self or others.

History: Subjective Reports

The psychotic patient may have a history of hospitalizations for psychosis and be taking antipsychotic medications. The psychotic may report hearing voices or believing that others can hear his/her thoughts or control those thoughts. The mood may be reported to be elevated (euphoria) or depressed. Hallucinations that are visual, tactile, olfactory (smell), or gustatory (taste) may also be reported.

Examination: Objective Findings

Some types of psychosis have a medical cause, and every patient should be carefully examined for medical conditions. In general, the patient with psychosis from a *medical* cause has disorientation, memory loss, short attention span, or fluctuating levels of consciousness. These signs are not usually seen in the psychosis that is primarily psychiatric.

Objective findings in psychosis include the following:

- *Appearance*: bizarre dress, odd mannerisms, inappropriate behavior
- *Speech*: talking to self, monotone
- *Thought flow*: lacking logical sequence
- *Affect*: mood appears inappropriate or blunted (flattened)
- *Perception*: false beliefs, confusion of internal reality with external reality
- *Reasoning*: lacking insight or judgment

EMT Treatment

The first concern is the safety of all present. The out-of-control psychotic person can be dangerous, especially if armed and paranoid. Disarming the person is a police responsibility.

If the hostile psychotic patient is aggressive and menacing, verbal restraint should be attempted before physical restraint.

- Emphasize the EMT identity and purpose as helpful and professional.
- Maintain a safe distance from the patient to avoid causing the patient to feel pressured or controlled. Move closer to the patient as rapport is established, but continue to maintain a buffer zone should the patient's behavior suddenly change. Avoid touching the patient until given permission.
- Always maintain an escape route should the patient become suddenly violent. When this is not practical, the EMT and other responders should have a plan to quickly request help and to work together to protect themselves from injury.
- Listen actively and indicate interest. "Not being heard" is a common precipitant of violent outbursts.
- Paraphrase and feedback to patient what is heard, especially reflecting back the patient's feelings. This helps to correct misunderstandings.

Physical restraint is indicated when verbal restraint is unsuccessful or the risk of violence is high. As indicated earlier in this chapter, it is the last resort.

- *Show of force*: A group is organized before confronting the patient. Specific limbs are assigned to each group member to control to avoid confusion.

The patient is confronted with the choice of the "easy" versus the "hard" way of accepting necessary transport and medical evaluation at the hospital.

- *Human restraint*: The patient's limbs and head are immobilized in a coordinated effort by the group on command of the team leader.
- *Mechanical restraint*: All four extremities and the waist are restrained. Padded leather restraints give better security than cloth and cause less injury to the patient.
- Observe carefully to avoid aspiration if the patient vomits while restrained.
- Prolonged restraint in the prone position must be avoided. This position may contribute to the risk of positional asphyxia. As soon as sufficient manpower and restraints are available, move the patient to a restrained supine position for transport.

Most psychotic patients are not violent or dangerous and need supportive therapy—reassurance and transport. Carefully explain your identity and purpose. Maintain a stance of concerned neutrality. Do not confront fantasies or illusions.

The psychotic patient who is not dangerous and refuses transport to the hospital presents a peculiar problem. In our society, one has the right to be different. However, many states have laws that allow psychotics who are "gravely disabled" (or other similar wording) to be treated against their will under provisions of an involuntary treatment act. States differ in who is empowered to carry out these laws—it may be local police, physicians, or specially trained mental health professionals. Physical restraint of these patients and transport by the EMT may be indicated (or prohibited). Understand and obey local policy.

EMT Special Considerations

The patient receiving antipsychotic drugs may present with a common side effect called *dystonic reaction*: involuntary contraction of the muscles in the head and neck. The patient appears oddly distorted, with facial grimacing and neck muscle contraction causing the head to tilt backward. There may be eye movement paralysis. The patient may also have drooling and difficulty in talking or swallowing. Dystonic reactions can be life threatening if air exchange is affected by laryngospasm (which occurs rarely). Ensure rapid provision of, or transport to, ALS services.

Geriatric Patients

Geriatrics is defined as "the branch of health care dealing with the problems of aging and the diseases of the elderly." The increasing proportion of people over the age of 65 and the increased activity of this group emphasize the need for the EMT to have additional knowledge of geriatrics. Aging is a natural process. The "aged" or elderly patient does, however, pose additional challenges for the EMT. These challenges can affect the EMT's ability to

- Effectively communicate with the patient
- Rapidly identify the emergently ill patient
- Properly conduct a detailed physical exam
- Utilize standard physiologic values and indicators in the assessment

Each of these challenges may be presented to the EMT by the elderly patient for a variety of reasons. In order to overcome these challenges, the EMT must be adequately prepared by anticipating them and having a plan of management.

■ COMMUNICATION

Communication with the elderly patient may be affected by a number of factors. These may include sensory losses, feelings of denial, and feelings of hopelessness.

With aging comes possible losses of or alterations to one's sensory functions. Hearing loss and vision deterioration are the two most common sensory changes observed. These changes directly affect communication between the EMT and the elderly patient. In addition to sensory changes, the elderly patient may be reluctant to communicate for other reasons. For example, the elderly male patient may not quickly volunteer information about his prostate problem to the EMT, particularly if the EMT is a woman. Communication may also be hampered by the patient's feelings about his/her illness. Some elderly patients choose to deny the possibility of chronic illness because this would be a recognition of aging. When the patient has been previously diagnosed as having a severe chronic disease or has been chronically ill, he/she may begin to experience feelings of hopelessness and depression.

To improve communications with the elderly patient, the EMT must recognize these potential patient concerns. Actions that may be taken to improve communications include the following:

1. Address the elderly patient in a formal manner, demonstrating respect.
   a. Polite introductions are always in order.

b. Use terms of respect such as Sir, Ma'am, Mr. Smith, or Miss Jones. If the patient introduces himself as Bob, then the assumption is made that the EMT may address the patient in this way.

c. Do not use terms of endearment such as "honey" or "sweetie." This may be viewed as disrespectful and may hamper all further efforts at effective communication.

d. Explain the reasons for actions to be taken ahead of time. For example, when listening to lung sounds, advise the patient that you will need to lift up the back of the shirt to listen to lung sounds.

e. Pay attention when the patient is speaking by using direct eye contact.

2. Look for evidence of hearing impairment, hearing aid use, or vision impairment.

a. Suggest that the patient put in his/her hearing aid before continuing with the assessment (in the nonemergent patient).

b. Speak louder but without shouting. This is especially important if the EMT has a normally soft voice.

c. Speak slowly and clearly.

d. The EMT may position himself/herself closer to the patient or closer to his/her "good ear." Caution must be observed to ensure that the patient is not immediately offended by an extremely close position.

e. Slower reflexes and thought processes require that the EMT allow sufficient time for the elderly patient to comprehend the question and develop a response.

3. Pay particular attention to modesty issues.

a. Modesty issues are important with all patients.

b. Professional mannerisms and a demonstrated concern for the patient's privacy will often place the patient at ease.

■ Physiologic Changes of Aging and the Focused History

Physiologic Changes

Clearly the most significant difference between caring for geriatric patients and other adult patients is recognizing the physiologic changes caused by aging. Many of the body's systems will experience functional changes, including the cardiovascular, respiratory, nervous, and musculoskeletal systems. These changes increase the likelihood of chronic illnesses and decrease the ability to compensate for traumatic injuries.

Cardiovascular System

■ Arteriosclerosis decreases the ability of the arteries to change diameter in response to an increased need for circulation.

- Hardening of the arteries increases peripheral vascular resistance, which may subsequently lead to hypertension and CHF.
- Aging of the heart may lead to an inability to maintain normal heart rates and adequate contraction strength.
- Overall, the elderly patient is often unable to effectively respond to increased oxygen demands with increased perfusion.
- The exam findings may include a heart rate or blood pressure inconsistent with the severity of the patient's illness or injury.

Respiratory System

- Aging decreases the elasticity of the lungs, which may be further compromised by years of smoking or COPD.
- The muscles used in respiration may be weaker while the chest wall is less flexible. These combine to decrease the tidal volume and increase the respiratory rate.
- A weak gag reflex and an inability to forcibly cough may increase the risk of aspiration and choking.
- Because of a weakened immune system, pneumonia is more common in the elderly compared to younger persons.
- Overall, the elderly patient is unable to effectively respond to increased oxygen demands with an increased minute ventilation.

Nervous System

- The sensory changes associated with aging include hearing impairment and vision loss as discussed earlier.
- The elderly patient may also experience alterations in memory, orientation, and mental abilities. These may range from occasional forgetfulness to diseases such as Alzheimer's disease.
- Nervous system changes may make assessment of the patient's current neurologic status a difficult task. The EMT should utilize a family member or friend to assist in defining the normal neurologic status of the patient.

Musculoskeletal System

- The elderly often experience a loss of muscle tone, bone strength, and flexibility. Osteoporosis further reduces bone strength.
- Kyphosis, a forward curvature of the spine, may be significant enough to interfere with effective ventilations.
- Often, a simple injury resulting from a low-mechanism event may lead to serious injury. For example, a fall from a standing position may result in a hip or pelvic fracture.
- The EMT must have a high index of suspicion for musculoskeletal injuries in the elderly even when minor mechanisms are involved.

Other Systemic Changes

- The elderly patient is prone to hypothermia or hyperthermia as a result of the decreased efficiency of the body's thermostat.
- Decreased renal function places the elderly patient at greater risk in the event of an accidental ingestion or overdose. Toxic levels of medications may occur more rapidly.

■ The decreased capability of the immune system coupled with the potential for inadequate nutritional intake make the elderly patient even less capable of responding to severe illness or injury.

Past Medical History

The elderly patient is much more likely to have a significant past medical history. The past history may include a variety of diagnosed illnesses, chronic symptoms, and an abundance of medications. Just as effective communication skills are needed in determining the chief complaint, similar skills will be needed in obtaining the past medical history. Many elderly patients will be unable to accurately recall the names of their chronic illnesses or the exact reasons specific medications are taken. In some cases, the past history is so extensive that much of it is irrelevant to the present illness or injury.

Some tips on obtaining an accurate past medical history include the following:

■ Begin with open-ended questions regarding the present medical condition: "For what illnesses is your doctor presently treating you?" Asking a more general question may result in a response that includes information from 20 years ago. While this may be useful, it is better to focus on present illnesses first.

■ If the patient has difficulty with this type of question, ask yes/no questions such as "Do you have diabetes? High blood pressure? Heart problems? Breathing problems?"

■ Ask questions regarding recent visits to a physician and recent hospitalizations. The reasons for these visits may provide information regarding the patient's medical conditions.

■ Inquire about the patient's medications. Although a great number of medications may be found in the patient's home, ask which medications the patient is currently taking.

■ When asking questions about the patient's medications, use simple, nontechnical language unless the patient has a medical background. Ask "Do you take this medication for your heart or blood pressure? Do you take this medicine to help you sleep?"

■ RECOGNIZING THE ACUTELY ILL OR INJURED ELDERLY PATIENT

As discussed previously, the elderly patient is less capable of effectively compensating when faced with a severe illness or injury. With this in mind, the emphasis on rapid assessment is even more critical. Medical conditions resulting in respiratory distress (COPD, asthma), cardiovascular distress (acute MI, shock, sepsis, or aortic aneurysm), or neurovascular disorders (hemorrhagic stroke) will not be tolerated well by the elderly patient. In the case of major trauma, the elderly patient's condition is likely to deteriorate rapidly. The mortality risk from multisystem trauma is three times greater at age 70 than at age 20.

The loss of effective compensatory mechanisms leaves little available time before definitive care must be provided to the elderly patient. The rapid assessment of the elderly patient who is in obvious distress or is traumatically injured is actually very similar to that of any other adult patient. The primary difference is in the evaluation of the assessment findings and the limited time available for the emergently ill or injured patient.

■ TREATMENT PRINCIPLES
Assessment of ABCDs

AIRWAY

Be alert for loose dentures that may occlude the airway. Remove all ■ loose dentures and secure them in a safe location as soon as possible.

Consider the decreased gag and cough ability, particularly in the pa- ■ tient with a decreased level of consciousness. Be prepared for vomiting by having suction equipment nearby.

BREATHING

■ Consider the poor minute ventilation of the elderly patient.

Since tidal volume may be impaired, the respiratory rate should be at ■ the upper end of the normal range. A rate of 12 or 14 breaths/min in an elderly patient may not be adequate.

Consider that pre-existing medical conditions can be easily aggravated ■ by even minor trauma in the elderly patient.

In the COPD patient, the poor elasticity of the alveoli combined with ■ the decreased flexibility of the chest wall may require a reduced volume during assisted ventilations.

The elderly patient may not be able to sustain an increased respiratory ■ rate for a prolonged period of time before exhaustion occurs. Exhaustion may quickly lead to respiratory failure.

Provide high-flow oxygen to the patient with respiratory distress. ■ Consider the need for immediate ventilatory assistance in the patient who is becoming tired or sleepy.

CIRCULATION

Since peripheral circulation may be poor in the elderly patient, use ■ central pulses (carotid) when peripheral pulses cannot be readily obtained.

Considering the cardiovascular effects resulting from aging, the compensatory mechanisms of increased heart rate and other adrenaline response signs may not be evident.

The EMT must be suspicious of findings such as a low or high blood pressure, or a fast or slow heart rate. Every attempt must be made to compare these readings to the patient's normal vital signs. The EMT must also consider the effect of medications taken as well as those that should have been taken but were not.

Position the patient as with any other patient. Place the hypotensive or extremely tachycardic patient supine with elevated lower extremities. Place the hypertensive patient in a sitting position or with the head slightly elevated.

Disability or Defibrillation

The extent of neurologic disability in the elderly patient may be difficult to assess. Pre-existing illness or stroke may make it virtually impossible to assess neurologic function. The EMT should enlist the assistance of a family member or friend to compare the present status to the patient's baseline.

In the pulseless patient, ventricular fibrillation is highly probable. The EMT trained in defibrillation must immediately use the AED to determine the presence of ventricular fibrillation.

The Nontrauma Patient

Obtaining A Focused History.

Focus on the chief complaint and the history of the present illness.

The EMT may need to redirect the patient in order to avoid discussion of presently irrelevant history.

Identify the present illnesses for which the patient is being treated or that have been diagnosed for the patient.

Identify the current medications for the patient.

Many elderly patients may receive regular home health care. In these cases, the EMT should consult with the home health care provider or his/her medical chart to obtain additional information.

Consider that most elderly patients will call for assistance only when they truly are ill or in pain.

Conducting a Focused Physical Examination

The purpose of the focused examination is to evaluate only those ■ systems related to the patient's complaints or the signs observed by the EMT.

■ Provide appropriate treatment as indicated by the examination.

   ■ Provide oxygen if this has not already been done.
   ■ Assist with medications such as nitroglycerin or bronchodilators (inhaler or nebulizer) when indicated and in the absence of contraindications.
   ■ Position the hypotensive, dizzy, or lightheaded patient in a supine position.
   ■ Assist ventilations when severe respiratory distress, pulmonary edema, or imminent respiratory failure are identified.
   ■ Gentle handling must be provided to the elderly patient because accidental musculoskeletal or soft tissue injury can easily occur.

Continue to reassess the patient because rapid changes may occur in ■ the elderly.

The Traumatically Injured Patient

In the general assessment used to identify the critically injured patient, consider the following factors:

   ■ *Mechanism*: Even mechanisms that appear to be minor can cause significant injury to the elderly patient. The likelihood of pelvic, hip, and other fractures from simple accidents such as falls is much greater.
   ■ *Compensatory mechanism*: Recall that the elderly patient may not be able to adequately compensate for even moderate blood losses or increases in oxygen demand.
   ■ *Pre-existing illness*: Consider the effect of pre-existing illnesses on the present injury. For example, pre-existing cardiac and respiratory illnesses further decrease the ability to compensate when traumatic injuries are present. Additionally, a pre-existing illness may be aggravated by the traumatic injury, resulting in a patient with both trauma and a medical illness requiring treatment.
   ■ *Medications*: Consider the effect of medications on the patient's symptoms and his/her ability to compensate. Medications may prevent the patient from accelerating his/her heart rate or may increase the likelihood of dehydration.
   ■ *Temperature regulation*: Recall that the elderly patient may have difficulty regulating his/her temperature. Avoid hypothermia, particularly when exposing the patient for a detailed examination.

The detailed examination of the elderly trauma patient is conducted in the same manner as with other adult trauma patients. Special considerations for the elderly patient include the following:

   ■ Treatment for specific injuries may need to be slightly modified.
   ■ The elderly patient's skeletal structure may not tolerate a traction splint without causing further injury. Additionally, it may be difficult to rule out

the presence of a pelvic or hip fracture, thus contraindicating the use of a traction splint.

■ The presence of a chronic cough and the decreased ability to cough forcefully may cause discomfort for the patient in the supine position.

■ The removal of dentures may increase the difficulty in obtaining an adequate face mask seal during ventilations.

■ When managing the traumatically injured elderly patient, bear in mind that his/her decreased compensatory mechanisms may result in rapid deterioration.

Terminal Illness and "Do Not Resuscitate" Orders

Although the elderly patient may have a terminal illness or a valid "Do Not Resuscitate" order, the EMT must continue to treat the non–cardiac arrest patient with respect and compassion. Recall that a "Do Not Resuscitate" order does not mean that EMS responders should not provide comfort measures and caring.

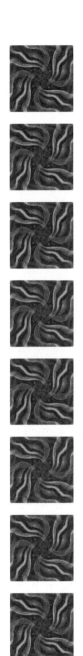

SECTION IV

PROCEDURES AND MEDICAL EQUIPMENT

The procedures in this section are included as refreshers for EMTs and other persons who are trained and certified in their use. Instructions with the illustrations are advised by the manufacturer of the device or are standards already accepted in the emergency care field by sources such as the American Heart Association. Local methods and procedures should supersede those indicated in this section.

19 Assessment

■ BLOOD PRESSURE MEASUREMENT*

Measurement of blood pressure (BP) with a sphygmomanometer and stethoscope can be reliable with proper technique or highly unreliable with improper technique. The principles are straightforward enough. An inflatable cuff is wrapped snugly around the arm and rapidly inflated beyond the systolic arterial pressure, blocking all flow through the artery. With stethoscope in place over the antecubital fossa (popliteal if using the thigh), the cuff is slowly deflated. The sound produced by the blood beginning to rush through the distorted artery as the cuff pressure falls below the systolic pressure marks that measurement (palpation of the radial or pedal pulses at this point marks the palpatory systolic pressure). The sound produced by the blood flowing through this distorted artery becomes abruptly muffled or disappears when the cuff pressure drops below the diastolic pressure (the artery is no longer distorted), and this marks that measurement. (No change in the pulse is palpable at this point, so that palpatory method yields only a systolic value.)

Another method similar to measuring BP by palpation involves the use of an instrument called a Doppler. This device uses a set of earpieces as with a stethoscope connected to a battery- or electricity-powered "box." The Doppler allows the user to hear the blood flowing through the artery as the systolic pressure is reached. As with the palpation method, the Doppler method does not allow the user to measure a diastolic pressure. It is extremely useful, however, when the blood pressure is difficult to obtain (assuming the ABCDs have already been managed.) More experienced EMTs may use the Doppler to listen for fetal heart sounds. Although the principles of blood pressure measurement are straightforward, errors of technique can occur that are related to the equipment, the patient, and the observer.

Equipment

The blood pressure cuff must be the proper size for the patient. It should cover roughly two thirds of the distance between the elbow and the shoulder. In smaller individuals, or children, if the choice is between a cuff that may be too small and one that may be too large, it is better to choose the larger of the two. The diameter of the arm

---

* From Macdonald, S. C., Butman, A. M., Wayne, M. A., et al.: Using Anti-Shock Trousers (MAST): A Guide for the EMT. Westport, CT, Emergency Training, 1982. Reprinted with permission of the publishers.

is also important—obese individuals will need a larger size. (If an oversized cuff is not available for a markedly obese individual, a palpatory systolic pressure can be obtained by applying the cuff on the forearm below the elbow.) Overall, if the cuff is too small, falsely high readings will result; if the cuff is too large, falsely low readings will result.

The cuff must be snugly applied around the arm. A loosely applied cuff will reduce the effective surface contact as the inflated cuff balloons, resulting in falsely high readings.

Anaeroid manometers are sturdy only to a certain point and should be calibrated yearly. This can be done simply with a mercury manometer by the use of a Y-connector.

The Patient

The patient's arm must be positioned at the level of the heart, such as in a normal supine or sitting position. If the arm is positioned below the level of the heart, falsely high readings will result; if above the heart, falsely low readings will result.

The patient should have minimal movement and should be asked to breathe normally. Movement can create additional noise heard by the stethoscope or Doppler, thereby interfering with the ability to hear the return of the arterial flow. Breath holding can create irregular and variable heart rates. The altered heart rate may also alter the blood pressure measurement. This is only a problem when the patient is purposefully breath holding or altering his/her respiratory pattern.

In some hypertensive patients, an auscultatory gap exists (a silent period between systolic and diastolic pressures) that can be misleading. This is why it is often recommended that determination of systolic pressure by palpation precede the auscultatory method. The gap may cover as much as 40 mm Hg and can lead to falsely low systolic estimations or falsely high diastolic estimations.

Quiet Korotkoff sounds (or weak pulses), such as those found in clinical shock, can lead to falsely low estimations of systolic pressure or falsely high estimations of diastolic pressure. Similar false readings may occur when the patient's heart rate is very slow (e.g., less than 60/min).

The Observer (Technique)

The speed of deflation must be roughly 3 mm Hg per second (range of 2 to 5). Too-rapid deflation can result in falsely low readings. A blood pressure cuff with a leaking bladder, gauge, or valve can cause rapid deflation. Use a properly functioning cuff to obtain an accurate BP measurement.

The stethoscope head must be placed firmly, but with as little pressure as possible, over the fossa. Heavy pressure will distort the artery, producing falsely low diastolic readings. Avoid holding the stethoscope head with the thumb. The strong pulse in the EMT's thumb may cause confusion or error if pulsations are amplified by the stethoscope.

The bounce of the aneroid gauge must be disregarded. The vibrations produced by the blood rushing through the distorted artery, which cause the audible sound, also cause the needle to bounce upward with each pulsation. The position of the needle before the bounce is the accurate reading.

Occasionally, the patient's blood pressure will be difficult to obtain. This difficulty may cause the EMT to doubt the findings of the BP measurement. At other times, the tension and excitement of the moment may add to the difficulty. These are not unusual occurrences, particularly for the newer, less experienced EMT. Avoid deflating the cuff and immediately reinflating to attempt another measurement. The two measurements are not likely to be the same. If the first attempt failed, consider using the other arm if possible. When the blood pressure is extremely difficult to obtain, the EMT must avoid the tendency to make repeated attempts. If after the second try the BP cannot be obtained, another EMT should attempt. After two attempts, repeated attempts by the same EMT are likely to reach the same result. These attempts only delay care. The experienced EMT may also conclude that the blood pressure cannot be obtained.

Other possible sources of error include those from viewing the gauge at an angle, too great a distance between the edge of the cuff and the stethoscope, the cuff bladder not being centered over the artery, sensory impairment, and, of course, inattention or carelessness.

Other Blood Pressure Tests

A clinical picture of shock may emerge in the initial assessment, but measurement of the systolic pressure yields a value greater than 90 mm Hg. This patient may be in the stage of compensatory shock, and the variant of blood pressure measurement called *postural signs* or *tilt test* is useful in this situation. Blood pressure that is normal in the supine position may drastically fall when the patient is elevated to either a sitting or a standing position. This condition, called *postural hypotension* or *orthostatic hypotension*, occurs because gravity makes the body do more work to maintain normal pressure when it is upright. This is the same phenomenon that occurs when one stands quickly after resting and feels dizzy. Blood pressure drops suddenly, and it takes a number of body mechanisms to readjust to the body's new position. The normal healthy person compensates quickly for the postural change. The patient in shock may be at the limit of his/her ability to compensate. To check for postural signs, the supine pulse and BP are recorded and the patient raised into a sitting position with feet dangling (assuming this is not contraindicated by specific injuries). After roughly 1 minute, the pulse and BP are rechecked. A 20-point change (increased pulse or decreased systolic) is taken as a positive tilt test. The test is also positive if the position change causes syncope, near-syncope, dizziness, or an altered mental status.

Another diagnostic test that can be of importance in the recognition of shock is the *capillary refill test*. This test quickly reveals whether the patient is significantly hypovolemic. When pressure is applied to the thumb, the flesh under the nail blanches. When the pressure is released, the flesh will appear normal in 2 seconds or less if the patient is normovolemic. If the capillary refill takes longer, the patient is probably hypovolemic. This can be a particularly useful test in revealing internal bleeding. Unfortunately, the capillary refill test does not work well in all persons. Some adults have poor peripheral circulation. This is often due to vascular disease but may be normal for some healthy patients. The capillary refill test is very effective, however, in children. With the exception of cold exposure, normally healthy children have good peripheral circulation.

■ USE OF THERMOMETERS

The medical thermometer is a device used to measure the heat of the body. It can be purchased calibrated in degrees Fahrenheit or Centigrade. Body temperature may be measured by one of three methods by placing a thermometer in the mouth (oral), in the rectum (rectal), or under the arm (axillary).

- The oral thermometer is held for 3 minutes under the patient's tongue with the lips closed, if possible. The temperature should not be taken for at least 10 minutes after ingestion of a hot or cold liquid. Oral thermometers are not advisable for infants, mouth breathers, or comatose or extremely ill patients.

- Rectal temperatures are obtained by inserting the thermometer in the anal canal to a depth of approximately 1 inch and allowing it to remain for 3 minutes. The thermometer should be lubricated using a water-soluble lubricant such as K-Y jelly.

- Axillary temperature is obtained by placing the thermometer for 3 to 5 minutes in the apex of the axilla with the patient's arm held close to the side of the body.

Before using the thermometer, be sure to "shake down" the fluid in it to a level a few degrees lower than normal body temperature. The normal temperature taken orally is 98.6°F (37°C). The rectal temperature is usually from 0.5°F to 1.0°F (0.25°C to 0.50°C) higher than the oral temperature and is the most accurate. Axillary temperatures are 0.5°F (0.25°C) lower than oral temperatures.

Because of concerns with disease transmission, many EMS systems use disposable paper strip "thermometers," thermometer cover slips, or tympanic membrane temperature devices. Tympanic thermometers function best when they are stored in an environment with a "normal" temperature. Storing these devices in a "cold" truck will likely result in inaccurate readings.

The term "fever" is used to describe a body temperature greater than 99.5°F. The term "hypothermia" describes a body temperature that falls below 95°F (35°C). When assessing body temperature for hypothermia, it is best to use a thermometer designed for this purpose (e.g., hypothermia thermometer). Most ordinary thermometers are not designed for low temperatures because they begin measuring temperatures above approximately 95°F. When using a tympanic thermometer, refer to the manufacturer's information to determine the lowest temperatures measured by the device.

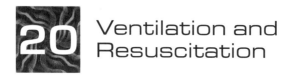

20 Ventilation and Resuscitation

■ GAG REFLEX

The gag reflex is an automatic reflex that closes the epiglottis over the opening to the trachea if a foreign substance, such as food or drink, is introduced. A patient who has a decreased level of consciousness, or who is unconscious because of trauma, excessive alcohol use, or excessive drug intake, loses the gag reflex and may aspirate food or liquid into the lung.

All patients with an altered level of consciousness or suspected neurologic impairment should have the presence of the gag reflex checked. The EMT should refrain from checking the gag reflex in the following patients:

- A traumatically injured patient with a suspected head injury
- A nontraumatically induced (e.g., stroke, ruptured aneurysm) closed head injury patient, particularly if the patient is hypertensive or has other signs of increasing intracranial pressure

To test a patient's gag reflex, place a blunt, thin object (wooden tongue depressor or oropharyngeal airway is most commonly used) on the tongue and carefully advance it to the posterior (back) of the oral pharynx. Often a reflex may be elicited by applying gentle downward pressure on the most posterior aspect of the tongue. If that is not successful, assume that a gag reflex is not present.

When checking for a gag reflex, it is not necessary to "jam" the testing device into the patient's mouth. The EMT must remain aware of the potential hazards of gag reflex checks. Careless use of the testing device may cause the patient to vomit. This could be disastrous for the patient who already has a decreased level of consciousness. Forceful or deep insertion of the tongue depressor may cause injury to the posterior oropharynx. Subsequent bleeding or swelling may add to the already existing airway concerns.

Pay close attention to the patient with a decreased or absent gag reflex. Use suction as required to reduce aspiration of secretions. Patients who are clearly unconscious or who have an absent gag reflex should receive further assessment and care by ALS personnel.

■ OROPHARYNGEAL AIRWAYS (OPA)

Oropharyngeal airways are used in unconscious patients to keep the airway open by preventing the tongue from falling back and occluding the airway. The initial steps in controlling the airway are:

318

Use the head tilt and chin lift method. When the potential for cervical spine injury exists, use the jaw thrust.

If effective ventilations cannot be delivered, reposition the airway and reattempt ventilations.

When effective ventilations can be delivered using airway positioning only, the insertion of the OPA may be delayed.

When manual positioning of the airway alone does not allow for effective ventilations, immediately insert an OPA in the unconscious patient.

OPAs come in several sizes and designs. Judge the correct size by measuring the distance between the corner of the mouth and the nearby earlobe (or from the patient's chin to the angle of the jaw). The OPA is inserted upside down, then rotated 180 degrees to its proper position as it is being inserted. The flanged end should ultimately rest against the lips or teeth. In young children, insert the OPA right side up, using caution to avoid pushing the tongue back.

The partially conscious patient will reject the airway, and when the gag reflex is present the person can vomit and aspirate. If the patient has any gag response to the airway, immediately remove it. Use caution if the level of consciousness is uncertain.

■ VENTILATION DEVICES

Pocket Mask

The use of the pocket mask by professional EMS responders has become exceedingly rare. This is largely due to the increased concern regarding the transmission of infectious disease and the increased availability of other manual ventilation devices (e.g., bag-valve or demand-valve mask). Pocket masks with a one-way valve or some type of filtration device are believed to effectively reduce the risk of infectious disease transmission during ventilations. First responders and laypersons who may perform CPR are more likely to use a pocket mask.

The pocket mask is a small collapsible plastic resuscitation mask. It is generally used with an OPA in the nonbreathing patient. Some come with oxygen inlets, allowing delivery of up to 50% oxygen. The pocket mask should have a one-way valve or adequate filtration device.

Use of the pocket mask allows a good sense of lung resistance/compliance, good visualization of the rise and fall of the chest, and good volumes. With the EMT positioned at the top of the patient's head (or to the side of the patient), the mask is held in place with two hands, allowing for a good seal to the patient's face.

The pocket mask should be considered an interim ventilation device for the EMT. The EMT must switch to a bag-valve mask or demand-valve mask using 100% oxygen as soon as one is available.

Bag-Valve Mask

The bag-valve mask may possibly be the most valuable piece of equipment used by the EMT. The well-trained EMT is extremely proficient in the use of the bag-valve mask.

The bag-valve mask is used for patients who are not breathing or who require assistance in breathing (Fig. 20–1A). It is useful to support respirations in patients who

- Have slow (<10 respirations/min) and/or shallow respirations
- Are becoming increasingly exhausted as a result of their respiratory distress
- Are experiencing respiratory distress that would benefit from positive pressure ventilation (e.g., pulmonary edema, flail chest)

Oxygen concentration can be varied from approximately 20% (without supplemental oxygen) to approximately 40% using a 10- to 12-L/min flow of supplemental oxygen. A concentration of 90–100% can be achieved with the addition of an oxygen reservoir (Fig. 20–1B). Today, most bag-valve masks used in the out-of-hospital setting are disposable and come with a built-in oxygen reservoir.

It is important to maintain a tight fit of face to mask in order to provide maximum efficiency. An OPA may be needed in conjunction with the bag-valve mask in unconscious patients to maintain proper

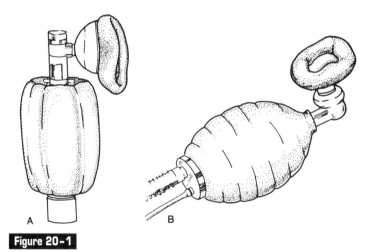

Figure 20–1

A, Bag-valve mask. *B*, Bag-valve mask capable of delivering 90 to 100% oxygen with secondary oxygen source and reservoir tubing or bag reservoir.

position of the tongue and ensure an open airway. When two EMTs are available, one can hold the mask in place to ensure a good seal while the other EMT maintains the head in the proper position and squeezes the bag. When only one EMT is available, the EMT should kneel above the patient's head, position the airway, use his/her knees to maintain the airway position, use one hand to maintain the mask seal, and squeeze the bag with the other hand.

The technique for use of the bag-valve mask is as follows:

■ The bag should be squeezed firmly (not forcefully) to deliver oxygen into the trachea and lungs. The supine patient's head should be placed in an extended "sniffing" position (except for patients with possible cervical spine injury). Watch for gastric distention caused by air forced into the stomach.

- Rapid, forceful ventilations increase the risk of gastric distention. In the adult, each ventilation should take about 1.5 to 2 seconds (1 to 1.5 seconds for pediatric patients). The ventilation should provide a steady flow of air.

- The volume of the ventilation should be limited by the observance of the chest beginning to rise. Ventilation beyond this point is normally not needed.

- In some patients, the ventilation delivery may be required to be forceful (e.g., partially obstructed airway, severe asthma, or COPD).

- Use extreme caution when providing positive pressure ventilation to the severe asthma or COPD patient, pneumothorax patient, and child/infant. Forceful ventilations, particularly those with large volumes, can create a pneumothorax or cause the progression of a pneumothorax to a tension pneumothorax.

■ When assisting the ventilations of the patient who is spontaneously breathing, the key to success is practice. Although many find this ventilation technique difficult to master, its use often yields dramatic results. The following are steps to aid in this procedure:

- First and foremost, explain to the patient each step as you proceed. Causing additional anxiety in the already agitated, hypoxic patient will only make the EMT's job of improving oxygenation more difficult.

- Attach a supply of oxygen to the bag-valve mask at a rate sufficient to keep the reservoir bag inflated (10 to 15 L/min is normally sufficient, including for those bag-valve masks that have a reservoir tube rather than a bag).

- The EMT should take a position directly behind the seated patient or above the supine patient's head.

- Using a properly sized face mask, place the mask near the patient's face. Gently squeeze the bag to ensure the patient can feel the air as it is blown across his/her face.

- Place the mask over the patient's nose and mouth, grasping the bony prominence of the chin with one or two fingers. Do not grasp on the soft area under the chin. Slowly ease the patient's head back to the EMT's chest while also tilting the head backward to open the airway.

- Squeeze the bag and ventilate (or have a partner perform this task).

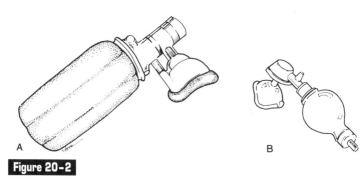

Figure 20-2

A and *B*, Bag-valve masks for infants and children. Pressure relief valves and smaller volume bags (*B*) protect lungs from overinflation.

- Begin to squeeze the bag as the patient begins to inhale. Stop squeezing the bag as the chest begins to rise. This requires close observation of the chest. Interpose additional ventilations if the patient's rate is too slow.
- If the patient is supine, use the steps for an apneic patient in addition to the steps above.

■ Special small bag-valve masks should be used with infants to prevent overinflation of their lungs (Fig. 20–2).

■ Closely monitor the patient's airway by continuously observing the mask for possible vomiting.

■ Suction vomit, blood, and extra secretions from the mouth and upper airway.

Demand-Valve Mask

The demand-valve mask can be used with essentially the same patients as the bag-valve mask. Its primary value is in the conscious patient who needs respiratory assistance.

Oxygen flow is triggered automatically by slight inspiratory pressure. Flow rates range from 100 to 150 L/min during inspiration. Flow ceases at a preset pressure limit of 40 mm Hg. This automatic triggering is clearly advantageous. However, the demand-valve mask has the disadvantage of delivering only dry, nonhumidified oxygen. Humidified oxygen is particularly useful for the asthma patient.

The high flow rate of the demand-valve mask can overcome the esophageal tone and inflate the stomach. This is a significant disadvantage because air in the stomach promotes vomiting, with the attendant risk of aspiration.

To assist ventilation with the demand-valve mask in the conscious hypoxemic patient, start by explaining the procedure to the patient.

Choose the appropriate mask size, and make a good seal with the thumb and fingers on the sides of the mask. Allow the patient's inspiratory effort to trigger oxygen flow. Gauge effectiveness by watching the chest expand.

The demand-valve mask can also be used to provide positive pressure ventilation for the unconscious hypoxemic patient who is not breathing. The manual override button allows the EMT to generate high pressures and fill the lungs even during CPR. Unfortunately, overinflation is a common complication, leading to gastric distention. Thus, the bag-valve mask is a better device for use during CPR.

■ OXYGEN DELIVERY DEVICES

The characteristics of the various oxygen delivery devices are compared in Table 20–1.

Venturi Mask

The Venturi mask is seldom used today in the out-of-hospital setting. The generally short transport times and the likelihood of a hypoxic patient make its use generally unnecessary for the EMT.

The Venturi mask is designed to deliver a fixed percentage of oxygen concentration (Fig. 20–3). This is accomplished by an adjustable flow rate dial or specific oxygen flow restrictors, which are inserted into the mask. The percentage of flow is not affected by the rate or depth of a patient's respirations. Oxygen percentages delivered normally are 24, 28, 35, and 40%.

Table 20–1	Flow Rates and Oxygen Concentrations of Oxygen Delivery Devices	
OXYGEN DELIVERY DEVICE	**FLOW RATE (L/MIN)**	**CONCENTRATION DELIVERED (% OXYGEN)**
Nasal cannula	1–2	24–28
	4–6	36–44
Venturi mask		
24%	4	24
28%	4	28
35%	8	35
40%	8	40
Simple face mask	6–10	35–55
Partial rebreather mask	6–10	40–60
Non-rebreather mask with reservoir	10–25	90–100

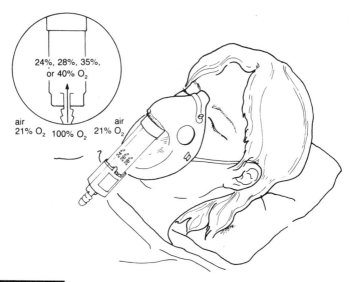

Figure 20-3

Venturi mask, in which 100% oxygen is mixed with room air, making accurate selection of oxygen concentration possible. The mask is especially useful in the treatment of patients with COPD.

Nasal Cannula

The nasal cannula is the most commonly used oxygen delivery device (Fig. 20–4). It is used for patients who:

- Are breathing spontaneously
- Are not in respiratory distress
- Require supplemental oxygen

It has the advantage of allowing the patient to talk. The patient usually does not feel smothered or claustrophobic.

A nasal cannula delivers from 20 to 40% oxygen concentration depending upon the oxygen flow rate (liters per minute). For example, 4 L/min is a routine setting, except for patients with COPD, who should initially be provided with 2 L/min.

The nasal cannula is not affected by mouth breathing, but the actual percentage of oxygen concentration is variable.

Simple Face Masks

Simple face masks may deliver 35 to 55% oxygen concentration (Fig. 20–5). They often give the anxious patient a feeling of suffocation. Face masks combine unused air in the upper airway and ambient air

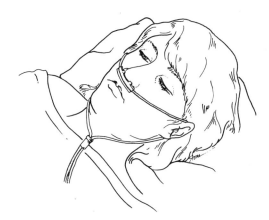

Figure 20-4

Nasal cannula.

with new oxygen. Flow rates of oxygen should be at least 6 L/min to exceed 20% oxygen (which is available in room air). The mask should have a tight seal for proper function.

Non-Rebreather and Partial Rebreather Masks

Non-rebreather-type masks contain an oxygen reservoir bag. Non-rebreather masks have two exhalation openings, each with a one-way valve. *Partial non-rebreather masks* have only one opening supplied with a one-way valve. The partial non-rebreather mask is more commonly used. The patient receives oxygen from the reservoir bag. It can deliver 90 to 100% oxygen (<100% is common because of poor mask-to-face seal).

The required flow rate is determined more by the volume inhaled by the patient with each breath. The flow rate should be set high enough to maintain an inflated reservoir bag (at least 10 L/min, usually 15 to 25 L/min). This is the oxygen delivery device of choice when high-flow oxygen is to be provided to the spontaneously breathing patient.

■ Suction Devices

A suction device should be capable of quickly removing blood, vomitus, or secretions from the upper respiratory system. Various portable devices are available; they may be hand or foot operated, or battery powered.

The suction device includes a plastic bag or bottle to trap the aspirate, flexible tubing, and "whistle tip" or Y-connector-type catheters of various sizes (Fig. 20–6A). Control over the amount of suction applied is achieved by placing a thumb over the open Y-connector (Fig. 20–6B).

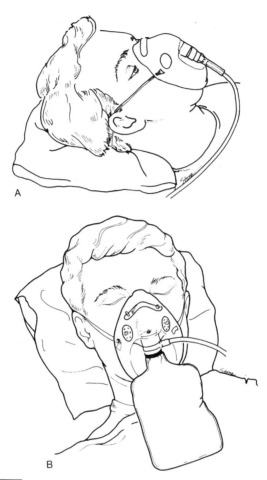

Figure 20-5

Face masks. *A*, Simple face mask. *B*, Face mask with oxygen reservoir for higher concentration of oxygen.

Proper suctioning technique can be ensured using the following steps:

■ Immediately turn the patient's head to the side. For patients with potential cervical spine injuries, tilt the backboard toward one side.

■ Select the proper catheter size for the size of the patient and for the type of secretions to be suctioned. Measure the length of catheter

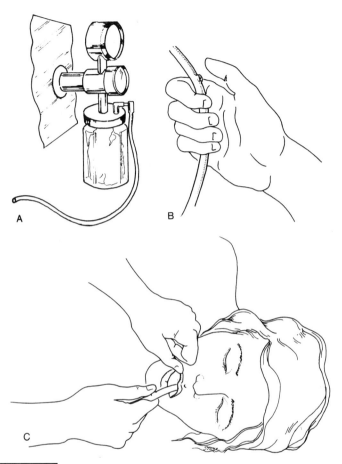

Figure 20-6

Suction. *A*, Typical wall-mounted vacuum suction device with a vacuum gauge and jar with a disposable plastic container. *B*, "Whistle tip" suction tip, thumb operated. *C*, Turn the patient's head to one side when possible, place the suction tip in one side of the patient's mouth, and do not suction for more than 15 seconds at a time.

to be inserted into the mouth in the same manner as measuring for an OPA.

Insert the tip of the catheter, but do not apply suction until the catheter is in the desired location (Fig. 20-6C). It is difficult to advance the catheter while suction is applied.

■ Do not suction the airway for periods of longer than 15 seconds, because the suction impedes the patient's ability to breathe. Occasionally, the EMT may encounter patients who must be suctioned for periods longer than 15 seconds because of continuous vomiting.

■ When the airway is cleared, ensure that the patient is adequately oxygenated. Provide high-flow oxygen or bag-valve mask assistance if needed.

■ Be careful not to cause additional gagging and vomiting during suctioning. *Note:* Suctioning may cause increased intracranial pressure if the patient has a head injury.

■ Clear secretions from the catheter using water or saline by applying suction until clear fluid reaches the trap.

Trauma Procedures

■ Antishock Trousers (MAST)

Antishock trousers, also called military antishock trousers (MAST) or pneumatic antishock garment (PASG), are a device designed to

- Increase the volume of blood to the heart, lungs, and brain of the patient in shock by decreasing the capacity of the circulatory system in the areas under the suit (legs and abdomen)
- Control internal and external hemorrhage in areas under the suit (particularly internal bleeding into the abdominal cavity)
- Serve as an effective splinting device for fractures of the pelvis and lower extremities

In theory, this device increases peripheral resistance, thereby reducing the normal blood flow to the extremities and causing improved blood flow to the more vital heart, lungs, and brain. *(It should be noted that recent studies question this method of action and the benefit of antishock trousers. Thus the indications for and use of this device are controversial. Some studies indicate that the improvement in blood pressure is short lived. Local policies and guidelines should be followed.)* In practice, this device probably provides the most benefit when transport times to definitive trauma management (e.g., surgery) are significantly extended, as in rural areas (particularly when ALS services are unavailable). In many parts of the nation, antishock trousers can be used only under immediate physician control (over a radio/telephone) or under the direction provided by written (standing) orders.

Use

Generally speaking, the trousers are applied to patients with the following conditions:

- A systolic blood pressure of less than 70 mm Hg and a pulse rate greater than 110/min with any multisystem trauma (involving the abdomen, pelvis, and/or lower extremities)
- A systolic blood pressure of less than or equal to 70 mm Hg with signs of shock (hypovolemic, neurogenic, anaphylactic)
- Nontraumatic bleeding and shock, but without chest pain (e.g., GI bleed, ectopic pregnancy, ruptured aortic aneurysm)
- Pelvic or complicated femur fractures
- Serious injury to lower extremities requiring direct pressure for control of hemorrhage.

Precautions

The use of antishock trousers is contraindicated in the presence of:

- Cardiogenic shock
- Traumatic or nontraumatic chest pain
- Pulmonary edema
- Trauma (blunt or penetrating) to any area of the chest, neck, or head when the bleeding cannot be controlled by direct pressure

In some cases, it would be best to avoid the use of MAST unless absolutely necessary as gauged by the patient's degree of shock and the transport time. Relative contraindications include:

- Hypotension resulting from hypothermia
- Burns on those areas normally covered by the trousers
- Pregnancy (the abdominal chamber inflation is the relative contraindication)
- Evisceration of the abdomen
- Impaled object in the abdomen, pelvis, or lower extremities
- Suspected tension pneumothorax
- Pediatric patients if the MAST are not capable of being shortened for the pediatric patient

However, if the patient's systolic blood pressure is still 70 mm Hg or less with signs of shock and without absolute contraindications, the EMT should contact medical control for possible permission to inflate the leg and/or abdominal chambers.

For the proper and safe operation of antishock trousers, the following precautions are vital:

- Avoid rapid/sudden deflation of the trousers once inflated, because this may cause irreversible shock. Deflation should never be attempted by EMTs in the field.
- Failure to inflate the chamber on the injured leg *first* may cause increased hemorrhage into the injured site.
- Continuous monitoring of vital signs, including respiratory status, is essential to providing safe treatment and preventing serious patient deterioration. Inflation of the abdominal section may interfere with effective ventilations resulting in respiratory distress.
- When using antishock trousers for femur fractures (midshaft), traction splints must go outside the trousers to prevent injuries to the skin.
- Monitor the tension of the trousers frequently to prevent undetected loss of air that could cause slow deflation. Be alert to changes in temperature and altitude because they can affect the pressure within the trousers as follows:
  - An increase in temperature will cause an increase in trouser pressure; a decrease in temperature causes a decrease in pressure.
  - An increase in altitude will cause an increase in pressure; a decrease in altitude causes a decrease in pressure.
- Watch for sharp objects that might puncture trousers.
- Do not create significant delays in transport in order to apply the trousers.

Application

Before applying antishock trousers, always perform the following steps:

■ Treat ABCD concerns first. Perform CPR, if required.

■ Administer high-flow oxygen. Assist ventilations if needed.

■ Check for and treat profuse bleeding.

■ With the patient in a supine position, assess vital signs, lung sounds, level and state of consciousness, and pupillary size and reaction to light.

■ Position the patient supine with the legs elevated to treat for shock. For the patient with suspected spinal injury, secure to a backboard and then elevate the foot of the board.

■ Remove the patient's clothing. Take actions to prevent hypothermia.

■ Complete the examination of the abdomen, pelvis, and legs. These areas will not be accessible for examination with the trousers in place.

■ Dress any severe wounds within the area to be covered by the trousers.

Apply the trousers by one of the following methods (Fig. 21–1):

1. *Quick Method:* Use this method ONLY in cases in which spinal injuries have first been ruled out (e.g., GI bleeding, ruptured ectopic pregnancy). The trousers are prefastened and quickly slipped over the legs and buttocks.
   a. Have all Velcro parts loosely fastened.
   b. One EMT slips his/her arms through the trouser's feet, sliding both hands and arms to the top opening of the trouser's legs.
   c. With his/her arms extending through the legs of the trousers, the EMT then grasps the top of the patient's feet so that the patient's toes are prevented from catching on the trousers.
   d. A second EMT then slips the trousers off his/her partner's arms and onto the patient's legs.
   e. The EMTs then move to opposite sides of the patient and, facing one another, gently but rapidly slide the abdominal chamber to just below the patient's rib margin.

2. *Standard Method:* The patient is moved onto the trousers and positioned so that the top of the abdominal chamber is just

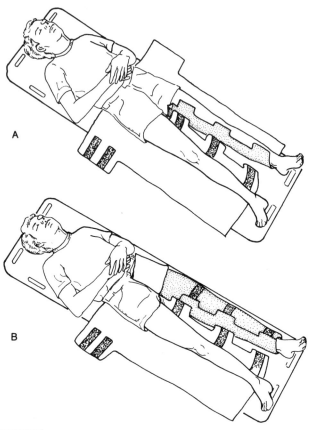

Figure 21–1

Antishock trousers. *A, B, C,* and *D,* Successive steps of log-rolling patient onto trousers and fastening first the legs and then the abdomen. *Illustration continued on opposite page*

below the rib margin. The Velcro strips are then adjusted and fastened.

3. *Backboard Method:* This method is used in serious trauma situations when a backboard is required for the treatment of suspected spinal injury and/or possible cardiac arrest. The trousers should be laid out on the backboard prior to positioning the patient. Use established backboard techniques to maintain proper spinal alignment. Use of a clam shell stretcher to position the patient onto the backboard would also be appropriate.

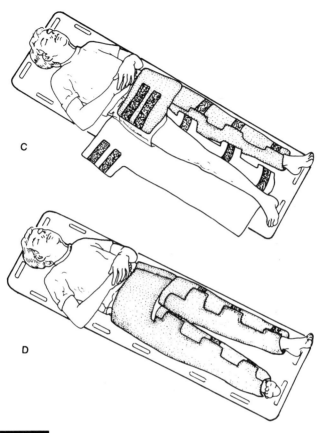

Figure 21-1

Continued.

4. *Center Fold Method*
   a. Lay out the trousers, rear or backside down, and undo the Velcro fasteners.
   b. Roll the bladders so they are all rolled toward the center point of the garment (legs to the middle and belly down).
   c. Grasp a substantial part of all of the bladders in one hand at the patient's crotch.
   d. Without releasing your hold, maneuver the trousers to a position below the patient's feet.
   e. Using an assistant, spread the patient's feet sufficiently for your hand and the bladders to be positioned at the patient's crotch.

      f. Position an EMT on each side of the patient, grasp the trousers at the top (where the top of the Velcro strap is secured) and work the trousers up under the patient's hips until the bladders are at the patient's crotch.

      g. Unroll the bladders into the appropriate positions and secure the Velcro straps.

After using one of the above methods to place the patient into the antishock trousers, complete the procedure with the following steps:

■ Attach the foot pump to the appropriate chamber access valve. (Leg chambers are inflated first, beginning with the severely injured leg when applicable. The abdominal chamber is inflated last.)

■ Make sure all stopcocks are closed.

■ Open the stopcocks to the leg chambers. (When one leg is severely injured, open only the stopcock for this trouser leg. After inflating this leg, then inflate the second leg.)

■ Using the foot pump, inflate the leg chambers.

■ Close the leg stopcocks and check lung sounds.

■ Open the abdominal stopcock.

■ Attach the foot pump to the abdominal chamber and inflate. Close the abdominal stopcock once inflation is complete.

■ The trousers are inflated until (this may vary with each manufacturer):

    ■ The pressure valves release automatically
    ■ The Velcro begins to appear to "tear away"
    ■ The pressure reaches approximately 100 mm Hg on the pressure gauge of the trousers

■ When the MAST are used for stabilization of leg or pelvic fractures, inflate only until the fractures are stabilized (as with a splint).

■ Once the trousers are inflated properly, the patient's pulse, respirations, blood pressure, lung sounds, and level of consciousness must be assessed and recorded every 5 minutes.

The primary goal of the EMT, when using antishock trousers, is to inflate the suit to a point where the patient displays a clinical response (improved level of consciousness, skin color, vital signs). Under most conditions, a blood pressure of 100 mm Hg systolic is adequate to maintain an acceptable clinical response. Blood pressures

over 100 mm Hg may cause renewed bleeding from injury sites and/
or additional complications of existing injuries.

■ WOUND CARE

Occlusive Dressings

An occlusive dressing is used in two different conditions: sucking
chest wound and abdominal evisceration. Materials that can be used
to make occlusive dressings include sterilized plastic wrap and sterile
Vaseline gauze. Although aluminum foil can also be used as an in-
sulator for the premature infant, it is difficult to work with to create
an occlusive dressing because it will not easily conform to the skin
surface.

■ OCCLUSIVE DRESSING FOR A SUCKING CHEST WOUND

■ Look for more than one penetrating wound on each side of the chest.

■ Size the dressing to be several times larger than the wound.

■ When more than one penetrating chest wound is found on a side of
the chest (one lung), seal all but the most anterior wound with
an occlusive dressing taped on four sides. Seal the most anterior wound
(or the only wound) at the end of a forced exhalation.

■ Tape on three sides. Leave the lowermost side (closest to the ground
or backboard) open to allow for possible drainage.

■ Use the same process if penetrating wounds are found on the other
side of the chest.

■ If only one side of the chest is affected, the patient may be placed
onto the injured side, if possible. When positive pressure ventilation
is needed, the patient must be placed in the supine position.

■ Observe carefully for the possible development of a tension pneumothorax. If tension pneumothorax is suspected, test by releasing
the seal on one side to see if air rushes out. If air is present, the occlusive
dressing must be removed for a short period to allow pressure release.
Reapply the occlusive dressing.

■ OCCLUSIVE DRESSING FOR ABDOMINAL EVISCERATION

■ Cover the eviscerated bowel completely with plastic wrap or aluminum foil. Place a dry, bulky dressing over this area to provide
stabilization.

■ Tape on four sides.

Extremity Splints

The management of fractures and dislocations is a challenge to patients and to common sense. There are few hard-and-fast rules.

Most musculoskeletal injuries are not life threatening. Exceptions include hemorrhage from open fractures, fractures to the thorax with insults to respiratory organs or large vessels, fractures to the pelvis, and fractures of the femur. However, the EMT must avoid concentrating on obvious fractures at the expense of neglecting the ABCDs.

Usually, the EMT has time to prepare a systematic approach to the problem and thus prevent additional injury to the surrounding tissue. The amount of time available will depend on the degree and severity of the total injuries. The multisystem trauma patient cannot afford to have significant time spent at the scene for splinting. Much of this may need to be done during transport if time permits.

The goal of the EMT is to stabilize, immobilize, and, if possible, realign the extremity(ies) to near-normal anatomic position.

There are numerous devices available for splinting (Figs. 21–2 through 21–4). When selecting a device for splinting, consider the following factors:

■ The location of the part to be stabilized.
  –Splint joint injuries with moldable splints (such as a ladder splint) in the position found.
  –Use traction devices for heavy-muscled long bones.
  –Splint to one joint above and one joint below the injured part.
■ The ease and comfort of application of the splint. Pillows and blankets are useful padding for simple rib fracture and ankle or foot injuries, and for elevation of extremity fractures during transportation. Vacuum splints, although extremely effective, can be slightly uncomfortable to a conscious patient.
■ Leave access to assess distal pulses (Fig. 21–5).
■ Pneumatic antishock trousers should be large enough to surround the pelvic girdle.

The EMT should adhere to the following rules of splinting:

Always work with a partner and predetermine the role each rescuer
■ will perform during treatment.

Figure 21-2

Air splints. *A*, EMT who is going to maintain traction of the fractured extremity should place the hand and arm inside the splint and grasp the wrist or ankle of the extremity to be splinted. *B*, With the extremity in proper alignment, slide splint from EMT's arm onto the fractured extremity. *C*, Maintain traction and alignment, and inflate the splint by mouth until it is moderately firm.

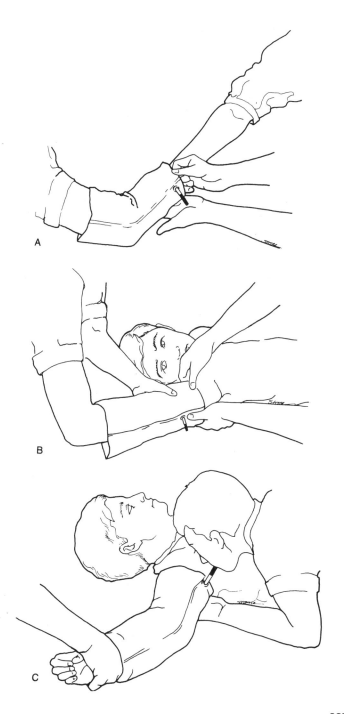

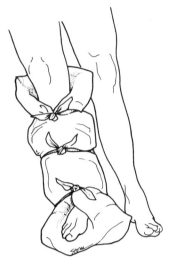

Figure 21-3

Pillow splint, an especially comfortable and stable method of splinting fractures of the ankles and feet.

■ Inform the patient of all treatment before beginning, including the possibility of when to expect pain.

■ Remove clothing, debris, jewelry, and boots/shoes.

■ Control hemorrhage with direct pressure, then elevation, and, if necessary, pressure to the appropriate pressure point.

■ Cover open wounds and exposed bones with sterile, dry dressings.

■ Assess arterial pulses, sensations, and movement distal to the site of injury, and record them.

■ Assemble necessary materials required for splinting. Place padding on the splint before beginning treatment.

■ Have your partner stabilize the joint above the splinting site. Gently apply traction in the direction of angulation. Move the limb very slowly to a normal anatomic position. It is not necessary to replace bone ends together. Align them parallel to each other. This does not apply to the splinting of injured joints (e.g., dislocations, sprains).

■ Reassess distal pulses, sensations, and movement after splinting is completed. If pulses or sensation have changed, do not reposition limb. Check the adequacy of traction. Record results, and advise the receiving physician of the time of loss of pulse or sensation.

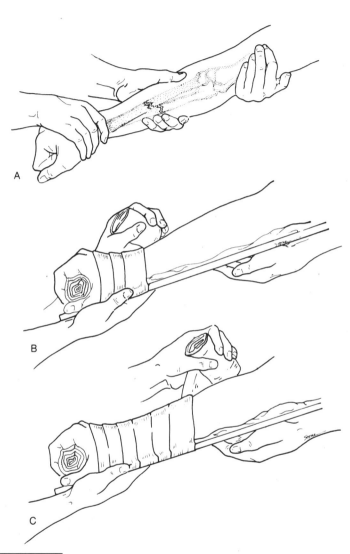

Figure 21-4

Board or ladder splint. *A*, Align fractured extremity with gentle traction. *B*, After padding the board to fill the contours of the arm, place splint along inside of forearm with roll of padding in palm of extremity. *C*, Secure extremity to splint with roll of bandage material.

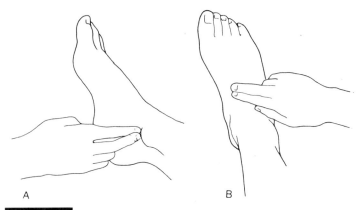

Figure 21-5

Pedal pulses. Distal pulses of lower extremities must be checked before and after splinting of fracture. *A*, Posterior tibialis pulse. *B*, Dorsalis pedis pulse.

■ The splint must immobilize at least one joint above and one joint below the fracture site.

■ Elevate the injured limb before transport.

Remember, when using air splints or MAST pants and moving from a cold to a warm environment or changing altitudes, that the pressure in the splint increases as the temperature and/or altitude increase.

Apply a sling and swath to injuries of the humerus and shoulder (Fig. 21–6). Support all splinted limbs to avoid sudden movement during transport.

Specific devices for splinting the lower extremity are shown in Figures 21–7 and 21–8. Traction splints are used primarily for mid-shaft femur fractures in which the following contraindications are *not* present:

■ Suspected fractures of the tibia and fibula
■ Suspected fracture/dislocation of the ankle or knee.
■ Suspected pelvic fracture or hip dislocation
■ Femur fracture involving the proximal portion (femoral head) or the distal portion.

Neck and Spine Immobilization

Injuries to the neck (cervical spine), midback (thoracic spine), and lower back (lumbar spine) may be subtle. The patient may complain of minor pain. Deformity may not be palpable. For this reason, it is vital for the EMT to get as clear a mental picture as possible of the mechanism and the force of the mechanism of injury.

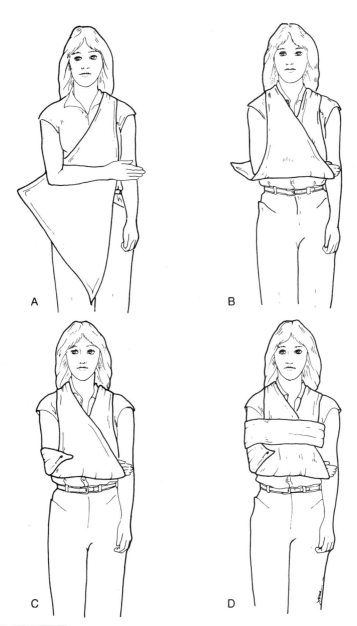

Figure 21-6

Sling and swathe used with injuries of the humerus and shoulder. *A*, Place patient's forearm across chest. *B*, Secure both ends of the sling with a knot in a comfortable position at the shoulder. *C*, Secure elbow flap of sling. *D*, Tie swathe around chest just tight enough to prevent arm from swinging away from patient's body.

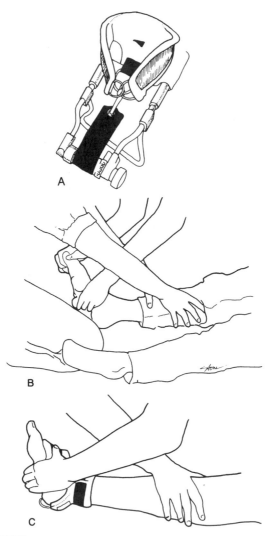

Figure 21-7

Applying a Hare traction splint. *A*, Proper position of the ankle hitch to the windlass. *B*, Remove shoe, sock, and all clothing from the fractured extremity. Assess for the presence of a distal pulse. Adjust the splint length to the patient's uninjured leg, including extra length for the windlass action. Open all splint straps. Place the splint alongside the patient's leg. *C*, Stabilize the fracture site while applying the ankle hitch. *D*, Apply traction by grasping the injured leg above the knee using both hands. *E*, Position splint in place firmly against the buttock and securely apply the ischeal strap. Use padding under the strap as necessary in the groin area. *Illustration continued on following page*

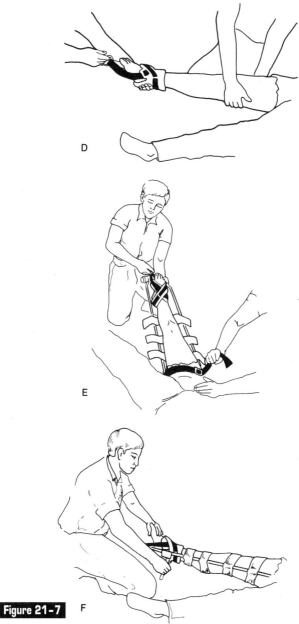

Figure 21-7   F

Continued   *F*, Attach the ankle hitch rings to the windlass and apply traction according to the patient's comfort. Secure all remaining leg straps, starting at the fracture site and working toward the ankle. Raise the stand to keep the heel off the surface.

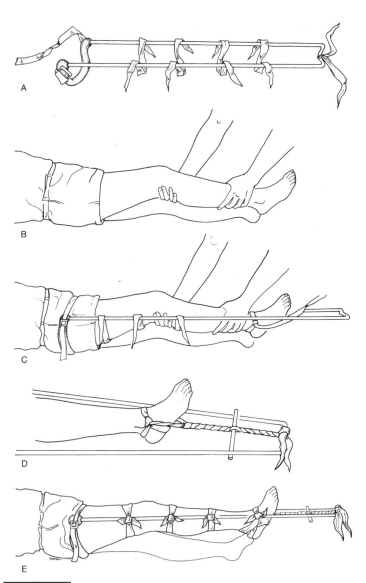

Figure 21-8

Thomas half-ring splint. *A*, Buckle of thigh strap is always positioned on outside of extremity. *B* and *C*, Follow the same steps to apply the splint as with the Hare splint, except that this splint does not have a built-in windlass and leg straps. Cravats are normally used for those purposes. *D*, Sample ankle strap and windlass. *E*, Splint in place.

General indications for use of a cervical collar (Fig. 20–9) and spine board immobilization include:

- All persons with traumatic head injuries and all unconscious trauma victims
- Any complaint of pain in any portion of the spine secondary to trauma
- Decreased sensation, numbness or tingling, or reduced or complete loss of motion of any or all extremities after trauma, even if it has resolved

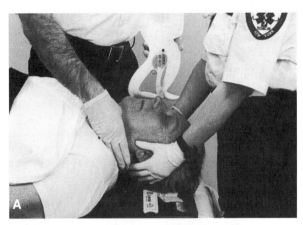

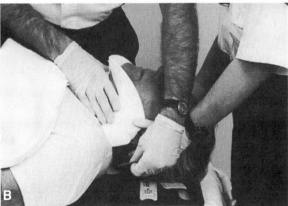

Figure 21-9

Cervical collar. *A,* Using both hands, placed on each side of the head, provide in-line cervical spine stabilization. Slide the collar under the patient's neck until the chin-support area is under the chin. The collar should be pulled snug and fastened closed. *B,* The head should be held stable during any movement of the patient until a cervical immobilization device or similar item is used to provide lateral support and to secure the head to the backboard. (From Henry, M.C. and Stapleton, E.R.: EMT Prehospital Care, 2nd ed. Philadelphia, WB Saunders, 1997, p. 565, reprinted by permission.)

- Palpable deformities or tenderness in any portion of the spine after trauma
- Lacerations and/or hematomas to the head from another moving object, or a blow to the head from a heavy or fast-moving source
- Deceleration injuries such as those resulting from a motor vehicle accident or fall
- A forceful blow to any portion of the spine
- Penetrating injuries occurring near the spine
- Diving injuries as well as unconscious submersion victims

There have been cases of patients with fractures of the spine that have gone unnoticed and were discovered hours later when severe symptoms began to develop. Often this circumstance can be avoided if EMT treatment is based upon the mechanism of injury. Rely on your initial impression: "If you think about the need for neck and spine immobilization, do it."

Cervical immobilization devices include commercially available hard collars, rolled blankets, and commercially available cervical immobilization devices. Cervical collars must be properly sized for the patient. Before applying any cervical immobilization device, the patient's neck must be stabilized manually:

- Align the head and neck along the long axis of the skeleton *before* assessing any other limb/injury.

- Should the patient's head/neck be rotated, provide initial stabilization, then rotate to anatomic position. Do not apply traction or pull on the head.

- Should the patient's head/neck be rotated and flexed or extended, first initiate in-line stabilization of the head. Next, rotate the head into a normal position (the result should be a forward-facing position with the neck and head in a neutral position).

Do not release manual stabilization of the neck until the patient has a cervical collar applied, is placed onto and secured to a backboard (or similar spinal immobilization device), and the head is secured to the backboard using a cervical immobilization device. When a cervical immobilization device is not available, use rolled towels along each side of the head. Secure the head to the backboard using a wide strip of adhesive tape across the forehead and attached to the backboard on each side.

When proper sizes of pediatric cervical collars are unavailable, the EMT may use a rolled blanket to create a "horse collar." The rolled blanket is curved to a U shape and placed around the child's head. The curve of the U rests on the superior surface of the head and the sides of the U are along each side of the child's head. This device and the child's head may then be secured to a backboard. In small children and infants, a folded towel may need to be placed under the child's shoulders and upper back to prevent neck flexion as a result of the large occiput.

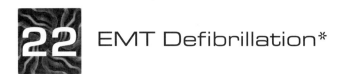

EMT Defibrillation*

> Note: *EMT defibrillation programs must have a medical director. EMTs trained in defibrillation can operate a defibrillator only under the authority of a physician.*

Defibrillation by EMTs was first demonstrated to be life saving in King County, Washington. Since that program began in 1978, survival from cardiac arrest has increased fourfold. As a result, hundreds of EMT defibrillation (EMT-D) programs have begun nationwide. Large amounts of data have been gathered to demonstrate the value of early defibrillation in the "chain of survival." Within the past few years, the American Heart Association proclaimed early defibrillation as the "standard of care" by stating, "Health care professionals with a duty to respond to a person in cardiac arrest should have a defibrillator available immediately or within 1 to 2 minutes." Defibrillation by EMTs can increase a community's survival rate from sudden cardiac arrest. Today, work is ongoing to demonstrate the ability to further improve the likelihood of resuscitation through early defibrillation programs using nontraditional first responders. This effort has been named public access defibrillation.

The rationale for EMT defibrillation is based on the following principles:

- The sooner a patient in ventricular fibrillation (VF) receives a defibrillatory shock, the greater the likelihood of successful resuscitation.

- The most frequent rhythm in out-of-hospital sudden cardiac arrest is VF. Up to 80% of persons with sudden cardiac arrest are in VF during the early minutes of their arrest. The percentage in VF declines with each passing minute. By 4 to 8 minutes after collapse, only 40 to 50% are still in VF. Those no longer in VF are in asystole (flatline) or pulseless electrical activity (PEA) and have virtually no chance of being resuscitated.

- Defibrillatory shocks, if provided soon enough, may be sufficient therapy to achieve a pulse and blood pressure. If, in addition, effective CPR has been administered, many resuscitated patients have virtually no long-term neurologic deficits.

EMT-D programs are likely to be most successful in communities in which bystander CPR occurs before the arrival of EMT-Ds and in which the average EMT-D response time is less than 6 minutes. CPR performed by bystanders appears to prolong the duration of VF and

---

*Portions of this chapter have been adapted from material generously provided by Richard O. Cummins, M.D., Medical Director of the King County, Washington, Early Defibrillation Program.

thus allows additional time for successful shocks by EMT-Ds. CPR, by itself, cannot restore a normal heart rhythm in the VF patient.

■ Ventricular Fibrillation

Ventricular fibrillation is a disorganized heart rhythm that cannot pump blood. Therefore, there is no pulse or blood pressure. The person is *clinically* dead. If the VF rhythm can be restored to a normal rhythm in minutes with a defibrillatory shock, the person can be saved. If the normal rhythm cannot be restored, the VF rhythm will deteriorate over minutes to an asystolic rhythm, from which the likelihood of resuscitation is very poor. The end result is a person who is *biologically* dead (no possibility of resuscitation).

VF usually occurs in persons with underlying heart disease. It frequently occurs in the setting of an MI or angina, but it can occur suddenly without any symptoms. The rhythm of VF does not come on gradually; it begins suddenly. Since there are no vital signs with this rhythm, the term "sudden cardiac death" is associated with it.

VF can also occur in persons with no heart disease. It may be seen in electric shock, drowning, and drug overdose or abuse (e.g., cocaine). Other frequently abused toxic substances that may increase the risk of VF are methamphetamines and inhaled hydrocarbons. "Huffing" of hydrocarbons, particularly metallic paints and halogenated hydrocarbons (Freons, Halons, and solvents), increases the irritability of the ventricles and the risk of VF.

■ EMT Defibrillation

EMT defibrillation programs use either manual or automated external defibrillators (AEDs). Advances in technology and the ease of training associated with automated defibrillators have significantly reduced the number of manual defibrillation–trained EMT-Ds.

Manual Defibrillation

In manual defibrillation programs, EMTs are trained to recognize VF on an ECG monitor and then must manually decide to charge and operate the defibrillator. Training in VF recognition is beyond the scope of this book. This chapter focuses on AED programs.

Automated External Defibrillation

In automated external defibrillation programs, EMTs operate devices that utilize a rhythm-analysis system. All AEDs are attached to the patient through two adhesive pads and connecting cables. These adhesive pads transmit the rhythm and deliver the electrical countershock. In addition, they allow continuous monitoring of patient contact to ensure proper connection and minimal impedance. External defibrillation devices are defined as "fully" automatic and "semiautomatic" (or "shock advisory") defibrillators.

"Fully" automatic defibrillators require only that the operator attach the defibrillator pads and turn on the device. The device immediately analyzes the rhythm and, if VF (or ventricular tachycardia above a preset rate) is present, the device will charge its capacitors and deliver a countershock.

"Semiautomatic" or "shock advisory" devices require additional operator steps, including pressing an "analyze" control to initiate rhythm analysis, and pressing a "shock" control to deliver the countershock. The shock control can only be activated when the device identifies a shockable rhythm and "advises" the operator to press the shock control. These devices never enter the analysis mode unless activated by the operator, and the final decision to deliver the shock remains in the hands of the human operator. Newer semiautomatic defibrillators are capable of being programmed to immediately begin analysis without activating the analysis mode. They continue to be termed "semiautomatic" since they still require operator activation of the shock delivery system when a shockable rhythm is detected.

All AEDs will shock certain types of ventricular tachycardia, if the rate is greater than preset values. All rescuers who operate automated defibrillators are trained to attach the device only to unconscious patients who are verified to be in cardiac arrest (without a pulse or normal respirations). With this approach, the operator serves as the "primary verification" system to confirm that a patient has had a cardiac arrest. In this clinical situation, with a nonbreathing, pulseless patient, electrical countershocks are indicated for the treatment of VF or fast ventricular tachycardia.

Operation of the Automated External Defibrillator

All AEDs require the same sequence of operation:

1. *Turn the power on and prepare the equipment.*
   a. In some systems, the operator must immediately begin providing a verbal report into a voice recording system.
   b. Verbalization of the steps of application often serves as an effective reminder to the operator.

2. *Attach the adhesive pads and patient cables.*
   a. With some newer defibrillation pad systems, pads are designed with integrated patient cables.
   b. For those without this design, the cables should be attached to the pads prior to application to the patient.

3. *Initiate analysis of the rhythm.*
   a. With some newer defibrillators, this is automatically accomplished by properly attaching the adhesive pads and cables to the patient.
   b. On other defibrillators, this step may only be required for the first of three sequential shocks.

    c. With all defibrillators, the operator must ensure that all patient movement has ceased before analysis begins.

4. *Deliver the shock, if indicated.*
    a. The shock must only be delivered after safely clearing the patient.
    b. If no shock is indicated, continue effective CPR in the unresponsive, pulseless patient.

Most EMT response teams will consist of at least two people. Once at the scene, one EMT performs as the defibrillator operator and the other is responsible for airway management and CPR. No other activities, including setting up oxygen delivery systems, suction equipment, intravenous lines, or mechanical CPR devices, take precedence over, or are performed prior to, rhythm analysis and defibrillation. The defibrillator operator concentrates on defibrillator operation, while the CPR provider attends to airway and chest compressions. EMTs must not touch the patient while the automated defibrillator analyzes the rhythm, charges the capacitors, and delivers the countershocks. Chest compressions and ventilation efforts must cease while the device is operating. This permits accurate analysis of the cardiac rhythm and prevents accidental shocks to the rescuer. With some defibrillators, the movements of CPR can cause the device to interrupt or stop its analysis process. The time between activating the rhythm-analysis system, which is when CPR must stop, and the delivery of a countershock will average 10 to 15 seconds. This time without CPR is a recognized exception to the American Heart Association guidelines, which recommend that CPR not be stopped for longer than 5 seconds. With AEDs, the positive effects of delivering an early defibrillatory shock outweigh the negative effects of temporarily stopping CPR.

For patients in continued VF after the first countershock, CPR may have to be interrupted for even longer periods to deliver the three recommended, sequential shocks. Even though the Standards for CPR and Emergency Cardiac Care accept a period of up to 1.5 minutes for diagnosing VF and delivery of three countershocks, all currently marketed automated defibrillators can deliver three countershocks in less than 45 seconds.

Delivery of the Shocks

The defibrillation pads are placed in position on the upper right sternal border and left lower ribs over the apex of the heart. The sternal pad (to which the white or negative cable is connected) is located immediately to the right of the sternum and just under the clavicle. The apex pad (to which the red or positive cable is connected) is located just under the margin of the left breast, laterally toward the left midaxillary line. Once the pads and cables are properly attached, all contact with the patient, including CPR, must be stopped so that accurate rhythm analysis may occur. Analysis of the rhythm takes from 5 to 15 seconds, depending on the brand of the automated defibrillator. If VF is present, the device will announce that a shock is indicated by a screen text message, a visual indicator, an audible tone, and often a voice-synthesized statement.

The defibrillator operator must always state loudly a "Clear the patient," message such as "I'm clear," "You're clear," "Everybody clear," or simply "Clear," before pressing the shock delivery control. In addition, the defibrillator operator should visually check the patient to ensure no one has inadvertently come in contact with the patient. Shock delivery should produce a sudden contraction of the patient's musculature. Most devices deliver 200 joules for the first shock. At least one new defibrillator, however, is designed to deliver a lower energy setting (>130 joules) using a different shock waveform.

After the first shock is delivered, do not restart CPR. Press the analyze control immediately to start another rhythm analysis cycle. If a shockable rhythm persists, the device will indicate this, and the "charging" and "shock indicated" sequence should be repeated for the second and third shocks.

Persistent Ventricular Fibrillation

The energy level of the second and third shock can range from 200 to 360 joules depending upon the AED's configuration. Some automated defibrillators are programmed to automatically increase the energy level to 200 to 300 joules on the second and to 360 joules for the third shock as well as any subsequent shocks.

If VF persists after three shocks, CPR should be resumed for 60 seconds. Then deliver another sequence of three "stacked" defibrillatory shocks after the appropriate analysis periods.

Persistent Ventricular Fibrillation after Six Shocks

Ventricular fibrillation rarely persists after six countershocks. Nevertheless, for the unusual occurrence of refractory VF after six countershocks, the following recommendations are made:

■ In tiered-response systems, the EMT should continue to deliver sets of three stacked shocks separated by 1 minute of CPR. This is continued until the patient is no longer in VF or until advanced cardiac life support (ACLS) responders arrive and direct otherwise.

■ In some EMS systems, paramedic response is unavailable or there will be long transport times to ACLS care. In such cases, it is reasonable to continue three stacked shocks, separated by 1 minute of CPR, until VF is converted to normal rhythm or until the device gives a message that shocks are no longer indicated. When paramedics are not available and there is a very short transport time to the nearest hospital or emergency facility, EMTs may be directed by medical control to stop shocking refractory VF after six shocks. In cases of long transport times to ACLS care, transporting with ongoing CPR is unlikely to result in a successful resuscitation for the VF patient. Studies have demonstrated the low probability of survival when sudden cardiac arrest victims are transported to a hospital with ongoing CPR.

AEDs can be left attached to the patient during transport in moving vehicles. They should never, however, be placed in analyze mode when the vehicle is moving. The movement of the transport vehicle may interfere with rhythm assessment, leading to a possibly inaccurate shock decision. If a patient deteriorates during transport and does require rhythm analysis and treatment, then the vehicle must be brought to a complete stop. In most cases, performing effective CPR in a rapidly moving ambulance is an extremely difficult task (except when mechanical CPR devices are used). Providing defibrillatory shocks in a rapidly moving motor vehicle also poses an increased potential for accidental shocks to EMS providers. Although the potential remains low with proper caution, there is little value in continuing the transport during defibrillation. The EMT-D's protocols must define when the EMT-D is no longer authorized to remain at the scene providing defibrillatory shocks, opting instead for rapid transport to a nearby hospital.

Refibrillation

If the patient regains a perfusing rhythm after countershocks, and then refibrillates, restart the treatment sequence from the beginning. Most AEDs that are configured to automatically increase energy levels will remain at the level programmed for the next shock. In these cases, the EMT-D should not change the energy setting by restarting the device. Instead, allow the AED to shock at its programmed energy level unless other procedures are required by the EMT-D's protocols. Whenever the "no shock indicated" message is received, check for a pulse and, if no pulse is found, resume CPR.

Three "no shock indicated" messages indicate a low probability that a shockable rhythm will be identified; therefore, the rhythm analysis periods should be repeated only after several minutes. However, AEDs with continuous patient monitoring systems may alert the operator to the possibility of a shockable rhythm. These devices prompt the operator with an audible "check patient" or "press analyze" message. When this prompt follows a "no shock indicated" analysis decision, the EMT-D should stop CPR, check for a pulse, and activate the analysis system. Newer defibrillators may be configured to automatically analyze the rhythm when a possible shockable rhythm is recorded. If the analysis identifies a shockable rhythm, the device will automatically charge and allow the operator to deliver a shock.

Application Criteria

AEDs should only be applied to patients who are in confirmed circulatory arrest (the absence of consciousness, normal respirations, and a carotid pulse). Although the new U.S. Department of Transportation EMT-B curriculum suggests application to those cardiac arrest patients over 12 years of age and weighing greater than 90 pounds, we suggest that application may be extended to patients over 8 years of age. This is consistent with current American Heart Association recommendations as well as those of many current AED manufacturers. The rationale for the lower age is based on the testing performed by the manufacturers with respect to AED rhythm interpretation and the risk/benefit assessment for the older child who may be in VF (although rarely). There is little chance of harm to the non-VF child (8 to 12 years old) but a significantly improved chance of resuscitation in the VF child. More work must be done to establish safe and effective means for first responder early defibrillation in children less than 8 years of age. As always, the EMT must follow the application criteria established by his/her medical director.

Postresuscitation Care

After successful defibrillatory shocks, the patient may become awake and responsive and/or may begin to breathe spontaneously. However, the patient may also remain in cardiac arrest without having a shockable rhythm even though the shocks successfully converted the patient's VF to an organized rhythm. When the defibrillatory shocks are unsuccessful, the patient may remain in a state of pulseless ventricular tachycardia or VF. In each event, overall patient care remains primary.

If the patient regains a pulse and blood pressure, the EMT must continue to support the patient with the following actions (ABCDs):

■ Properly position the patient and maintain the airway.

- ■ Ensure that the airway is clear. Suction as needed.
- ■ In the very rapid resuscitation, placement of the patient in the recovery position (lateral recumbent) may be appropriate, assuming spontaneous ventilations are present and adequate.

■ Without delay, assist ventilations and provide supplemental oxygen, if available.

- ■ If the ventilatory rate and/or depth are inadequate, assist the patient with bag-valve mask ventilations and 100% oxygen.
- ■ Assess the lung sounds for pulmonary edema or rhonchi. In these cases, the patient may benefit from positive pressure ventilation regardless of the spontaneous ventilatory rate and depth.
- ■ When the ventilatory rate and/or depth are adequate (typically found in patients with EMT-witnessed arrests and others with extremely short arrest times), provide high-flow oxygen using a partial or non-rebreather mask.

■ Assess perfusion.

- ■ A hypotensive postarrest patient may have experienced sufficient myocardial damage to prevent adequate cardiac output. Continued CPR may be necessary in the unconscious, hypotensive postarrest patient.
- ■ Continue to monitor other vital signs. This must be done frequently, particularly in the unconscious patient.

■ Monitor closely for the return of VF and cardiac arrest.

- Be prepared to quickly reassess the patient.
- Do not remove the AED from the patient until another defibrillator is available for use by the next level of care (e.g., paramedics, emergency department).
- Should the patient become unresponsive and pulseless, immediately return to the steps of analysis and defibrillation as needed.

■ Quickly perform a detailed physical exam and continue ongoing assessments.

- Once the patient's VF is resolved, perform a rapid, detailed physical exam.
- The physical exam should look for potential trauma occurring after the cardiac arrest (e.g., head injury from a fall), airway and breathing complications, or blood pressure abnormalities.
- Use other responders to assist in obtaining a focused history as well as a past medical history.
- Continuously reassess the patient, including ABCs and vital signs.

■ Perform additional treatment and prepare for transport.

- Provide treatment for serious trauma identified in the physical exam.
- Trauma treatment may even include cervical spine immobilization, positive pressure ventilations and positioning for blood pressure management (foot end of backboard elevated for shock or head end elevated for severe hypertension).
- For ease of movement, a backboard or other similar patient movement device should be used to place the patient on the stretcher. This device will also be helpful when moving the patient at the hospital.

■ Continue patient care while awaiting the arrival of the ALS team or transporting.

- Be attentive to the ABCDs.
- Notify the incoming ACLS responders or the receiving hospital of critical patient information.
- Always be watchful for the return of VF!

■ STANDING ORDERS FOR EMT-Ds

The following are standing orders for EMT-Ds using AEDs in King County, Washington. The standing orders for manual external defibrillation by EMTs are not included, because this function is not within the scope of this book. These standing orders are provided as an example only.

Standing Orders for Patient Treatment for King County EMS Personnel Trained in Early Defibrillation

Scope

These Standing Orders direct the use of both automated and manual external defibrillators operated by currently certified and authorized King County EMS Defibrillation Providers.

Purpose

The purpose of these orders is to direct the prompt defibrillation of patients who have confirmed circulatory arrest due to ventricular fibrillation.

Authorization

In the event of a full cardiac arrest in King County, Washington, the Defibrillation Provider is authorized to perform the following:

I. Immediately upon arrival, verify respiratory and circulatory arrest by the absence of: consciousness, normal respirations and a carotid pulse.

II. Initiate CPR and defibrillation protocols.

III. GENERAL DEFIBRILLATION PROTOCOL. King County EMS Defibrillation Providers are authorized to deliver electric shocks with a defibrillator to patients whose ECG rhythm is VF. This should be done as quickly as possible, with a minimum interruption of CPR. Exact sequencing details may vary as long as the following overall goals are realized:

    A. VF is *shocked repeatedly* and as *rapidly* as possible.
    B. *Effective CPR* is performed and *interrupted for a minimum time.*
    C. *Overall patient care and safety* are never neglected.

IV. ASSESSMENT. Assess/analyze the ECG rhythm for the presence of ventricular fibrillation (VF):

    A. Turn the defibrillator power on and begin a verbal report.
    B. Immediately attach the defib pads with cables to the patient's chest.
    C. Clear patient to analyze/assess the patient's rhythm.

V. TREATMENT ALGORITHM FOR AUTOMATED EXTERNAL DEFIBRILLATION.

    1. Assess ABCs. If not breathing, begin ventilations. If no pulse, then . . .
    2. Perform effective CPR until AED is attached.
    3. Clear the patient.
    4. Activate the analyze mode.

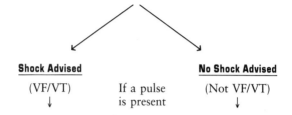

Shock Advised		**No Shock Advised**
(VF/VT)	If a pulse	(Not VF/VT)
↓	is present	↓

5. Deliver Three Stacked Shocks.

- Clear patient. Shock at 200 joules.
- Clear patient. Analyze. If shock advised, then . . .
- Clear patient. Shock at 200 joules.
- Clear patient. Analyze. If shock advised, then . . .
- Clear patient. Shock at 360 joules.

↓

6. Pulse Check/CPR/Pulse Check.
- Check pulse. If no pulse, then . . .
- Perform CPR for 15 seconds.
- Check pulse again. If no pulse, then . . .

↓

7. Deliver Three Stacked Shocks

- Clear patient. Analyze. If shock advised, then . . .
- Clear patient. Shock at 360 joules.
- Clear patient. Analyze. If shock advised, then . . .
- Clear patient. Shock at 360 joules.
- Clear patient. Analyze. If shock advised, then . . .
- Clear patient. Shock at 360 joules.

↓

5. Pulse Check/CPR/Pulse Check.
- Check pulse. If no pulse, then . . .
- Perform CPR for 15 seconds.
- Check pulse again. If no pulse, then . . .

↓

6. Analyze (2nd time)
- Clear patient.
- Analyze.
- If no shock indicated, then . . .

↓

7. Pulse Check/CPR/Pulse Check
- Check pulse. If no pulse, then . . .
- Perform CPR for 60 seconds
- Check pulse again. If no pulse, then . . .

↓

8. Pulse Check/CPR/Pulse Check.
- Check pulse. If no pulse, then . . .
- Perform CPR for 60 seconds.
- Check pulse again. If no pulse, then . . .

↓

9. Repeat Shocks and CPR.

- Alternate sets of up to 3 stacked shocks at 360 joules with effective CPR at 60-second intervals as long as VF persists.

8. Analyze (3rd time).
- Clear patient.
- Analyze.
- If no shock indicated, then . . .

↓

9. Pulse Check/CPR/Pulse Check
- Check pulse. If no pulse, then . . .
- Perform CPR until arrival of paramedics or the presence of VF.
- Check pulse every 1 to 3 minutes.

↓

If a pulse is present,
- Check the airway and breathing.
- Assist respirations; provide oxygen.
- Check the blood pressure.
- Proceed with other patient care.

NOTES

A. If VF recurs at any time, return to the VF protocol with shocks.

B. If VF has occurred anytime, continue analyzing the pulseless patient after every few minutes of CPR even if 3 "no shock advised" prompts are received.

C. If the patient is <u>never in VF</u> and three consecutive "no shock advised" prompts are received, continue effective CPR until paramedics arrive.

D. From the beginning of the resuscitation, the defib tech must take charge of the scene and patient care.

E. The "check patient" prompt indicates the patient <u>may now be in a shockable rhythm</u>. If the last analysis was a "no shock advised," the defib tech may assume there is a change in the patient's rhythm, stop CPR, check pulse, clear patient, and begin analysis.

F. Time and equipment permitting, record a paper strip when "no shock advised" prompt is received.

Appendix

A. CLINICAL GUIDELINES

1. NON–CARDIAC ARREST PATIENT.   In events other than cardiac arrest, the defib tech shall examine the patient, obtain vital signs and administer oxygen *before* initiating the use of the ECG monitor with monitoring electrodes. Each *Manual Defib provider* must be currently King County Manual Defib certified and authorized in order to place the ECG monitor on a non–cardiac arrest BLS patient (after the exam, vital signs, and oxygen). The *Automated Defib provider* may monitor a non–cardiac arrest patient. However, this can be done **ONLY**: (1) when on an ALS response with paramedics responding; (2) after completing the primary survey, obtaining vital signs, and providing appropriate treatment for ABCs; and (3) after applying ECG monitoring electrodes. *Defib Pads are not to be applied to non–cardiac arrest patients.*

2. **Carotid Pulse Check.**   In an unconscious, unresponsive patient, always check for a carotid pulse (absence of a femoral pulse does not confirm cardiac arrest).

3. **Communication.**   Verbal communication is to be ongoing throughout the event, describing the resuscitation as things occur. The cassette tape shall continue to record until pramedics arrive and specifically direct the defib tech to discontinue the tape recording, or until the patient is transported and care is assumed by hospital staff.

4. **No Prescribed Period of Initial CPR.**   Upon arrival at the scene and verification of cardiac arrest, the defibrillation EMT/ first responder shall proceed immediately with the defibrillation protocols outlined in these Standing Orders (after properly positioning the patient and working environment if necessary).

5. **No Excessive Interruptions of CPR.**   If delays in CPR of 5 seconds or more are encountered (e.g., vomiting, safety issue), resume CPR as soon as possible until the problem is resolved. Once the issue is resolved, reassess the patient and continue with the defib Standing Orders. Delays in CPR of more than 5 seconds are permitted only during rhythm assessment/analysis and shock delivery. *In particular, do not delay CPR while checking to see if a rhythm is producing a pulse. PULSE CHECKS SHOULD TAKE NO MORE THAN 5 SECONDS. IF NO PULSE IS FOUND IN 5 SECONDS, RESUME CPR IMMEDIATELY.*

6. **Blood Pressure Less Than 60 mm Hg.**   If the patient's systolic blood pressure after resuscitation is less than 60 mm Hg, and the patient remains unconscious, continue CPR. Do not stop chest compressions just because the heart has started to beat. The heartbeat may be inadequate to perfuse the patient but still may provide a pulse. Do not depend on touch to measure the blood pressure—it is notoriously inaccurate. Instead, use a blood pressure cuff.

7. **Rapid Defibrillation.**   The first shock should be delivered within 60 seconds of the provider's arrival at the patient's side. This time is typically started when the patient is determined to be pulseless (i.e., when the defib tech is authorized to power the defibrillator and apply to the patient). <u>For the defib tech</u>, defibrillation is the highest

priority in a cardiac arrest. It takes precedence over basic CPR, ventilations, suctioning, history taking, verbal updates, or to troubleshooting problems with the tape cassette or ECG paper. For the CPR technician, maintaining the airway, providing effective ventilations, and performing effective CPR are the highest priorities.

8. Documentation Submittal. Tape recordings are required for all cardiac arrest patients in whom CPR is started with a few exceptions (*CPR is required before defibrillator attachment*). The tape recording and Medical Report form must be submitted to King County EMS within 4 days of the cardiac arrest event. Tape recordings and, if applicable, paper strip recordings, are also required for all pediatric cardiac arrests.

B. Special Patient and Pediatric Guidelines

1. Pediatric Arrest. For children less than 8 years of age, verify cardiac arrest and begin effective CPR. As soon as possible, attach the defibrillator using monitoring electrodes only. Immediately after attachment, cease CPR and patient movement for a 10-second pulse check. Record the ECG during this interval on the cassette tape and paper (LifePak 250 or First Medic 710 only). After 10 seconds, resume effective CPR. During all 5-second pulse checks, ensure the cassette and paper tape recordings are made without motion. *Do not analyze or shock a cardiac arrest patient who is less than 8 years of age.* For children over 8 years of age, follow the standard defibrillation protocols.

2. Hypothermic Arrest. The hypothermic heart in VF (<85°F core temp.) does not respond to defibrillation. Since field body core temperatures are not available, defibrillation should not be withheld under the assumption that the heart is hypothermic. Analyze/assess the rhythm and, if the rhythm is VF, deliver up to 3 shocks in presumed hypothermic cardiac arrest. If VF persists after 3 shocks, stop defibrillation attempts. Resume CPR and rewarming.

3. Traumatic Arrest. Defibrillation is ineffective in the true traumatic cardiac arrest. If major blood loss/major trauma is obvious, initiate basic life support. Rhythm assessment and defibrillation have low priority in cardiac arrest due to trauma. If major blood loss/major trauma is not obvious, approach the patient as usual and initiate defibrillation protocols.

4. Automatic Internal (Implanted) Cardiodefibrillators (AICD). These devices have a limited number of shocks. The patient may still be in VF/VT after the AICD has exhausted its programmed therapies or its battery. If it appears the patient's AICD has delivered a shock, wait 1 minute from the time of the shock before attaching the external defibrillator and proceeding with the defibrillation Standing Orders. During the one-minute wait, continue with CPR and other resuscitation measures.

C. Safety in Defibrillation

1. Everyone, including the defib tech, must be clear of the patient when delivering the defib shock. The defib tech *must visually and verbally clear the patient prior to the shock*. Clearing of the patient is also required prior to rhythm analysis/assessment.
2. Ensure defib pads/paddles are in firm contact with the patient's skin. If necessary, shave excessive hair. If the patient is wet or sweaty, dry off the chest before attempting to apply pads or defibrillate.
3. Remove any creams, patches, and/or ointments from the chest (e.g., nitro patch, paste). Do not take the time to identify which type of cream/ointment/patch is on the patient.
4. Some agencies may have to transport patients to emergency facilities. If it is necessary to deliver a shock while transporting the patient, the defib tech shall proceed in the following manner:
   a. Bring the vehicle to a complete stop. Assure there is no motion affecting rhythm analysis.
   b. Reassess the rhythm to ensure that artifact is not mistakenly identified as VF.
   c. Assure the safety of all personnel. *Defibrillation hazards increase* in an area of limited space or when metal objects are close by.

■ Avoiding the Common Pitfalls

Even the most experienced defibrillation provider occasionally falls victim to the common pitfalls of resuscitation. Identifying these pitfalls and constantly striving to avoid them will be in the EMT-D's best interests. The following is a list of some common pitfalls along with suggested steps to avoid them.

Pitfall.   Focusing solely on the delivery of shocks.

Avoidance.   The focus must remain on resuscitation, not just defibrillation. All the elements of the chain of survival fit together to improve the victim's chance of successful resuscitation. For example, the value of CPR to successful defibrillation should not be forgotten. The defibrillator operator should delegate the responsibility for airway management and effective CPR to other team members. The EMT-D must be able to step back and look at the big picture. Every aspect of the resuscitation needs to be performed to the best of each team member's abilities. Even after converting VF to an organized rhythm, there is much patient care remaining to be done.

Pitfall.   Losing control of the scene (or not having it to begin with).

Avoidance. From the beginning of the resuscitation, the EMT-D operating the defibrillator must remain in charge of all patient care unless another on-scene responder with higher training is supervising and directing the EMT-D. Chaos often occurs when a team leader is not managing the resuscitation and effectively communicating with his/her team members. The EMT-D must be able to ensure that every aspect of the resuscitation is being performed well. This includes effective airway management and CPR, rapid defibrillation, scene safety, requests for additional resources, and all other patient care issues. Leadership, however, does not always mean dictating orders. Rather, it describes the ability to guide all team members toward the accomplishment of a specific mission. In this case, the mission is a successful resuscitation from sudden cardiac death.

PITFALL. Believing that training consists only of knowing how to operate the defibrillator and deliver shocks.

Avoidance. Learning how to operate the defibrillator and delivering shocks is actually the simplest part of the entire process. In the King County area, children as young as 11 years of age have been trained to operate an AED. The difficulty for the EMS provider is the integration of defibrillation with all the other aspects of resuscitation. Rapid assessment, CPR, airway management, safety, protocol adherence, and postresuscitation care must all be managed by the EMT-D. Consequently, effective training incorporates these aspects of resuscitation into the training scenario. Training should allow the EMT-D to demonstrate his/her ability to

- Properly operate the defibrillator
- Adhere to protocol directives
- Perform equipment troubleshooting
- Ensure safety
- Ensure effective CPR and airway management
- Adapt to special patients and situations
- Provide proper post resuscitation care

PITFALL. When the resuscitation is not going very well, panicking and losing control of the scene.

Avoidance. When this occurs, there are two common causes. First, training may have been insufficient or inadequate. Truly understanding the protocol sequences and putting them into practice in a training setting on a frequent basis will often solve this problem. This, of course, does not ensure that every aspect of the resuscitation will go well. Instead, it provides the EMT-D with instinctive reactions that are not adversely affected by those little things that frequently go wrong at an emergency scene. Frequent practice incorporating "problems" and adverse conditions at a scene will better prepare the EMT-D for these types of resuscitations.

Second, this situation may occur because the EMT-D has forgotten the number one rule of resuscitation: "Treat the Patient!" The EMT-D must keep in mind that the AED is another tool that can be used to achieve the goal of successful resuscitation from sudden cardiac arrest. Although the AED is a powerful and effective tool for the EMT-D, successful resuscitation will require all the skills of the EMT-D and his/her team. When in doubt as to what is the next step, think about the goals of resuscitation (from VF and non-VF) and treat the patient.

■ Public Access Defibrillation

Today, out-of-hospital defibrillation is primarily provided by first responders within local fire and EMS agencies. Across the United States, there is a move toward increasing the availability of AEDs. This effort, largely supported by the American Heart Association, should improve the chance of resuscitation for sudden cardiac arrest victims by decreasing the time to defibrillation. This movement has been termed "public access defibrillation" (PAD). In some ways, this term may be misconstrued for something it is not. The basic idea is to provide defibrillators that could be used by minimally trained persons who are not traditional first responders (not paid or volunteer fire or EMS providers). For example, the defibrillator may be placed in a high-rise building for use by specially trained persons (targeted responders) such as security officers.

Already, new defibrillators have been designed that are simpler to use, lightweight, easy to maintain, and less expensive than the AEDs used in recent years. Efforts are also underway to enact legislative changes that would address issues such as liability and would encourage PAD. Commercial airlines and police departments have already demonstrated the efficacy of this idea.

The movement toward training nontraditional first responders in the use of AEDs will certainly affect the EMT-D. The EMT-D and his/her EMS agency can improve the quality of this new aspect of the EMS system by taking an active role in the development of PAD programs. Coordination between developing PAD programs and local EMS providers is essential. Common issues for discussion during coordination efforts include

■ Equipment compatibility and familiarization
■ Protocol changes (if needed)
■ Role definitions
■ Opportunities for training and drilling together

The EMT-D may be a valuable resource to local organizations considering PAD programs. He/she should recognize the tremendous value offered to the community by early CPR and early defibrillation through PAD programs. Active participation by experienced EMT-Ds will only serve to enhance the quality of this new addition to the EMS system.

23 Pharmacology for the EMT

Increasingly, EMTs are being trained and directed to provide specific medications when indicated. The addition of medications to the EMT's treatment plan is most valuable when the therapeutic effect of the medication is dependent on early administration by first responders, and when ALS responders are delayed or unavailable. This is similar to the rationale for training EMTs and other first responders in the use of AEDs. In both cases, the failure of the first responder to provide early intervention creates a high likelihood of further deterioration of the patient's illness.

As with defibrillation, the EMT must understand the indications, contraindications, potential adverse effects, and medical directives for the proper use of medications. The number and types of medications available to the EMT will vary depending on local medical control. Although the number of available medications may be limited, the EMT may also assist the patient with his/her own medications. Medications typically administered by the EMT (see Table 23–1), as well as those for which the EMT provides assistance, are discussed in this chapter. Additional medication information may also be found in Appendix A.

■ MEDICAL CONTROL

Before treating a patient with medications, the EMT must completely understand the directives of his/her medical control. The EMT is allowed to administer or assist with the administration of medications only when authorized by his/her designated medical director or medical control. The medical director may provide these directives in a variety of forms, including the following.

STANDING ORDERS. In this case, the EMT's medical director will provide written directives and procedures for the use of medications. These directives and procedures must be followed exactly as written. Standing orders should include the indications, contraindications, and methods of administration for each medication.

GUIDELINES. In some agencies, the EMT medical director may simply provide written guidelines for the use of medications. These guidelines may allow some deviation based upon specified criteria. For example, the guidelines may allow the EMT to consider assisting the patient with his/her nitroglycerin when signs and symptoms of cardiac-related pain are present. These guidelines would not require

Table 23-1 Specific Medications Commonly Administered (Including Assisted Administration) by the EMT

Drug	Indications for Use	Side Effects and Contraindications	Administration and Dosage	Safety Notes and Other Information
Oxygen	Oxygen is provided to increase the concentration of oxygen inspired by the patient. It functions by increasing the oxygen available for transport to the tissues. It is provided to the patient whose illness or injury has created an increased demand for oxygen. Examples include shock, COPD, pulmonary edema, and apnea.	There are no true contraindications for oxygen administration. The most significant side effect is the potential for decreasing the respiratory drive in the COPD patient. This potential effect is disregarded when the patient is in respiratory distress.	Oxygen is delivered as an inhaled gas using a nasal cannula, face mask, bag-valve mask, or demand-valve mask. The dose varies with each delivery device and ranges from 2 to 25 L/min.	Oxygen is considered a hazardous material because it is an oxidizer and readily supports combustion. Keep away from hydrocarbons and ignition sources.
Glucose (Insta-Glucose)	Oral glucose is provided to the *conscious* hypoglycemic patient in order to raise the blood glucose level. Examples include hypoglycemic and insulin shock patients.	Providing glucose to the nonhypoglycemic patient may elevate the blood glucose level. This is a lesser risk than the hypoglycemic patient continuing to lower his/her glucose level, resulting in unconsciousness. Oral glucose is contraindicated in the patient with a decreased level of consciousness who is unable to control his/her airway.	Glucose is administered in a gel solution by placing the gel in the patient's mouth (cheek). It should be allowed to be initially absorbed in the mouth rather than swallowed. A small amount of the glucose gel is placed in the mouth at one time.	Assure the patient is awake and able to maintain his/her airway.

Medication				
Aspirin	Aspirin is provided to the patient suspected of having an acute MI. It is administered to reduce the risk of further clotting.	Aspirin is contraindicated in the patient who is hypersensitive to aspirin. It is also contraindicated in children with flu-like symptoms. The single dose provided by the EMT should not result in any possible side effects associated with chronic aspirin use.	In the prehospital setting, aspirin is often administered in the form of chewable tablets. The dosage will vary depending on the physician's experience. Typically 1–4 chewable baby aspirins, or 1 adult strength tablet, are sufficient (325 mg).	Assure the patient is awake, upright, and able to maintain his/her airway. Although aspirin is not included in the EMT curriculum, many systems allow its administration.
Nitroglycerin (Nitrostat, Nitrolingual spray)	The EMT may assist a patient with nitroglycerin when he/she is experiencing pain or discomfort consistent with previous angina episodes. The nitroglycerin serves to dilate the blood vessels, including the coronary arteries.	Nitroglycerin should not be administered to patients who are hypotensive. It also should not be given to the obvious acute MI patient or bradycardic patient without physician consultation. Side effects of nitroglycerin include a headache and decreased blood pressure. The EMT should ensure the nitroglycerin has been prescribed to the patient (i.e., the medication does not belong to someone else).	Nitroglycerin is typically prescribed for angina to patients in a spray or tablet form. The common dosage is 0.4 mg/tablet or metered spray.	The EMT must avoid holding a nitroglycerin tablet in his/her bare hand for a prolonged period of time. Skin absorption of nitroglycerin by the EMT may cause a headache or dizziness.

Table continued on following page

Table 23-1 [Continued]

Drug	Indications for Use	Side Effects and Contraindications	Administration and Dosage	Safety Notes and Other Information
Epinephrine (EpiPen)	Epinephrine is administered to patients experiencing a severe allergic reaction or anaphylactic reaction. The EMT may assist the patient in providing the self-administration. The epinephrine functions by countering the effects of bronchiole constriction and blood vessel dilation. This in turn improves blood pressure and respiratory difficulty.	When severe anaphylaxis is present, there are no real contraindications to the use of epinephrine. Nearly all patients are likely to experience side effects, including tremors, agitation, palpitations, and restlessness. Cardiac arrhythmias, including ventricular fibrillation, may be generated by the use of epinephrine. Patients with a history of hypertension or heart disease or who take antidepressant medications are at risk for other adverse effects.	The autoinjectable epinephrine is packaged with a fixed amount of drug. This amount in the package may vary between 0.2 and 1.0 mg. The typical dosage is 0.2–0.5 mg. Read the label carefully to ensure the patient administers the correct dosage.	If possible, have a defibrillator and/or cardiac monitor available. ALS must be requested or met if available.
Bronchodilators (Proventil, Ventolin, Alupent, Metaprel, Terbutaline, Brethaire)	Bronchodilators are administered to patients experiencing acute or chronic disease of the bronchioles. Typically, these patients have asthma or COPD. The EMT may assist the patient in self-	The patient who is unable to adequately ventilate on his/her own will not be able to properly use an inhaler or nebulizer. He/she requires ventilatory assistance. Side effects of bronchodilators include tachycardia, tremors,	Metered dose inhalers deliver a set dose with each puff. Medications for nebulized administration are prepackaged in single doses, although some may require the	The EMT must ensure the patient is properly using the inhaler or nebulizer to maximize effectiveness.

	administration of these medications. Bronchodilators function by dilating the narrowed or constricted bronchioles.	restlessness, agitation, palpitations, hypertension, and cardiac arrhythmias.	addition of a saline diluent.	
Syrup of ipecac	Syrup of ipecac induces vomiting. It is primarily used in accidental ingestions, poisonings, and overdoses.	Do not administer ipecac to patients with any of the following: altered mental status; seizures; pregnancy; acute MI; or ingestion of corrosives, petroleum products, antiemetics, strychnine, tricyclic antidepressants, or cocaine. When short transport times to the hospital are present or the time since ingestion has been prolonged, ipecac may not be necessary in the prehospital setting.	Ipecac is administered in the following dosages: Adult: 2 tablespoons (30 ml) Child: 1 tablespoon (15 ml) Infant: 1–2 teaspoons (5–10 ml) Follow with 2 to 4 glasses of water or clear liquid.	The EMT must ensure the patient is capable of maintaining his/her own airway. If the patient's level of consciousness is decreasing at all, the ipecac should not be given. Contact medical control before administering.
Activated charcoal	Activated charcoal absorbs and neutralizes many chemical substances. It is used in specific ingestions.	Do not administer activated charcoal prior to ipecac administration. The induced vomiting must be complete before administering charcoal. Because of its taste, many patients are reluctant to take the charcoal.	Charcoal is administered using 2 tablespoons (30 ml) in a glass of water. A sweetened slurry is available for children.	Contact medical control before administering.

the EMT to encourage the patient to use his/her nitroglycerin but would provide the EMT with that option.

ON-LINE MEDICAL CONTROL. In other agencies, the EMT may be required to contact (usually by radio or telephone) his/her designated medical control agency or person. After discussing the patient and the need for specific medication administration or assistance, the EMT will receive approval or denial to continue with the medication.

■ TERMINOLOGY AND ADMINISTRATION

Drug Names

Medications are referred to by their generic or trade names. *Generic names* are not specific to a manufacturer. They provide a simple way of identifying the drug (e.g., oral glucose). *Trade names* are names developed by a manufacturer for its particular products. They often have some resemblance to the generic name for ease of identification (e.g., Insta-Glucose).

Indications, Contraindications, and Side Effects

An *indication* is a sign, circumstance, or condition in which a medication may be provided to the patient in order to yield a specific treatment effect. The indications for use of a medication are those patient circumstances or conditions for which the medication may provide benefit. A *contraindication* is a condition or circumstance in which the administration of a medication may result in a harmful effect or unreasonable side effect. Medications are not administered when a contraindication is present. Since medications often affect many body systems, undesired effects may also occur when medications are administered. *Side effects* are undesirable but expected effects of a medication.

Action and Dosage

The *action* of a medication is the accomplishment of a desired effect or the effect itself. Since medications often have multiple effects, those that are undesirable are referred to as side effects. The *dosage* of the medication refers to the amount administered over a specified period of time. The dosage administered is the minimum amount necessary to achieve the desired effect (action).

Routes of Administration

Medications may be administered in a variety of ways. The method chosen depends upon the specific drug, the available form of the drug, and, in some cases, the desired rapidity of onset of action.

Routes of administration include intravenous, intramuscular injection, subcutaneous injection, inhalation, sublingual, and oral. The EMT-B may administer or assist in the administration of medications using any of these routes except the intravenous route.

Administration Specifics

INTRAMUSCULAR INJECTION

- This method provides a rapid absorption of the medication into the body and is a relatively simple task to learn.
- The EMT is unlikely to use this route of administration unless he/she is assisting a patient with an injection of epinephrine (e.g., autoinjectable epinephrine) for anaphylaxis.
- Once the intramuscular injection of epinephrine is administered by the patient, the EMT must closely monitor and continuously reassess the patient. When the patient is an adult, the EMT should have a defibrillator available in the unlikely event that the patient develops a lethal arrhythmia.

INHALATION

- This method provides a fairly rapid absorption, with fewer systemic effects.
- It is limited to certain drugs capable of being administered in this form. For the EMT, these drugs include oxygen and inhaled bronchodilators.
- Inhalation also requires that the patient be capable of properly using the inhaler or nebulizer. The patient must be ventilating adequately in order for inhaled bronchodilators to be used. The poorly ventilating patient must have ventilatory assistance rather than medication assistance.
- The EMT may assist the patient in using his/her own inhaled bronchodilators for relief of asthma or COPD.
  - Proper use of the inhaler or nebulizer is critical to obtaining the full effect of the medication.
  - When using a metered-dose inhaler, the patient usually tests the inhaler by activating it once into the air. He/she then places his/her mouth over the inhaler mouthpiece, creating a good seal. Holding the inhaler upright, the patient takes a deep breath and simultaneously activates the inhaler. If possible, the patient should attempt to hold his/her breath for a brief period (a few seconds).
  - When using a nebulizer, the patient places the medication into the nebulizer cup. After completing the assembly, the nebulizer is powered on. If functioning properly, the nebulizer should create a mist from the mouthpiece. Holding the nebulizer assembly upright, the patient places his/her mouth securely over the mouthpiece and inhales through his/her mouth. The patient should attempt to breathe in deeply and hold his/her breath for a brief period (a few seconds). The nebulizer may be powered by an air or oxygen device.
  - Coughing after using an inhaler or nebulizer is to be expected.
- The inhaler must contain a medication prescribed for acute episodes of respiratory difficulty (e.g., albuterol [Ventolin, Proventil], metaproterenol [Alupent]). Medications prescribed for daily use will not provide relief to the patient (e.g., triamcinolone [Azmacort], cromolyn [Intal]).

SUBLINGUAL ADMINISTRATION

- This method normally provides relatively rapid absorption.
- It is limited to certain drugs and requires an awake patient.
- The EMT may assist a patient in the use of his/her prescribed nitroglycerin. The EMT must assure that the nitroglycerin is prescribed for the patient, and not for another family member or friend.
- Nitroglycerin should not be administered to a patient who is hypotensive. In the setting of bradycardia, nitroglycerin should be used with caution.
- Procedures for administration include:
  - The patient must be sitting, semireclined, or supine. He/she must not suddenly sit up or stand for a few minutes following the nitroglycerin administration.
  - The patient should place one nitroglycerin tablet under his/her tongue. He/she should not swallow the tablet.
  - The EMT may ask the patient if the nitroglycerin seems to burn under the tongue as a means of assessing the potency of the medication. Nitroglycerin potency is affected by age, temperature, and moisture.
  - Nitroglycerin may also be prescribed in a spray form. The administration is provided by spraying the nitroglycerin under the tongue.
  - Nitroglycerin administration should be ceased if the patient becomes hypotensive or dizzy.
  - Nitroglycerin paste or patches normally are not used for the initial relief of anginal pain.

ORAL ADMINISTRATION

- This is the simplest route of administration; however, it is also the slowest.
- This route is limited to awake patients when administering specific medications. For the EMT, these medications will likely include oral glucose, aspirin, activated charcoal, and syrup of ipecac.
- When aspirin is administered, it should be in the chewable tablet form. Providing drinking water for the administration of nonchewable aspirin is not very practical in a transport vehicle. Syrup of ipecac and activated charcoal also require drinking water or clear liquids.
- Oral glucose is not initially swallowed by the patient. Rather, glucose is absorbed readily when placed in the cheek of the mouth. Although it may be swallowed, absorption may be more rapid via the membranes in the mouth rather than the GI tract.
- No medications should be placed in the mouth of a patient who cannot completely manage his/her own airway. The risk of aspiration is too great. In the case of the hypoglycemic diabetic (insulin shock), the patient should receive ALS care or immediate transport to a hospital emergency department.

■ SUMMARY

Although the administration of these or other medications may be included in the EMT's training, the authorization to administer medications to a patient must be provided by the EMT's medical director or medical control. Medication administration without such authorization is outside the EMT's scope of practice. The EMT should receive additional information and training when medication administration (other than oxygen) is to be part of his/her duties. As always, the EMT must follow local protocols and training directives.

Appendix A
Commonly Prescribed Drugs

■ GENERAL DRUG TYPES AND HOW THEY WORK

The majority of the emergent patients to which the EMT is called will have an illness or complaint related to a cardiac, respiratory, seizure, diabetes, or overdose emergency. With this in mind, this appendix provides information regarding commonly prescribed medications. For each general category of medications, the basic function of the drug, common examples, and potential adverse effects are listed. Keep in mind that the information contained in this appendix is not complete and provides a very small amount of detail. However, a basic understanding of commonly prescribed drugs may assist the EMT in learning some of the patient's past medical history as well as the potential for adverse effects in the event of an overdose.

Antihypertensive Drugs

Usually, drugs for hypertension are a mixture of two or more, or a combination of, drugs from the three basic categories used to reduce hypertension. The type of drug used is determined by the severity of the hypertension as well as the patient's overall medical history and general health.

VASODILATORS

- Vasodilators directly affect the muscles in the arterial walls and relax them, thereby reducing blood pressure.
- Trade names include Capoten, Prinivil, Vasotec, Minipress, Cardura, and Norvasc. (Generic names for these and other drugs mentioned in this appendix can be found in Table A–1, at the end of the appendix.)
- Adverse effects vary. Overdoses may lead to hypotension, orthostatic hypotension, dizziness, and tachycardia.

DIURETICS

- Diuretics reduce blood pressure by reducing fluid volume in the vascular system. (Some patients refer to these as "water pills.")
- Trade names include Lasix, Esidrix, Bumex, Aldactone, Hydrochlorothiazide, and Dyrenium.
- Adverse effects are relatively similar. Diuretics may lead to electrolyte imbalance, dehydration, and altered action of other drugs.

CENTRAL NERVOUS SYSTEM ANTAGONISTS

- CNS antagonists affect various parts of the CNS, which in turn cause a relaxation of the muscles in the blood vessels.
- Trade names include Catapres, Serpasil, Esimil, Tenormin, Lopressor, and Inderal.
- Adverse effects vary. Severe rebound hypertension may occur if medication is withdrawn abruptly (Catapres, Inderal). Hypotension and fatigue may occur.

Cardiac (Heart) Drugs

These drugs have a direct effect on the heart and the heart's electrical conduction system. Many of these drugs are prescribed for various medical illnesses including hypertension.

ANTIARRHYTHMICS

- Antiarrhythmics correct irregularities in the electrical impulses that cause the heart to beat in even cycles. Often the irregularity is a condition causing the heart to beat too fast or causing the heart to have extra beats.
- Trade names include Pronestyl, Inderal, Quinidex, Isoptin, Cardizem, Lanoxin, and Cordarone.
- Adverse effects can be very severe. Overdoses can lead to slow heart rates, hypotension, and cardiac arrest.

DIGITALIS FAMILY

- This special drug category has the effect of increasing the force of the heart's contractions and slowing the heart rate, thereby making the heart a more efficient pump.
- The most common trade name is Lanoxin.
- Adverse effects can become severe. Overdoses of Lanoxin can lead to slow heart rates, hypotension, and cardiac arrest.

ANTIANGINAL DRUGS

- Drugs in various categories such as the nitrate group (i.e., nitroglycerin) cause a relaxation of the arteries supplying the heart, thereby providing an increase in blood and oxygen to the heart. The drug Inderal is often used for its ability to slow down the heart rate, reducing the requirement for extra oxygen by not allowing the heart to increase its activity.
- Trade names include Nitro-Bid, Nitrostat, Nitro-Dur, and Isordil for the nitrates group. Other drugs include Inderal, Cardizem, and Procardia.
- Adverse effects of nitrates typically include headaches and orthostatic hypotension. Other antianginal drugs may also cause slow heart rates, hypotension, and dizziness. Overdoses may be severe due to extreme hypotension or extreme slowing of the heart rate.

Bronchodilators

Patients with chronic respiratory diseases such as asthma and COPD may have medications prescribed for use on a regular basis and others for use in cases of acute respiratory distress. Although most of these drugs fall into the category of bronchodilators, a few of the medications prescribed for regular use fall into other classifications, such as steroids.

- Bronchodilators cause relaxation of the bronchial muscles. Other drugs for chronic respiratory disease are used to decrease bronchial inflammation and/or to prevent the release of agents that cause inflammation.
- Trade names of bronchodilators include Proventil, Ventolin, Alupent, Atrovent, Primatene Mist, Maxair, Theo-Dur, Dilor, and Aminophylline. Other drugs for chronic respiratory disease include Beclovent, Aerobid, Azmacort, and Intal.
- The most common adverse effects of bronchodilators are increased heart rate, nervousness, and headache. Overuse, particularly with existing cardiac disease, may cause increased work of the heart, leading to additional acute cardiac complaints.

Diabetes Drugs

Patients with diabetes who are being treated with medications typically are prescribed insulin replacement or oral hypoglycemic drugs. Insulin replacement drugs are administered to the patient by daily subcutaneous injections.

- *Insulin replacement drugs* are used in patients who have a significant insulin production deficiency and therefore cannot produce the insulin required to maintain glucose control. *Oral hypoglycemic* drugs are prescribed to patients who have a decreased release of insulin and who are unable to control glucose levels through dietary methods.
- Examples of insulin replacement drugs include regular insulin (Novolin R, Humulin R), semilente, NPH insulin (Humulin N, NPH), insulin in zinc suspension (Humulin L, Lente, Novolin L), ultralente, and regular and NPH mixture (Novolin 70/30). Oral hypoglycemic drugs include Orinase, Glucotrol, Micronase, DiaBeta, Glucophage, and Diabinese. Some patients may also have glucagon for use by the patient, family, or EMS provider in an emergent hypoglycemic setting (glucagon can increase the blood glucose level).
- The single most common adverse effect of insulin replacement and oral hypoglycemic drugs is hypoglycemia (low blood sugar level). Overdoses of both types of drugs can be severe and life threatening if not treated promptly.

Anticonvulsants

Anticonvulsants are used to suppress seizures by reducing the "excitability" of neurons in the brain. Although an attempt is made to treat the seizure disorder with a single drug, multiple anticonvulsants may be prescribed if necessary.

- Anticonvulsants treat convulsions (seizures) by reducing the "excitability" of neurons in the brain.
- Trade names of anticonvulsants include Tegretol, Dilantin, Depakote, Klonopin, Neurontin, and Luminal.

- Adverse effects include drowsiness and CNS depression. Overdoses can result in severe CNS depression or unconsciousness. Dilantin overdoses may also cause cardiac arrhythmias and hypotension.

Antihistamines

Antihistamines are used to counteract the stuffy, runny nose; itchy eyes; and scratchy throat caused by the release of the body chemical histamine (immune response). This release is common with allergic and anaphylactic reactions.

- Antihistamines are used to relax bronchial muscles and inhibit vasodilation as well as increased capillary "leaking" resulting from an allergic reaction (immune response).
- Trade names include Benadryl, Tavist, Seldane, Claritin, and Vistaril.
- Adverse effects vary with the sedative effect of the drug. Effects include drowsiness, aggravation of asthma, and hypotension. Overdoses are likely to cause lethargy, unconsciousness, and hypotension.

Analgesics

Analgesics are used to relieve severe to mild pain. Analgesics may be classified into groups such as strong analgesics, mild analgesics, and antipyretics (fever reducing).

Strong Analgesics

- Strong analgesics are in the narcotic family. Trade names include MS Contin, Percodan, Dilaudid, Demerol, and Talwin.
- Adverse effects include nausea and vomiting, constipation, drug dependence, and drowsiness. Effects may be severe, particularly in overdoses, leading to respiratory depression, reduced gag reflex, inability to cough, decreased level of consciousness, hypotension, and seizures.

Mild Analgesics: Narcotic Containing

- Mild analgesics are a weaker form of narcotics. Trade names include Codeine Sulfate and Darvon. These may be found in combination with other analgesics (e.g., Tylenol with codeine.)
- Adverse effects include nausea, vomiting, and drowsiness. Overdoses may produce effects similar to those of strong analgesics, including CNS depression, convulsions, and respiratory depression.

Mild Analgesics: Antipyretics

- Although used for mild pain relief, some of these drugs are often used for other effects, including fever reduction and anti-inflammatory, and anti-clotting effects. Drugs within this group are often referred to as nonsteroidal anti-inflammatory drugs (NSAIDs). Examples include aspirin (Ecotrin), acetaminophen (Tylenol), ibuprofen (Advil, Motrin), naproxen (Aleve), and indomethacin (Indocin).
- The most common adverse effect of these drugs is related to GI upset and possible GI bleeding (with long-term use; excludes acetaminophen). Aspirin

is not recommended for children with flu-like symptoms, because there is an increased risk of Reye's syndrome. Overdose of aspirin may cause ringing in the ears (tinnitus), dizziness, fever, hyperventilation, and an altered level of consciousness. Massive overdoses of ibuprofen may cause coma, renal failure, seizures, and cardiorespiratory arrest. Generally, patients who overdose on NSAIDs are asymptomatic with the exception of GI upset. Significant overdoses of acetaminophen may result in damage to the liver.

Psychotropic Drugs

These drugs have been found to be useful in managing day-to-day stress by relieving the symptoms of psychiatric disorders. Psychotropic drugs are separated into three categories: antianxiety drugs, antidepressant drugs, and antipsychotic drugs.

ANTIANXIETY DRUGS

- Anxiety neurosis is characterized by panic, apprehension, tension, and fatigue. Antianxiety drugs include the benzodiazepines, such as Valium, Librium, Serax, and Equanil.
- Adverse effects include drowsiness, drug dependence, and behavioral disinhibition. Overdoses may lead to respiratory depression and decreased level of consciousness.

ANTIDEPRESSANT DRUGS

- Depressed patients are brooding, suffer feeling of extreme helplessness, and tend to be self-critical. They often experience fatigue, loss of appetite, headache, and decreased concentration. Antidepressant drugs generally fall into the categories of tricyclic antidepresssants, monoamine oxidase (MAO) inhibitors, and others.
- Trade names of tricyclic antidepressants include Elavil, Tofranil, Sinequan, Norpramin, Pamelor, and Anafranil. Adverse effects include sedation and hypotension. Overdoses may be severe and lethal. Effects of overdoses include fast heart rate, decreased level of consciousness, cardiac arrhythmias, hypotension, seizures, and cardiac arrest.
- Trade names of MAO inhibitors include Parnate, Nardil, and Marplan. Adverse effects include overstimulation of the CNS and orthostatic hypotension. Overdoses may present with agitation, hallucinations, increased temperature, and seizures. May cause hypertensive crisis if the patient eats fermented food/drink (e.g., dairy and yeast products, wine) or takes amphetamine-like drugs such as those found in diet pills or cold medicines.
- Trade names of other antidepressants include Prozac, Desyrel, Zoloft, Paxil, Ludiomil, and Wellbutrin. Adverse effects vary but may include nausea, headache, and agitation. These antidepressants are not as toxic as are tricyclic antidepressants.

ANTIPSYCHOTIC DRUGS

- Antipsychotic drugs are divided into three categories: the phenothiazines, the butyrophenones, and the thioxanthenes. Because of their side effects, these drugs are saved for the most severe situations. Antipsychotic drugs have direct effect on the brain to control paranoid or schizophrenic disorders.

- Trade names of phenothiazines include Thorazine, Mellaril, Prolixin, Compazine, and Stelazine. Adverse effects include orthostatic hypotension and acute dystonic reactions (abnormal muscle tone, often presenting as an enlarged tongue with interference with normal speech and swallowing).

- Trade names of thioxanthenes include Navane and Taractan. Adverse effects may include hypotension, but to a lesser degree than phenothiazines.

- One trade name of the butyrophenones is Haldol. This drug is also used to treat Tourette syndrome and behavioral problems in children. Adverse effects include sedation and potentially dramatic dystonic reactions.

■ COMMONLY USED MEDICATIONS AND THEIR INDICATIONS

Table A–1 is an alphabetical list by brand name and generic name (in capital letters) of the most commonly used drugs, the usual indications for use, and the basic families from which they are derived. Only the medicines that are used on a long-term basis are included. Short-term or occasionally used drugs such as antibiotics, hormones, birth control pills, and medicines for colds have been excluded. Also, many of these drugs have been selected to assist the EMT to recognize pertinent chronic disease by the medicine taken by the patient. The medicines in the table are usually potent and have serious side effects when not used as prescribed. This table of drugs is established from a list of drugs used over the entire United States. EMTs should become familiar with the drugs more commonly used in their own communities.

Drug	Indications for Use	General Drug Type
ACETAMINOPHEN	Tylenol, Datril	Pain, fever, inflammation	Mild analgesic
ACETAZOLAMIDE	Diamox	Seizures, glaucoma	Weak diuretic
ACYCLOVIR	Zovirax	Herpes	Antiviral drug
Adapin	DOXEPIN	Depression	Tricyclic antidepressant
Aerobid	FLUNISOLIDE	Asthma	Anti-inflammatory
ALBUTEROL	Proventil, Ventolin	Asthma, COPD	Bronchodilator
Aldactazide	SPIRONOLACTONE + HYDROCHLOROTHIAZIDE	High blood pressure	Potassium-sparing diuretic
Aldactone	SPIRONOLACTONE	High blood pressure	Potassium-sparing diuretic
Aldomet	METHYLDOPA	High blood pressure	Used in combination with other hypertensive medications
Aldoril	METHYLDOPA + HYDROCHLOROTHIAZIDE	High blood pressure	Diuretic with CNS relaxant of vascular system
ALLOPURINOL	Zyloprim	Gout, high uric acid blood level	Prophylactic for gout
ALPRAZOLAM	Xanax	Anxiety	Tranquilizer
Alupent	METAPROTERENOL	Asthma	Bronchodilator
Aminophylline	—	Asthma	Bronchodilator
AMIODARONE	Cordarone	Cardiac arrhythmia	Antiarrhythmic
AMITRIPTYLINE	Elavil, Triavil	Depression	Tricyclic antidepressant
AMLODIPINE	Norvasc	Hypertension	Vasodilator

Table continued on following page

379

Table A-1 (Continued)

	Drug	Indications for Use	General Drug Type
AMOXAPINE	Asendin	Depression	Antidepressant
Anafranil	CLOMIPRAMINE	Depression	Tricyclic antidepressant
Anaprox	NAPROXEN	Pain, inflammation, arthritis	Non-narcotic, nonsteroidal analgesic
Anhydron	CYCLOTHIAZIDE	High blood pressure	Diuretic
Antivert	MECLIZINE	Vertigo	Antihistamine
Apresoline	HYDRALAZINE	Essential hypertension	Vasodilator
Artane	TRIHEXYPHENIDYL	Parkinson's disease	Synthetic antispasmodic—works like atropine
Asendin	AMOXAPINE	Depression	Antidepressant
Atarax	HYDROXYZINE	Nausea, vomiting, anxiety, tension	Antihistamine
ATENOLOL	Tenormin	Angina, hypertension	Beta-adrenergic blocker—action is to slow heart rate
Ativan	LORAZEPAM	Anxiety, for sleep	CNS tranquilizer
Atrovent	IPRATROPIUM	COPD	Bronchodilator
Azmacort	TRIAMCINOLONE	Asthma	Anti-inflammatory
Azolid	PHENYLBUTAZONE	Arthritis, other inflammations	Anti-infammatory
BECLOMETHASONE	Vanceril, Beclovent	Asthma	Anti-inflammatory
Beclovent	BECLOMETHASONE	Asthma	Anti-inflammatory
Benadryl	DIPHENHYDRAMINE	Allergic reaction	Antihistamine
Benemid	PROBENECID	Gout, high uric acid blood level	Prophylactic for gout
Bentyl	DICYCLOMINE	Nausea and vomiting	Anticholinergic

Drug	Indication	Classification
BENZTROPINE / Cogentin	Parkinsonism	Anticholinergic
Blockadren / TIMOLOL MALEATE	Angina, hypertension	Beta-adrenergic blocker—action is to slow heart rate
Brethine / TERBUTALINE	Asthma	Bronchodilator
Bricanyl / TERBUTALINE	Asthma	Bronchodilator
BUMETANIDE / Bumex	Hypertension	Diuretic
Bumex / BUMETANIDE	Hypertension	Diuretic
BUPROPION / Wellbutrin	Depression	Antidepressant
Butazolidin / PHENYLBUTAZONE	Arthritis	Short-term anti-inflammatory
Calan / VERAPAMIL	Effort angina, coronary artery spasm, paroxysmal atrial tachycardia (PAT)	Calcium channel blocker
Capoten / CAPTOPRIL	Hypertension	Antihypertensive
CAPTOPRIL / Capoten	Hypertension	Antihypertensive
CARBAMAZEPINE / Tegretol	Seizure	Anticonvulsant
Cardioquin / QUINIDINE	Cardiac arrhythmia	Antiarrhythmic
Cardizem / DILTIAZEM	Angina	Calcium channel blocker
Cardura / DOXAZOSIN	Hypertension	Vasodilator
Catapres / CLONIDINE	High blood pressure	Neuroeffector vasodilator
CHLORDIAZEPOXIDE / Librium	Anxiety	Tranquilizer
CHLORPROMAZINE / Thorazine	Psychosis	Antipsychotic (phenothiazine)
CHLORPROPAMIDE / Diabinese	Diabetes	Oral hypoglycemic
CHLORPROTHIXENE / Taractan	Psychosis	Antipsychotic (thioxanthene)
CHLORTHALIDONE / Hygroton	Congestive heart failure, hypertension	Diuretic
CHLORTHALIDONE + RESERPINE / Regroton	CHF, high blood pressure	Diuretic

Table continued on following page

Table A-1 (Continued)

DRUG	DRUG	INDICATIONS FOR USE	GENERAL DRUG TYPE
CHLOROTHIAZIDE	Diuril, Diupres	High blood pressure	Vasodilator
CIMETIDINE	Tagamet	Ulcer disease	Histamine H_2 receptor antagonist
Claritin	LORATADINE	Allergic reaction	Antihistamine
CLEMASTINE	Tavist	Allergic reaction	Antihistamine
Clinoril	SULINDAC	Arthritis	NSAID
CLOMIPRAMINE	Anafranil	Depression	Tricyclic antidepressant
CLONAZEPAM	Klonopin	Seizures	CNS depressant
CLONIDINE	Catapres	High blood pressure	Neuroeffector vasodilator
CLORAZEPATE	Tranxene	Anxiety	CNS tranquilizer
Cogentin	BENZTROPINE	Parkinsonism	Anticholinergic
ColBenemid	COLCHICINE	Gout	Prophylactic for gout
COLCHICINE	ColBenemid	Gout	Prophylactic for gout
Compazine	PROCHLORPERAZINE	Nausea, psychosis	Antipsychotic (phenothiazine)
Cordarone	AMIODARONE	Cardiac arrhythmia	Antiarrhythmic
Corgard	NADOLOL	Angina, hypertension	Beta-adrenergic blocker—action is to slow heart rate
Coumadin	WARFARIN	Post-CVA, blood clot	Anticoagulant
CROMOLYN	Intal	Asthma	Inhibits the release of histamines
CYCLANDELATE	Cyclospasmol	Nighttime leg cramps, thrombophlebitis	Vasodilator
CYCLOBENZAPRINE	Flexeril	Muscle spasms, pain	Smooth muscle relaxor
Cyclospasmol	CYCLANDELATE	Nighttime leg cramps, thrombophlebitis	Vasodilator
CYCLOTHIAZIDE	Anhydron	High blood pressure	Diuretic

CYPROHEPTADINE	Periactin	Colds, allergies	Phenothiazine
Dalmane	FLURAZEPAM	Insomnia	Benzodiazepine
Darvocet	PROPOXYPHENE NAPSYLATE	Pain	Mild analgesic, mild narcotic
Darvon	PROPOXYPHENE	Pain	Mild analgesic, mild narcotic
Darvon-N	PROPOXYPHENE NAPSYLATE	Pain	Mild analgesic, mild narcotic
Datril	ACETAMINOPHEN	Pain, fever, inflammation	Analgesic
Deltasone	PREDNISONE	Asthma, arthritis	Anti-inflammatory
Depakote	DIVALPROEX	Seizures	Anticonvulsant
Demerol	MEPERIDINE	Severe pain	Strong narcotic (opiate)
DESIPRAMINE	Norpramin	Depression	Tricyclic antidepressant
Desyrel	TRAZODONE	Depression	Antidepressant
DiaBeta	GLYBURIDE	Diabetes	Oral hypoglycemic
Diabinese	CHLORPROPAMIDE	Diabetes	Oral hypoglycemic
Diamox	ACETAZOLAMIDE	Seizures, glaucoma	Diuretic
DIAZEPAM	Valium	Seizures, anxiety	Benzodiazepine, CNS tranquilizer
DICYCLOMINE	Bentyl	Nausea, vomiting	Anticholinergic
DIFLUNISAL	Dolobid	Pain, inflammation, arthritis	Non-narcotic, nonsteroidal analgesic
DIGOXIN	Lanoxin	CHF, cardiac arrhythmia	Antiarrhythmic
Dilantin	PHENYTOIN	Seizures	Anticonvulsant
Dilaudid	HYDROMORPHONE	Severe pain	Strong narcotic (opiate)
Dilor	DIPHYLLINE	Asthma	Bronchodilator
DILTIAZEM	Cardizem	Effort angina, coronary artery spasm	Calcium channel blocker
DIPHENHYDRAMINE	Benadryl	Allergic reaction	Antihistamine
DIPHENOXYLATE	Lomotil	Diarrhea	Antidiarrheal anticholinergic
DIPYRIDAMOLE	Persantine	Cardiac chest pain	Antianginal

Table continued on following page

Table A-1 (Continued)

Drug		Indications for Use	General Drug Type
DISOPYRAMIDE	Norpace	Cardiac arrhythmia	Antiarrhythmic
Diuril, Diupres	CHLOROTHIAZIDE	High blood pressure	Vasodilator
DIVALPROEX	Depakote	Seizures	Anticonvulsant
Dolene	PROPOXYPHENE	Pain	Mild analgesic, mild narcotic
Dolobid	DIFLUNISAL	Pain, inflammation, arthritis	Non-narcotic, nonsteroidal analgesic
Donnatal	PHENOBARBITAL + HYOSCAMINE + ATROPINE + SCOPOLAMINE	Stomach spasm	Anticholinergic
Doriden	GLUTETHIMIDE	Insomnia	Nonbarbiturate sedative-hypnotic
DOXAZOSIN	Cardura	Hypertension	Vasodilator
DOXEPIN	Adapin, Sinequan	Depression	Antidepressant
Dyazide	HYDROCHLOROTHIAZIDE + TRIAMTERENE	High blood pressure	Diuretic
DYPHYLLINE	Dilor	Asthma	Bronchodilator
Dyrenium	TRIAMTERENE	High blood pressure	Potassium-sparing diuretic
Edecrin	ETHACRYNIC ACID	High blood pressure	Diuretic
Elavil	AMITRIPTYLINE	Depression	Tricyclic antidepressant
Elixophylline	THEOPHYLLINE	Asthma	Bronchodilator
ENALAPRIL	Vasotec	Hypertension	ACE inhibitor
Enduron	METHYCLOTHIAZIDE	CHF	Diuretic
EPHEDRINE/THEOPHYLLINE	Marax	Asthma	Bronchodilator
Equanil	MEPROBAMATE	Anxiety, tension, promotes sleep	Tranquilizer

384

Esidrix		Diuretic
Esimil		Neuroeffector vasodilator
ETHACRYNIC ACID	High blood pressure	Hypnotic
ETHCHLORVYNOL	High blood pressure	Sedative-hypnotic
ETHOSUXIMIDE	Insomnia	Anticonvulsant
HYDROCHLOROTHIAZIDE	High blood pressure	
GUANETHIDINE	High blood pressure	
Edecrin	High blood pressure	
Placidyl	Insomnia	
Zarontin	Petite mal seizures	
PIROXICAM	Pain, inflammation, arthritis	Non-narcotic, nonsteroidal analgesic
FENOPROFEN	Arthritis	NSAID
Feosol	Iron deficiency	Iron
FERROUS SULFATE	Iron deficiency	Iron
Feldene		
Nalfon		
FERROUS SULFATE		
Fiorinal	Pain	Analgesic
Flagyl	Vaginal infection	Antiprotozoal, antibacterial
Flexeril	Muscle spasms, pain	Smooth muscle relaxor
FLUNISOLIDE	Asthma	Anti-inflammatory
FLUOXETINE	Depression	Antidepressant
FLUPHENAZINE	Psychosis	Antipsychotic (phenothiazine)
FLURAZEPAM	Insomnia	Benzodiazepine
FUROSEMIDE	High blood pressure, CHF	Diuretic
Aspirin combination		
METRONIDAZOLE		
CYCLOBENZAPRINE		
Aerobid		
Prozac		
Prolixin		
Dalmane		
Lasix		
GABAPENTIN	Seizures	Anticonvulsant
SULFAMETHOXAZOLE	Urinary tract infection	Sulfa drug
GLIPIZIDE	Diabetes	Oral hypoglycemic
Glucophage	Diabetes	Oral hypoglycemia
GLIPIZIDE	Diabetes	Oral hypoglycemic
GLUTETHIMIDE	Insomnia	Nonbarbiturate sedative-hypnotic
GLYBURIDE	Diabetes	Oral hypoglycemic
GUANETHIDINE	High blood pressure	Neuroeffector vasodilator
Neurontin		
Gantanol		
Glucotrol		
Metformin		
Glucotrol		
Doriden		
DiaBeta, Micronase		
Ismelin, Esimil		

Table continued on following page

385

Table A-1 (Continued)

DRUG		INDICATIONS FOR USE	GENERAL DRUG TYPE
Halcion	TRIAZOLAM	Insomnia	Hypnotic
Haldol	HALOPERIDOL	Psychosis	Antipsychotic (butyrophenone)
HALOPERIDOL	Haldol	Psychosis	Antipsychotic (butyrophenone)
HYDRALAZINE	Apresoline	High blood pressure	Vasodilator
HYDROCHLOROTHIAZIDE	Esidrix, Hydrodiuril, Oretic	High blood pressure, CHF	Diuretic
HYDROCHLOROTHIAZIDE + TRIAMTERENE	Dyazide	High blood pressure	Diuretic
Hydrodiuril	HYDROCHLOROTHIAZIDE	High blood pressure, CHF	Diuretic
HYDROMORPHONE	Dilaudid	Severe pain	Strong narcotic (opiate)
Hydropres	RESERPINE + HYDROCHLOROTHIAZIDE	High blood pressure	Neuroeffector vasodilator
HYDROXYZINE	Vistaril, Atarax	Nausea, vomiting, anxiety, tension	Antihistamine
Hygroton	CHLORTHALIDONE	CHF, high blood pressure	Diuretic
IBUPROFEN	Motrin	Arthritis	NSAID
Imavate	IMIPRAMINE	Depression	Antidepressant
IMIPRAMINE	Imavate, Tofranil, SK-Pramine	Depression	Antidepressant
Inderal	PROPRANOLOL	Angina, cardiac arrhythmia, hypertension	Beta-adrenergic blocker—action is to slow heart rate
Indocin	INDOMETHACIN	Arthritis	NSAID
INDOMETHACIN	Indocin	Arthritis	NSAID

INSULIN	Ilentin, Lente Semilente, Ultralente NPH, NPH Ilentin, Protamine, Humulin R, Humulin N, Novolin 70/30, Novolin L, Zinc Insulin	Diabetes	Insulin replacement
Intal	CROMOLYN	Asthma	Inhibits the release of histamines
IPRATROPIUM	Atrovent	COPD	Bronchodilator
Ismelin	GUANETHIDINE	High blood pressure	Neuroeffector vasodilator
ISOCARBOXAZID	Marplan	Depression	MAO inhibitor
Isoptin	VERAPAMIL	Effort angina, coronary artery spasm, PAT	Calcium channel blocker
Isordil	ISOSORBIDE DINITRATE	Angina	Antianginal (nitrates), vasodilator
Isosorb	ISOSORBIDE DINITRATE	Angina	Antianginal (nitrates), vasodilator
ISOSORBIDE DINITRATE	Isordil, Isosorb, Sorbitrate	Angina	Antianginal (nitrates), vasodilator
ISOXSUPRINE	Vasodilan	Chronic organic brain disease	Vasodilator
K-Dur	POTASSIUM CHLORIDE	Potassium replacement	Potassium supplement
K-Lyte	POTASSIUM CHLORIDE	Potassium deficiency	Potassium supplement
Klonopin	CLONAZEPAM	Seizures	CNS depressant
LABETALOL	Normodyne, Trandate	Hypertension	Beta blocker
Lanoxin	DIGOXIN	CHF, cardiac arrhythmia	Antiarrhythmic
Lasix	FUROSEMIDE	CHF, high blood pressure	Diuretic
LEVOTHYROXINE	Synthroid	Hypothyroidism	Thyroid hormone
Librium	CHLORDIAZEPOXIDE	Anxiety	Antianxiety drug
LISINOPRIL	Prinivil, Zestril	Hypertension	ACE inhibitor
Lomotil	DIPHENOXYLATE	Diarrhea	Antidiarrheal anticholinergic
Lopressor	METOPROLOL	High blood pressure	Beta blocker

Table continued on following page

Table A-1 (Continued)

Drug		Indications for Use	General Drug Type
LORATADINE	Claritin	Allergic reaction	Antihistamine
LORAZEPAM	Ativan	Anxiety, for sleep	CNS tranquilizer
Ludiomil	Ludiomil	Depression	Antidepressant
Luminal	Luminal	Seizure	Anticonvulsant, sedative
MAPROTILINE	Ludiomil	Depression	Antidepressant
Marax	EPHEDRINE + HYDROXYZINE + THEOPHYLLINE	Asthma	Bronchodilator, sedative
Marplan	ISOCARBOXAZID	Depression	MAO inhibitor
Maxair	PIRBUTEROL	Asthma	Bronchodilator
MECLIZINE	Antivert	Vertigo	Antihistamine
Mellaril	THIORIDAZINE	Psychosis	Antipsychotic (phenothiazine)
MEPERIDINE	Demerol	Severe pain	Strong narcotic (opiate)
MEPROBAMATE	Equanil, Miltown	Anxiety, tension, promotes sleep	Tranquilizer
Metahydrin	TRICHLORMETHIAZIDE	High blood pressure	Diuretic
METAPROTERENOL	Alupent	Asthma	Bronchodilator
Metformin	Glucophage	Diabetes	Oral hypoglycemia
METHIMAZOLE	Tapazole	Hyperthyroidism	Inhibits synthesis of thyroid hormones
METHYCLOTHIAZIDE	Enduron	CHF	Diuretic
METHYLDOPA	Aldomet	High blood pressure	Used in combination with other hypertensive medications
METHYLDOPA + HYDROCHLOROTHIAZIDE	Aldoril	High blood pressure	Diuretic with CNS relaxant of vascular system

METHYLPHENIDATE	Ritalin	Narcolepsy, hyperactivity	CNS stimulant
METOLAZONE	Zaroxolyn	High blood pressure	Diuretic
METOPROLOL	Lopressor	High blood pressure	Beta blocker
METRONIDAZOLE	Flagyl	Vaginal infection	Antiprotozoal, antibacterial
Micronase	GLYBURIDE	Diabetes	Oral hypoglycemic
Miltown	MEPROBAMATE	Anxiety, tension, promotes sleep	Tranquilizer
Minipress	PRAZOSIN	Hypertension	Beta-adrenergic blocker—action is to slow heart rate
MORPHINE	MS Contin	Severe pain	Strong narcotic (opiate)
Motrin	IBUPROFEN	Arthritis	NSAID
MS Contin	Morphine	Severe pain	Strong narcotic (opiate)
Mysoline	PRIMIDONE	Seizure	Anticonvulsant
NADOLOL	Corgard	Angina, hypertension	Beta-adrenergic blocker—action is to slow heart rate
Nalfon	FENOPROFEN	Arthritis	NSAID
Naprosyn	NAPROXEN	Arthritis	NSAID
NAPROXEN	Naprosyn, Anaprox	Arthritis	NSAID
Naqua	TRICHLORMETHIAZIDE	Hypertension	Diuretic
Nardil	PHENELZINE	Depression	MAO inhibitor
Navane	THIOTHIXENE	Psychosis	Antipsychotic, thioxanthene
Neurontin	GABAPENTIN	Seizures	Anticonvulsant
NIFEDIPINE	Procardia	Effort angina, coronary artery spasm	Calcium channel blocker
Nitro-Bid, Nitrostat	NITROGLYCERIN	Cardiac chest pain	Antianginal
Nitro-Dur	NITROGLYCERIN	Cardiac chest pain (angina)	Nitro paste chest pad
Normodyne	LABETALOL	Hypertension	Beta blocker

389

Table continued on following page

Table A-1 *(Continued)*

	DRUG	INDICATIONS FOR USE	GENERAL DRUG TYPE
Norpace	DISOPYRAMIDE	Cardiac arrhythmia	Antiarrhythmic
Norpramin	DESIPRAMINE	Depression	Tricyclic antidepressant
NORTRIPTYLINE	NORTRIPTYLINE	Depression	Tricyclic antidepressant
Norvasc	AMLODIPINE	Hypertension	Vasodilator
Oretic	HYDROCHLOROTHIAZIDE	High blood pressure, CHF	Diuretic
Orinase	TOLBUTAMIDE	Diabetes	Antidiabetic
Oxalid	OXYPHENBUTAZONE	Arthritis, rheumatoid spondylitis	Anti-inflammatory, analgesic (potent)
OXAZEPAM	Serax	Anxiety, insomnia	Tranquilizer
OXYCODONE	Percodan	Severe pain	Strong narcotic (opiate)
OXYPHENBUTAZONE	Oxalid, Tandearil	Arthritis, rheumatoid spondylitis	Anti-inflammatory (dangerous drug)
Pamelor	NORTRIPTYLINE	Depression	Tricyclic antidepressant
PAPAVERINE	Pavabid	Arterial spasm	Vasodilator
Paregoric	—	Diarrhea	Narcotic (opiate)
Parnate	TRANYLCYPROMINE	Depression	MAO inhibitor
PAROXETINE	Paxil	Depression	Antidepressant
Pavabid	PAPAVERINE	Arterial spasm	Vasodilator
Paxil	PAROXETINE	Depression	Antidepressant
PENTAZOCINE	Talwin	Severe pain	Strong narcotic (opiate)
PENTOXIFYLLINE	Trental	Claudication	Hemorrheologic
Percodan	OXYCODONE	Severe pain	Strong narcotic (opiate)
Periactin	CYPROHEPTADINE	Colds, allergies	Phenothiazine

Persantine	DIPYRIDAMOLE	Antianginal
PHENELZINE	Nardil	MAO inhibitor
PHENOBARBITAL	Luminal	Anticonvulsant, sedative
PHENYLBUTAZONE	Azolid, Butazolidin	Anti-inflammatory
PHENYTOIN	Dilantin	Anticonvulsant
PINDOLOL	Visken	Beta-adrenergic blocker—action is to slow heart rate
PIRBUTEROL	Maxair	Bronchodilator
PIROXICAM	Feldene	Non-narcotic nonsteroidal analgesic
Placidyl	ETHCHLORVYNOL	Sedative-hypnotic
POTASSIUM	Slow-K, K-Lyte, K-Dur	Potassium supplement
PRAZOSIN	Minipress	Vasodilator
PREDNISONE	Deltasone	Anti-inflammatory
PRIMIDONE	Mysoline	Anticonvulsant
Prinivil	LISINOPRIL	ACE inhibitor
Pro-Banthine	PROPANTHELINE BROMIDE	Anticholinergic
PROBENECIDE	Benemid	Prophylactic for gout
PROCAINAMIDE	Pronestyl	Antiarrhythmic
Procardia	NIFEDIPINE	Calcium channel blocker
PROCHLORPERAZINE	Compazine	Antipsychotic (phenothiazine)
Prolixin	FLUPHENAZINE	Antipsychotic (phenothiazine)
PROPOXYPHENE NAPSYLATE	Darvon-N, Darvocet	Mild analgesic, mild narcotic
Proloid	THYROGLOBULIN	Thyroid hormone
Pronestyl	PROCAINAMIDE	Antiarrhythmic
PROPANTHELINE BROMIDE	Pro-Banthine	Anticholinergic

Table continued on following page

391

Table A-1 (Continued)

DRUG		INDICATIONS FOR USE	GENERAL DRUG TYPE
PROPOXYPHENE	Darvon, Dolene, SK-65	Mild pain	Narcotic
PROPRANOLOL	Inderal	Angina, hypertension, cardiac arrhythmia	Beta-adrenergic blocker—action is to slow heart rate
PROPYLTHIOURACIL	—	Hyperthyroidism	Inhibits synthesis of thyroid hormones
Proventil	ALBUTEROL	Asthma, COPD	Bronchodilator
Prozac	FLUOXETINE	Depression	Antidepressant
Quibron	THEOPHYLLINE	Asthma	Bronchodilator
Quinaglute	QUINIDINE	Cardiac arrhythmia	Quinine (controls potassium)
Quinidex	QUINIDINE	Cardiac arrhythmia	Quinine (controls potassium)
QUINIDINE	Quinaglute, Quinidex, Cardioquin	Cardiac arrhythmia	Quinine (controls potassium)
RANITIDINE	Zantac	Ulcer disease	H₂ receptor blocker
Regroton	CHLORTHALIDONE + RESERPINE	CHF, high blood pressure	Diuretic
RESERPINE	Serpasil, Sandril, Regroton, Hygroton	High blood pressure	Diuretic, vasodilator
RESERPINE + HYDROCHLOROTHIAZIDE	Hydropres	High blood pressure	Neuroeffector vasodilator
RESERPINE + HYDROFLUMETHIAZIDE	Salutensin	High blood pressure	Diuretic, vasodilator
Ritalin	METHYLPHENIDATE	Narcolepsy, hyperactivity	CNS stimulant
Salutensin	RESERPINE + HYDROFLUMETHIAZIDE	High blood pressure	Diuretic, vasodilator

Sandril	RESERPINE	CHF, high blood pressure	Diuretic, vasodilator
SECOBARBITAL	Seconal	Insomnia	Barbiturate
Seconal	SECOBARBITAL	Insomnia	Barbiturate
Seldane	TERFENADINE	Allergic reaction	Antihistamine
Ser-Ap-Es	RESERPINE + HYDRALAZINE + HYDROCHLOROTHIAZIDE	High blood pressure	Diuretic, vasodilator
SERTRALINE	Zoloft	Depression	Antidepressant
Serax	OXAZEPAM	Anxiety, insomnia	Tranquilizer
Serpasil	RESERPINE	High blood pressure	Diuretic, vasodilator
Sinequan	DOXEPIN	Depression	Antidepressant
SK-65	PROPOXYPHENE	Mild pain	Narcotic
SK-Pramine	IMIPRAMINE	Depression	Antidepressant
Slow-K	POTASSIUM	Potassium deficiency	Potassium supplement
Sorbitrate	ISOSORBIDE DINITRATE	Angina	Antianginal (vasodilator)
SPIRONOLACTONE	Aldactone	High blood pressure	Potassium-sparing diuretic
SPIRONOLACTONE + HYDROCHLOROTHIAZIDE	Aldactazide	High blood pressure	Potassium-sparing diuretic
Stelazine	TRIFLUOPERAZINE	Psychosis	Antipsychotic (phenothiazine)
SULFAMETHOXAZOLE	Gantanol	Urinary tract infection	Sulfa drug
SULINDAC	Clinoril	Arthritis	NSAID
Synthroid	LEVOTHYROXINE	Hypothyroidism	Thyroid hormone
Tagamet	CIMETIDINE	Ulcer disease	Histamine H_2 receptor antagonist
Talwin	PENTAZOCINE	Severe pain	Strong narcotic (opiate)
Tandearil	OXYPHENBUTAZOLE	Arthritis	Anti-inflammatory (extremely toxic)
Tapazole	METHIMAZOLE	Hyperthyroidism	Inhibits synthesis of thyroid hormone
Taractan	CHLORPROTHIXENE	Psychosis	Antipsychotic (thioxanthene)

Table continued on following page

393

Table A-1 (*Continued*)

	DRUG	INDICATIONS FOR USE	GENERAL DRUG TYPE
Tavist	CLEMASTINE	Allergic reaction	Antihistamine
Tegretol	CARBAMAZEPINE	Seizure	Anticonvulsant
Tenormin	ATENOLOL	Angina, hypertension	Beta-adrenergic blocker—action is to slow heart rate
Brethine, Bricanyl	TERBUTALINE	Asthma	Bronchodilator
Seldane	TERFENADINE	Allergic reaction	Antihistamine
Theo-Dur	THEOPHYLLINE	Asthma	Bronchodilator
Quibron, Elixophylline, Theo-Dur	THEOPHYLLINE	Asthma	Bronchodilator
Marax	THEOPHYLLINE + EPHEDRINE + Hydroxyzine	Asthma	Bronchodilator, sedative
Mellaril	THIORIDAZINE	Psychosis	Antipsychotic (phenothiazine)
Navane	THIOTHIXENE	Psychosis	Antipsychotic (thioxanthene)
Thorazine	CHLORPROMAZINE	Psychosis	Antipsychotic (phenothiazine)
Proloid	THYROGLOBULIN	Hypothyroidism	Thyroid hormone
Tigan	TRIMETHOBENZAMIDE	Control of nausea and vomiting	Antiemetic
Blockadren	TIMOLOL MALEATE	Post-MI, hypertension	Beta-adrenergic blocker—action is to slow heart rate
Tofranil	IMIPRAMINE	Depression	Antidepressant, tranquilizer
Tolinase	TOLAZAMIDE	Diabetes	Oral hypoglycemic
Orinase	TOLBUTAMIDE	Diabetes	Oral hypoglycemic
Tolectin	TOLMETIN	Arthritis, pain	Anti-inflammatory
Tolectin	TOLMETIN	Arthritis, pain	Anti-inflammatory

Generic	Brand	Indication	Class
TOLAZAMIDE	Tolinase	Diabetes	Oral hypoglycemic
LABETALOL	Trandate	Hypertension	Beta blocker
CLORAZEPATE	Tranxene	Anxiety	Tranquilizer
TRANYLCYPROMINE	Parnate	Depression	MAO inhibitor
TRAZODONE	Desyrel	Depression	Antidepressant
PENTOXIFYLLINE	Trental	Claudication	Hemorrheologic
TRIAMCINOLONE	Azmacort	Asthma	Anti-inflammatory
TRIAMTERENE	Dyrenium	High blood pressure, CHF	Potassium-sparing diuretic
AMITRIPTYLINE	Triavil	Depression	Tricyclic antidepressant
TRIAZOLAM	Halcion	Insomnia	Hypnotic
TRICHLORMETHIAZIDE	Metahydrin, Naqua	CHF, hepatic cirrhosis	Diuretic
TRIFLUOPERAZINE	Stelazine	Psychosis	Antipsychotic (phenothiazine)
TRIHEXYPHENIDYL	Artane	Parkinson's disease	Synthetic antispasmodic, works like atropine
TRIMETHOBENZAMIDE	Tigan	Nausea and vomiting	Antiemetic
ACETAMINOPHEN	Tylenol	Pain, fever, inflammation	Mild analgesic
DIAZEPAM	Valium	Anxiety, seizures	Benzodiazepine
BECLOMETHASONE	Vanceril	Asthma	Anti-inflammatory
ISOXSUPRINE	Vasodilan	Chronic organic brain disease	Vasodilator
ENALAPRIL	Vasotec	Hypertension	ACE inhibitor
ALBUTEROL	Ventolin	Asthma, COPD	Bronchodilator
VERAPAMIL	Calan, Isoptin	Effort angina, coronary artery spasm, PSVT	Calcium channel blocker
PINDOLOL	Visken	Angina, hypertension	Beta-adrenergic blocker—action is to slow heart rate

Table continued on following page

Table A-1 *(Continued)*

Drug	Indications for Use	General Drug Type
Vistaril HYDROXYZINE	Anxiety, nausea, vomiting, tension	Antihistamine
WARFARIN Coumadin	Post-CVA, blood clot	Anticoagulant
Wellbutrin BUPROPION	Depression	Antidepressant
Xanax ALPRAZOLAM	Anxiety	Tranquilizer
Zantac RANITIDINE	Ulcer disease	H_2 receptor blocker
Zarontin ETHOSUXIMIDE	Petit mal seizures	Anticonvulsant
Zaroxolyn METOLAZONE	High blood pressure	Diuretic
Zestril LISINOPRIL	Hypertension	Angiotensin inhibitor
Zoloft SERTRALINE	Depression	Antidepressant
Zovirax ACYCLOVIR	Herpes	Antiviral drug
Zyloprim ALLOPURINOL	Gout, high uric acid blood level	Prophylactic for gout

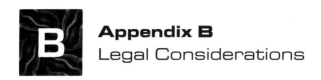

Appendix B
Legal Considerations

Legal action against members of the health professions increases each year. The EMT should be aware that he/she is included in this group and should understand the type of circumstance that could result in legal action against him/her. Fortunately, legal action against EMTs is uncommon. However, this should not cause the EMT to be less mindful of the potential for litigation as a result of his/her EMS actions.

Maintaining a professional, compassionate, considerate attitude is the best way to prevent the patient and/or family members from becoming unhappy with the treatment provided. The discontented patient is the one most likely to institute legal action. Patients will often overlook certain mistakes in treatment if they feel that the health professional has a general attitude of genuine concern and truly has their best interests in mind, regardless of the circumstances. Above all, the EMT must provide the best, most appropriate care within the limits of his/her training and medical authorization to substantially reduce the risk of future litigation.

■ FOUR ELEMENTS OF A LEGAL ACTION

Duty

In a suit, the plaintiff (person who is suing) must prove the duty of the person or agency to perform actions involving him/her.

- If it is the duty of the EMT to provide transport of an ill patient, it is also the duty of the EMT to take all reasonable precautions to protect the patient and others on the street by avoiding reckless and/or careless handling of the vehicle so as not to cause additional harm to the patient or others.
- It is the duty of the EMT to provide the appropriate care whenever necessary, according to the standards by which he/she is certified, as long as he/she is identifiable by virtue of uniforms, patches, marked vehicles, and so on. The EMT's actions are compared to a standard of care generally determined by local EMS practices, protocols, medical directives, and training.
- During off-duty hours, care is provided by the EMT according to the best judgment of the EMT at the time. Although many states have "Good Samaritan" laws, the element of liability still exists regardless of the good intentions of the off-duty EMT.
- EMTs under the influence of drugs or alcohol should consider the consequences of a possibly impaired ability to function normally. Such reckless behavior places the patient, the EMT, and the EMS system at risk for potential harm.

Breach of Duty

EMTs who fail to perform expected actions, or whose actions exceed the training and skills for which they are certified, would be considered in breach of duty. For example, EMTs performing intravenous therapy, endotracheal intubation, and so on when not certified to perform these actions are in breach of duty.

Damage or Harm

The harm or damage must be proved to have occurred. Without actual damage or harm, the clinical error or omission of the EMT is primarily a professional issue rather than a legal issue.

Proximate Cause

The EMT must be proved to be the proximate cause of the damage or injury. The EMT's action (error) or omission must be responsible in some way for direct or indirect causation of the harm experienced by the patient.

- Rib fractures occurring while CPR is being given to a patient without respirations and who is pulseless would not usually be considered a case of proximate cause.
- Injuries during treatment that could have been prevented by normal prudent care by the EMT are cause for a charge of proximate cause.

■ DOCUMENTATION

The EMT often spends a great deal of time completing patient medical reports and unusual incident reports. Medical reports are typically completed for each response to which the EMT is dispatched. Occasionally, the EMT must also document the details of an unusual incident, such as suspected child abuse, a suspicious death, or accidental injury to a patient.

Concise, truthful, and complete field medical reports of patient examination and treatment must be an absolute priority of the EMT once the patient's care has been completed. Well-documented patient care also demonstrates concern and professionalism.

- Patient reports should include accurate subjective statements made by the patient, the patient's family, or witnesses without subjective embellishment by the EMT. Pertinent positives and negatives identified in the history should be documented in the report.
- Objective statements included in the report must be based on known facts, observations, and examination results (negative and positive). Objective statements must remain pertinent to the patient's medical or emotional problems.
- A logical approach to the examination and treatment often demonstrates the professionalism and competency of the EMT. The report must also include the treatment actions performed by the EMT as well as the results, if any, of these actions.
- When abbreviations are used, they should be those generally recognized by the medical profession (see Appendix E). As a general rule, the report should

be written so that the EMT will not have difficulty reciting specifics of the incident years afterward.

Occasionally, special situations will require additional documentation. For example, incidents involving major crimes may require additional documentation of information obtained or learned by the EMT. The EMT may be requested to testify in a court proceeding related to the incident (death inquest, criminal or civil trial). Other incidents that may benefit from additional documentation include

- Incidents resulting in an accidental injury to the patient
- Incidents of accidental clinical error or omission
- Incidents involving suspected criminal acts (child abuse, domestic violence, rape)
- Suspicious deaths

The EMT will appear most professional in a court proceeding if he/she is able to accurately testify based upon detailed documentation.

A commonly encountered special situation involves the patient's refusal of treatment or transportation. Many EMS systems have a procedure for documenting patient refusals. At a minimum, the EMT should document (in the patient report)

- The advice given to the patient (e.g., advised to allow bandaging and splinting and transport to the hospital)
- The patient's refusal of treatment and/or transportation
- The risks and concerns discussed with the patient

All details of a patient refusal should be noted in the report. This information could be placed in a brief statement at the end of the report. The EMT completing the report should sign the statement, have the patient sign the statement, and, if at all possible, have a witness sign the statement. Although these steps will not guarantee legal protection, they do demonstrate the EMT's good faith efforts to properly care for the patient.

■ PATIENT CONSENT FOR TREATMENT

State and local laws regarding emergency consent of minors and the patient's right to refuse treatment should be explicitly understood. Local law officers are an excellent source of precise information concerning this subject. Read the law. Do not rely on word of mouth.

Most states have implied consent laws for emergency settings by which minors may be treated without parents or guardians available for consent, and for patients who are not mentally capable of making their own decisions (permanently or temporarily). For example, a disoriented diabetic refusing medical treatment is probably not able to properly make this decision at the present time. When an injured minor requiring medical treatment is allowed to refuse such treatment, the EMT may also be at risk for legal action. Often, assistance from law enforcement officers can be extremely valuable when the patient is adamantly refusing necessary care. The EMT must keep in mind that the adult patient who appears mentally competent at the time has the right to refuse treatment.

Special care must be exercised when physical force and/or restraints are considered, so as to avoid the act of false imprisonment of the patient. Any injury inflicted on the patient during the course of treatment or transportation against the will of the patient may be legal grounds for suit against the responsible EMT.

A significant risk of forcible restraint is that the patient may be critically injured in the process. Numerous cases across the United States have been reported in which a restrained person died as a result of "positional asphyxia." Although rare, this typically occurs when law enforcement officers restrain a person being taken into custody. It can occur, however, when EMTs restrain a patient. Positional asphyxia occurs as a result of several factors that combine to inhibit the patient's ability to ventilate. These factors include

- Neck restraints or choke holds—these can injure the trachea or surrounding soft tissue.
- Prone positioning—this position places weight on the abdomen and chest, possibly inhibiting the ability to ventilate.
- Aspiration—combined with the prone position and intoxication, the restrained patient is at an increased risk for vomiting.
- Physical exertion—the patient is using a tremendous amount of energy to fight the restraint, which causes an increased demand for oxygen.

To avoid injury to the restrained patient and to the EMS providers, the EMT should take the following steps:

- Place the patient in a supine or lateral recumbent position once control of the patient is gained.

- Monitor the airway and ventilations closely, particularly in the lethargic and/or intoxicated patient.

- Restrain the patient's arms and legs. One method is to secure the arms and legs to a backboard or stretcher. The arms are secured in a straightened position along the body. Restraining one arm over the head for a prolonged period may cause serious shoulder injury.

- Secure the patient and backboard (if used) to the stretcher during transport.

- Before transporting, ensure that the patient does not have any hidden weapons or sharps on his/her person.

- Avoid the particularly dangerous areas of the patient (mouth, hands, and knees). These are weapons the patient may still use.

- If the patient is spitting, biting, or threatening the EMT with these actions, place a surgical mask or oxygen face mask (with supplied oxygen) on the patient.

■ PATIENT WISHES

Advance Directives

Many patients today are communicating their wishes regarding long-term care and care in the event of sudden death. This is commonly observed in the patient with a terminal illness. Many states have recently enacted laws allowing adult patients to refuse ALS therapies and/or CPR. These laws often have what are referred to as "Do Not Resuscitate" (DNR) or "No CPR" orders. In these cases, the patient signs a legal document that must be honored by the EMS provider. A common method of communicating this involves the use of a standard form and an identifying bracelet. These items are intended to be available or visible to the EMT in the event of a cardiac arrest. In addition, such legislation typically describes methods for rescinding the advance directive.

The EMT must be knowledgeable of state laws regarding advance directives and "No CPR" directives. *Regardless of the advance directive, the EMT must keep in mind that a patient wish to have no CPR does not mean that no care is provided. The EMT must continue to provide all care that provides basic comfort and treatment.* Emotional support and concern for the patient and family members continue to be the EMT's responsibility in situations of terminal illness or advance directives.

Confidentiality

All patients desire to have information related to their care and treatment managed in a confidential manner. Some states have enacted legislation that prohibits the dissemination of specific information (typically related to sexually transmitted diseases) under nearly any circumstance. The EMT must be knowledgeable of state laws regarding specific aspects of confidentiality. For the most part, a patient's medical information must be kept confidential and provided only to other health care providers who have a need to know the information. For the EMT, this includes advanced-level prehospital care personnel and hospital medical personnel. Care must also be taken to assure the confidentiality of patient reports (written, verbal, and radio reports).

■ LEGAL REPORTING

The EMT will frequently encounter situations involving suspected criminal activity. Although much of the information obtained when treating a patient may be considered confidential (part of the patient and health care provider relationship), most states have requirements for the reporting of specific crimes. These requirements vary from state to state, however, common examples include child abuse or neglect, domestic violence, rape, assault, and gunshot wounds. The

EMT is ethically, if not legally, obligated to report crimes that injure or harm other persons, particularly suspected child abuse, domestic violence, and assault, and persons whose behavior is self-destructive. The EMT should be knowledgeable of state laws regarding the legal reporting of suspected crimes.

■ SUMMARY

It is not the intent of this appendix to scare the EMT into thinking that everyone he/she treats is looking for a reason to institute legal action. Instead, it is a reminder that the law does not provide a "blank check" to health care professionals just because they are involved in assisting with medical emergencies.

As a general rule, if EMTs treat their patients as though the patients were their own family members, then they will provide the appropriate level of concern and treatment and will avoid situations that may cause legal action.

It is vital that EMTs be familiar with all legal positions regarding the field EMT in their working areas. Consider these steps in avoiding legal action:

- Provide timely, effective medical care within the scope of your level of training and medical direction.
- Provide quality medical care free of errors and omissions to the greatest extent possible.
- Comply with all legal requirements of consent, refusal, confidentiality, and legal reporting.
- Maintain accurate, truthful, and complete records and documentation.

Appendix C
Fahrenheit-Centigrade Conversion Table

FAHRENHEIT DEGREES	CENTIGRADE DEGREES
32	0
41	5
50	10
68	20
77	25
86	30
95	34.97
96	35.52
97	36.08
98	36.63
98.6	36.96
99	37.19
100	37.74
101	38.30
102	38.85
103	39.41
104	39.96
105	40.52
106	41.07

TO CONVERT °F TO °C
Subtract 32, then multiply by 5/9 or 0.555

TO CONVERT °C TO °F
Multiply by 9/5 or 1.8, then add 32

Appendix D
Universal Anatomic Positions

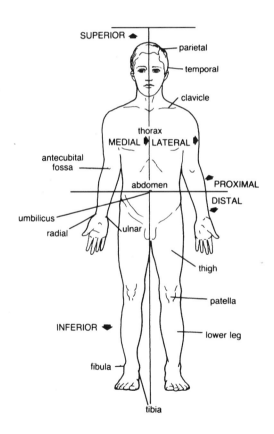

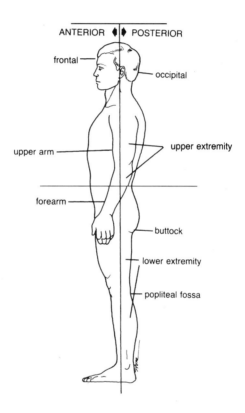

ANTERIOR ◆|◆ POSTERIOR

frontal

occipital

upper arm

upper extremity

forearm

buttock

lower extremity

popliteal fossa

Appendix E
Abbreviations

ā	before
abd	abdomen/abdominal
amb	ambulance
AMI	acute myocardial infarction
A/O	alert and oriented
AOB	alcohol on breath
ASAP	as soon as possible
ax	axillary
@	at
bid	two times a day
bilat	bilateral
BP	blood pressure
c̄	with
cap	capsule
c/c	chief complaint
cl	clear
CNS	central nervous system
c/o	complaining of
conj	conjugate
C-spine	cervical spine
diff	difficulty
DOA	dead on arrival
dsg	dressing
Dx	diagnosis
ECG	electrocardiogram
E&R	equal and reactive
est	estimated
ETOH	ethyl alcohol
ext	extremity
F&D	fixed and dilated
fx	fracture
GI	gastrointestinal
GCS	Glasgow Coma Scale
GSW	gunshot wound
H/A	headache
HEENT	head, eyes, ears, nose, throat

Hg	mercury
Ht	height
HTN	hypertension
Hx	history
jt	joint
Ⓛ	left
lac	laceration
lg	large
liq	liquid
LLQ	left lower quadrant
LOC	level of consciousness
L-spine	lumbar spine
LUQ	left upper quadrant
MCA	motorcycle accident
med(s)	medicine(s)
mg	milligrams
min	minute
ml	milliliter
ML	midline
mm	millimeter
mod	moderate
M = R	mid, equal, reactive
multi	multiple
MVA	motor vehicle accident
NC	nasal cannula
neg	negative
NKA	no known allergies
NPO	nothing by mouth
NROM	normal range of motion
N&V	nausea and vomiting
o	no/none
occ	occasional
OD	overdose
p̄	past/after
P	pulse
P.D.	police department
PE	pulmonary embolus
P.E.	physical examination
ped	pedestrian
pHx	past history
pMHx	past medical history
PMD	private medical doctor
PND	paroxysmal nocturnal dyspnea

po	by mouth
poss	possible
POV	privately owned vehicle
prn	as needed
prox	proximal
pt	patient
qid	four times a day
®	right
re	regarding
req	request
RLQ	right lower quadrant
R/O	rule out
Rt	routine
RUQ	right upper quadrant
Rx	treatment
s̄	without
sl	slight
sm	small
SOB	short(ness) of breath
ss	half
S-spine	sacral spine
STH	said to have
STHH	said to have had
STHB	said to have been
SW	stab wound
Sx	sign/symptom
T	temperature
Tab	tablet
TB	tuberculosis
TIA	transient ischemic attack
tid	three times a day
T-Spine	thoracic spine
Tx	transport
unc	unconscious
unk	unknown
URI	upper respiratory infection
UTI	urinary tract infection
WD/WN	well-developed/well-nourished
WNL	within normal limits
wt	weight
y/o	year old

+	plus, positive
=	equal
−	negative
×	times
≈	approximately
1°	primary, first degree
2°	secondary, second degree
3°	third degree
♂	male
♀	female
↑	increasing up, above
→	carry thought on
↓	decreasing, down, below
>	greater than
<	less than
/	per
	supine
	semireclining
	sitting
	standing

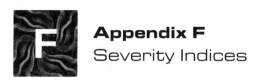

Appendix F
Severity Indices

■ **TRAUMA SEVERITY INDICES**

Table F-1   Revised Trauma Score Variable Breakpoints

Glascow Coma Scale	Systolic Blood Pressure (mm Ha)	Respiratory Rate (per Minute)	Coded Value
13–15	>89	10–29	4
9–12	76–89	>29	3
6–8	50–75	6–9	2
4–5	1–49	1–5	1
3	0	0	0

*From Champion, H.R., et al.: A revision of the trauma score. J. Trauma 29:623, 1989;
© 1989 by the Williams & Wilkins Co., Baltimore.

Table F-2   Summary of Data*

Sum of RTS Coded Variables (T-RTS)	Number of Patients	Per Cent Survivors
12	1,375	0.995
11	222	0.969
10	116	0.879
9	64	0.766
8	51	0.667
7	33	0.636
6	27	0.630
5	22	0.455
4	36	0.333
3	9	0.333
2	7	0.286
1	4	0.250
0	134	0.037

*From Champion, H.R., et al.: A revision of the trauma score. J. Trauma 29:623, 1989;
© 1989 by the Williams & Wilkins Co., Baltimore.

■ Apgar Score

The Apgar score is useful in evaluating the status of the infant. The Apgar score should be determined immediately after birth and 5 minutes after delivery. This score is determined by assessing the appearance, pulse, reflexes, and respiration of the infant according to Table F–5.

A score of 7 to 10 indicates adequate function of the infant. A score of 4 to 6 indicates moderate depression. Infants with scores less

Table F–3   Nelson Scale for Children*

	Score†		
Variable	0	1	2
Respiratory effort	Labored or absent	Some distress	No distress
Skin color	Cyanotic	Pale, flushed, mottled	Normal
Activity	Delirium, stupor, coma	Lethargy	Normal
Play	Refused to play	Decreased	Normal
Temperature (°F)	<97.4, >104	101.1–104	97.4–101

*Scale developed by Dr. Kathleen Nelson in 1975 at Yale University School of Medicine, New Haven, CT.
†10 points is not sick; 8 or 9 is moderately sick; 7 points or less is very sick.

Table F–4   Pediatric Trauma Score*
(Check One Category for Each Component)

	Category		
Component	+2	+1	−1
Size	≥20 kg	10–20 kg	<10 kg
Airway	Normal	Maintainable	Unmaintainable
Systolic BP†	≥90 mm Hg	90–50 mm Hg	<50 mm Hg
CNS	Awake	Obtunded/LOC	Coma/decerebrate
Open Wound	None	Minor	Major/penetrating
Skeletal	None	Closed fracture	Open/multiple fractures
			Sum _____ (PTS)

*From Tepas, J.J.: Emergency Medical Services for Children; Report of the Ninety-Seventh Ross Conference on Pediatric Research. Columbus, OH, Ross Laboratories, 1989, p. 66; reprinted by permission.
†If proper size BP cuff not available, BP can be assessed by assigning

  +2: Pulse palpable at wrist
  +1: Pulse palpable at groin
  −1: No pulse palpable

Table F-5   Apgar Score

	SCORE		
SIGN*	0	1	2
A: Appearance (color)	Blue, pale	Body pink, extremities blue	Completely pink
P: Pulse (heart rate)	Absent	<100	>100
G: Grimace (reflexes)	No response	Grimace	Cough, sneeze
A: Activity (muscle tone)	Limp	Some flexion of extremities	Active motion
R: Respiration	Absent	Slow, irregular	Strong cry

*Each sign is evaluated individually and scored from 0 to 2 at both 1 and 5 minutes of life. The final score at each time is the sum of the individual scores.

than 4 will often require resuscitation. Remember that babies are often blue or extremely pale 1 minute after delivery, with flaccid muscles and poor respirations; hence it is important to reassess the infant's score at 5 minutes after delivery.

■ LEVEL OF CONSCIOUSNESS

Table F-6   Glascow Coma Scale

Eyes	Open	Spontaneously	4
		To verbal command	3
		To pain	2
	No response		1
Best motor response	To verbal command	Obeys	6
	To painful stimulus	Localizes pain	5
		Flexion—withdrawal	4
		Flexion—abnormal (decorticate rigidity)	3
		Extension (decerebrate rigidity)	2
		No response	1
Best verbal response		Oriented and converses	5
		Disoriented and converses	4
		Inappropriate words	3
		Incomprehensible sounds	2
		No response	1
TOTAL			3–15

The Glasgow Coma Scale, based on eye opening and verbal and motor responses, is a practical means of monitoring changes in level of consciousness. If response on the scale is given a number, the responsiveness of the patient can be expressed by the sum of the figures. The lowest score is 3; the highest is 15.

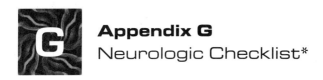

Appendix G
Neurologic Checklist*

■ INSTRUCTIONS

Record the vital signs in Unit I. If the patient can talk, check (√) one appropriate box in each of Units II, III, and IV. An oriented patient should know his name, age, and the like. A moan can be checked as "garbled" speech. If the patient is unable to talk, check (√) "none" in Unit III and one appropriate box in Unit V. In an "inappropriate" response, the patient is not effective in removing the painful stimulus; when "decerebrate," the extremities reflexly extend and/or hyperpronate. In Unit VI, draw the size and shape of each pupil and check (√) for a reaction to light. Under Unit VII, normal strength is scored as "4," slight weakness "3," a 50 percent reduction in strength "2," marked weakness and without spontaneous movement "1," and complete paralysis "0."

Unit	Time					
I Vital signs	Blood pressure					
	Pulse					
	Respirations					
	Temperature					
II Conscious and	Oriented					
	Disoriented					
	Restless					
	Combative					
III Speech	Clear					
	Rambling					
	Garbled					
	None					
IV Will awaken to	Name					
	Shaking					
	Light pain					
	Strong pain					
V Nonverbal reaction to pain	Appropriate					
	Inappropriate					
	"Decerebrate"					
	None					
VI Pupils	Size on right					
	Size on left					
	Reacts on right					
	Reacts on left					
VII Ability to move	Right arm					
	Left arm					
	Right leg					
	Left leg					

*Reproduced courtesy of American College of Surgeons.

Appendix H
Helmet Removal*

The varying sizes, shapes, and configurations of helmets necessitate some understanding of their proper removal from victims of motorcycle or other recreational accidents. The rescuer who removes a helmet improperly might inadvertently aggravate cervical spine injuries. Additionally, the failure to remove the helmet may cause further injury to the patient and make the EMT's job more difficult.

The use of helmets in a variety of recreational and motorized two- or three-wheeled vehicles has dramatically increased over the past few years. Initially, many states mandated the wearing of helmets for motorcyclists. Today, some cities have also mandated the use of helmets for bicyclists. Helmets are also used in a variety of recreational activities, including football, hockey, motocross, auto racing, kayaking, and, occasionally, roller-blading and skate boarding. Regardless of the use or type of helmet, the EMT must understand the reasoning for removing a helmet along with the proper procedures for accomplishing this task.

In general, the EMT should remove the helmet of an injured person when doing so would provide proper spinal alignment and immobilization on a backboard, or when the airway must be accessed. For example, the failure to remove a motorcycle or bicycle helmet would cause neck flexion. This flexion may cause further injury to the cervical spine or interfere with the ability to maintain an open airway. For this reason, the EMT should remove all motorcycle and bicycle helmets. Conversely, football and hockey helmets should not automatically be removed. The protective pads worn by these players cause slight elevation of the body when placed on a backboard. Removal of the helmet would cause significant neck extension. For these types of helmets, when protective pads are also being worn by the patient, the EMT should remove the helmet only to access the head or airway. In some cases, this may not even be necessary. The face mask of the helmet may be removed (cut), allowing some access to the face and airway. Helmets used without protective shoulder pads, such as those used by kayakers, should be treated as bicycle helmets and removed.

■ TYPES OF HELMETS

Helmet Removal

These procedures apply to the removal of helmets covering the entire face and head, typically used by motorcyclists.

---

*Reproduced with permission of the American College of Surgeons.

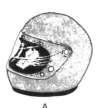

A

Full face coverage—motorcycle,
auto racer

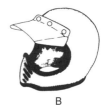

B

Full face coverage—motocross

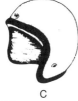

C

Partial face coverage—motorcycle,
auto racer

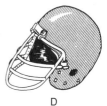

D

Football

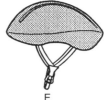

E

Light head protection—bicycle.

1. One rescuer applies in-line stabilization of the cervical spine by placing his/her hands on each side of the helmet with the fingers on the patient's mandible. This position prevents slippage if the strap is loose.
2. The second rescuer cuts or loosens any straps at the chin and neck. The first rescuer continues to maintain stabilization.
3. The second rescuer then places one hand on the mandible at the angle, with the thumb on one side and the long and index fingers on the other. With the other hand, the second rescuer applies pressure from the occipital region. This maneuver is intended to maintain cervical spine alignment and stabilization. Traction should not be applied. The first rescuer may now turn over the task of stabilization to the second rescuer.
4. The first rescuer, at the top of the head, removes the helmet. Four factors should be kept in mind:
   ■ The helmet is egg shaped, and, therefore, must be expanded laterally to clear the ears.
   ■ If the helmet provides full facial coverage, glasses must be removed first.

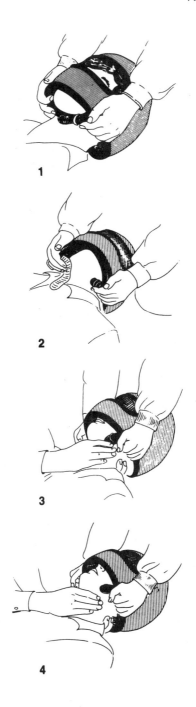

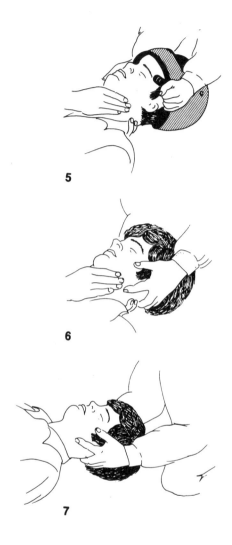

- If the helmet provides full facial coverage, the nose will impede removal. To clear the nose, the helmet must be tilted backward and raised over it.
- Some helmets contain air bladders that must be deflated to allow removal of the helmet.

5. Throughout the removal process, the second rescuer maintains cervical stabilization from below in order to prevent flexion, extension, or lateral movement of the spine.

6. After the helmet has been removed, the rescuer at the top of the head replaces his/her hands on either side of the patient's head to take over the task of cervical spine stabilization.
7. In-line stabilization of the cervical spine is maintained from above until the patient is placed on a backboard (or other spinal immobilization device), has a cervical collar applied, and has been immobilized with a cervical immobilization device.

■ SUMMARY

The helmet must be maneuvered over the nose and ears while the head and neck are stabilized.

- In-line stabilization is maintained from above.
- In-line stabilization is transferred below with pressure on the jaw and occiput.
- The helmet is removed.
- In-line stabilization is re-established from above.

When in doubt as to whether or not the helmet should be removed, consider the following factors:

1. *Is the patient seriously ill or injured?* If yes, remove the helmet quickly and carefully. When advanced airway management techniques are required at the scene or hospital, the helmet will be removed anyway.
2. *Is the airway compromised in any way? Are injuries to the face being worsened by the inability to access the injury?* If yes, then remove the helmet quickly and carefully.
3. *Are bulky protective pads (e.g., shoulder pads) being worn by the patient?* If yes, then removal of the entire helmet should only occur if access to the airway or head is absolutely required. Doing this will typically require removal of the pads also. If no pads are worn, then removal of the helmet must occur to maintain proper spinal alignment. Consider removing the face mask when this is possible and provides sufficient access.

Appendix I
Medical Device Problem Reporting Program

EMTs frequently use medical equipment and devices in providing emergency care. Occasionally, these devices may fail or malfunction leading to concern for potential patient injury. In 1990, the U.S. Congress enacted the Safe Medical Devices Act (SMDA) in an effort to improve the reporting of medical device problems. The final Medical Device Reporting (MDR) rule, effective in July 1996, includes requirements for "user facilities" to report medical device problems. The MDR rule does define ambulances and rescue services as "user facilities" and requires these services to report medical device problems.

The Food and Drug Administration (FDA) is responsible for overseeing the MDR program. The specific FDA requirements are beyond the scope of this appendix. The following is a summary of the requirements and an overview of reporting requirements for EMS agencies. The information provided in this section is based upon 21 CFR Part 803, "Medical Device Reporting," effective April 11, 1996, and "Medical Device Reporting for User Facilities," Food and Drug Administration, U.S. Department of Health and Human Services, April 1996. The EMT or EMS agency should review these publications for specific details and requirements.

■ DEFINITIONS

- *Medical device*—any item that is used for the diagnosis, treatment, or prevention of a disease, injury, or other condition and is not a drug or biologic. All items used in medical practice that are not drugs or biologics are generally considered devices.

- *Device user facility*—a hospital, ambulatory surgical facility, nursing home, outpatient diagnostic facility, or outpatient treatment facility that is not a "physician's office." Outpatient treatment facilities include ambulance providers, rescue services, and home health care groups.

- *Malfunction*—a failure of a device to meet its performance specifications or to perform as intended.

- *"Caused or contributed to"*—A device may have "caused or contributed to" a patient's death or serious injury, if the death or serious injury was or may have been attributed to the device or the device may have been a factor in the death or serious injury because of device failure; malfunction; improper or inadequate device design, manufacture, or labeling; or user error.

- *MDR reportable event*—an event during which a user facility becomes aware of information that reasonably suggests that a device has or may have caused or contributed to a death or serious injury. User facilities are encouraged, but are not required, to report malfunctions that do not result in a death or serious injury. User facilities should report the malfunction to the manufacturer.

■ REPORTING AND COMPLIANCE REQUIREMENTS FOR EMS PROVIDERS

The FDA has determined that "ambulances and rescue services" fall within the definition of "user facility" because they are outpatient treatment facilities. The FDA is concerned that the risks posed by potential device malfunctions in the EMS setting are of a critical nature. EMS providers should completely understand the FDA's definition of "becomes aware" of an MDR event. According to the FDA, "A user facility 'becomes aware' of an MDR reportable event when medical personnel, who are employed by or formally affiliated with the facility, acquire information that reasonably suggests that a reportable event has occurred." Essentially, the FDA considers the EMS agency aware of the event once one of the agency's personnel (e.g., an EMT) has information suggesting an adverse event.

Each EMT and EMS agency should review the specific definitions and requirements contained in the sources noted at the end of this appendix. Table I–1 summarizes the MDR requirements affecting most EMS providers.

■ ADDITIONAL INFORMATION AND FORMS

Printed Information

Additional information may be obtained by mail or through the Internet. FDA forms 3500A (see Fig. I–1) and 3419 as well as the "Medical Device Reporting for User Facilities" manual are available

- *From the Internet at*: http://www.fda.gov
- *As printed materials from*: National Technical Information Service, Springfield, VA 22161; telephone (703) 487-4650

Submitting Forms

Identify each report and envelope with the name of the report (e.g., semiannual report or user facility report). MDR and semiannual reports should be sent to

> Food and Drug Administration
> Center for Devices and Radiological Health
> Medical Device Reporting
> P.O. Box 3002
> Rockville, MD 20847-3002

In the event the EMS provider believes that a public health emergency exists, the provider should contact the FDA at

> FDA Emergency Operations Branch
> Office of Regional Operations
> (301) 443-1240

Table I-1 Summary of MDR Reporting and Compliance Requirements for an EMS Agency (User Facility)

REQUIREMENT	REPORTING TO	TIME CONSTRAINT
Reportable event resulting in death	FDA and the device manufacturer (Form 3500A)	Report within 10 work days
Reportable event resulting in serious injury	The device manufacturer (Form 3500A); report to the FDA if the manufacturer is unknown	Report within 10 work days
Submit semiannual reports of MDR deaths and serious injuries	FDA	These reports must be submitted by January 1 and July 1 (for the preceding 6-month period); submittal is not required if no individual reports were submitted to the FDA or manufacturers during the reporting period
Designate a facility contact person	The FDA will conduct correspondence regarding an MDR with this person	NA
Maintain MDR event files (all records related to an adverse event whether reported or not)	Must be accessible to FDA employees at reasonable times	Records must be kept for 2 years from the date of the event
Develop and implement written procedures for reporting adverse medical device events	Must be accessible to FDA employees at reasonable times	Must be maintained by the user facility

For use by user-facilities,
distributors and manufacturers for
MANDATORY reporting

MEDWATCH
THE FDA MEDICAL PRODUCTS REPORTING PROGRAM

Form Approved: OMB No. 0910-0291 Expires: 12/31/94
See OMB statement on reverse

Mfr report #

UF/Dist report #

Page ____ of ____

FDA Use Only

A. Patient information

1. Patient identifier	2. Age at time of event: or _____ Date of birth:	3. Sex ☐ female ☐ male	4. Weight ___ lbs or ___ kgs

In confidence

B. Adverse event or product problem

1. ☐ Adverse event   and/or   ☐ Product problem (e.g., defects/malfunctions)

2. Outcomes attributed to adverse event (check all that apply)

☐ death _____ (mo/day/yr)
☐ life-threatening
☐ hospitalization – initial or prolonged

☐ disability
☐ congenital anomaly
☐ required intervention to prevent permanent impairment/damage
☐ other: _____

3. Date of event (mo/day/yr)	4. Date of this report (mo/day/yr)

5. Describe event or problem

6. Relevant tests/laboratory data, including dates

7. Other relevant history, including preexisting medical conditions (e.g., allergies, race, pregnancy, smoking and alcohol use, hepatic/renal dysfunction, etc.)

C. Suspect medication(s)

1. Name (give labeled strength & mfr/labeler, if known)

#1

#2

2. Dose, frequency & route used #1 #2	3. Therapy dates (if unknown, give duration) from/to (or best estimate) #1 #2

4. Diagnosis for use (indication) #1 #2	5. Event abated after use stopped or dose reduced #1 ☐ yes ☐ no ☐ doesn't apply #2 ☐ yes ☐ no ☐ doesn't apply

6. Lot # (if known) #1 #2	7. Exp. date (if known) #1 #2	8. Event reappeared after reintroduction #1 ☐ yes ☐ no ☐ doesn't apply #2 ☐ yes ☐ no ☐ doesn't apply

9. NDC # – for product problems only (if known)

10. Concomitant medical products and therapy dates (exclude treatment of event)

D. Suspect medical device

1. Brand name

2. Type of device

3. Manufacturer name & address	4. Operator of device ☐ health professional ☐ lay user/patient ☐ other:

6. model # _____ catalog # _____ serial # _____ lot # _____ other #	5. Expiration date (mo/day/yr) 7. If implanted, give date (mo/day/yr) 8. If explanted, give date (mo/day/yr)

9. Device available for evaluation?   (Do not send to FDA)
☐ yes   ☐ no   ☐ returned to manufacturer on _____ (mo/day/yr)

10. Concomitant medical products and therapy dates (exclude treatment of event)

E. Initial reporter

1. Name, address & phone #

2. Health professional? ☐ yes ☐ no	3. Occupation	4. Initial reporter also sent report to FDA ☐ yes ☐ no ☐ unk

FDA

Submission of a report does not constitute an admission that medical personnel, user facility, distributor, manufacturer or product caused or contributed to the event.

FDA Form 3500A (6/93)

Figure I-1

Individual Adverse Event Report (FDA Form 3500A). *Illustration continued on following page*

Medication and Device Experience Report
(continued)

Refer to guidelines for specific instructions

Submission of a report does not constitute an admission that medical personnel, user facility, distributor, manufacturer or product caused or contributed to the event.

U.S. DEPARTMENT OF HEALTH AND HUMAN SERVICES
Public Health Service • Food and Drug Administration

Page ____ of ____

FDA Use Only

F. For use by user facility/distributor–devices only

1. Check one
☐ user facility ☐ distributor

2. UF/Dist report number

3. User facility or distributor name/address

4. Contact person

5. Phone Number

6. Date user facility or distributor became aware of event (mo/day/yr)

7. Type of report
☐ initial
☐ follow-up # ____

8. Date of this report (mo/day yr)

9. Approximate age of device

10. Event problem codes (refer to coding manual)
patient code ___ — ___ — ___
device code ___ — ___ — ___

11. Report sent to FDA?
☐ yes ____ (mo/day/yr)
☐ no

12. Location where event occurred
☐ hospital ☐ outpatient diagnostic facility
☐ home ☐ ambulatory surgical facility
☐ nursing home
☐ outpatient treatment facility
☐ other: ____ specify

13. Report sent to manufacturer?
☐ yes
☐ no (mo/day/yr)

14. Manufacturer name/address

G. All manufacturers

1. Contact office – name/address (& mfring site for devices)

2. Phone number

3. Report source (check all that apply)
☐ foreign
☐ study
☐ literature
☐ consumer
☐ health professional
☐ user facility
☐ company representative
☐ distributor
☐ other:

4. Date received by manufacturer (mo/day/yr)

5.
(A)NDA # ____
IND # ____
PLA # ____
pre-1938 ☐ yes
OTC product ☐ yes

6. If IND, protocol #

7. Type of report (check all that apply)
☐ 5-day ☐ 15-day
☐ 10-day ☐ periodic
☐ Initial ☐ follow-up # ____

8. Adverse event term(s)

9. Mfr. report number

H. Device manufacturers only

1. Type of reportable event
☐ death
☐ serious injury
☐ malfunction (see guidelines)
☐ other: ____

2. If follow-up, what type?
☐ correction
☐ additional information
☐ response to FDA request
☐ device evaluation

3. Device evaluated by mfr?
☐ not returned to mfr.
☐ yes ☐ evaluation summary attached
☐ no (attach page to explain why not) or provide code:

4. Device manufacture date (mo/yr)

5. Labeled for single use?
☐ yes ☐ no

6. Evaluation codes (refer to coding manual)
method ___ — ___ — ___
results ___ — ___ — ___
conclusions ___ — ___ — ___

7. If remedial action initiated, check type
☐ recall ☐ notification
☐ repair ☐ inspection
☐ replace ☐ patient monitoring
☐ relabeling ☐ modification/adjustment
☐ other: ____

8. Usage of device
☐ initial use of device
☐ reuse
☐ unknown

9. If action reported to FDA under 21 USC 360i(f), list correction/removal reporting number:

10. ☐ Additional manufacturer narrative and/or **11.** ☐ Corrected data

The public reporting burden for this collection of information has been estimated to average one-hour per response, including the time for reviewing instructions, searching existing data sources, gathering and maintaining the data needed, and completing and reviewing the collection of information. Send your comments regarding this burden estimate or any other aspect of this collection of information, including suggestions for reducing this burden to:

Reports Clearance Officer, PHS
Hubert H. Humphrey Building, Room 721-B
200 Independence Avenue, S.W.
Washington, DC 20201
ATTN: PRA

and to:
Office of Management and Budget
Paperwork Reduction Project (0910-0291)
Washington, DC 20503

Please do NOT return this form to either of these addresses.

FDA Form 3500A - back

Figure I-1

Continued

Questions and FDA Contact

Specific questions regarding medical device reporting should be sent to the FDA (include your name, return address, phone number, and fax number, if applicable) at

Food and Drug Administration
Center for Devices and Radiological Health
Division of Surveillance Systems (HFZ-530)
Medical Device Reporting (MDR) Inquiries
1350 Piccard Drive
Rockville, MD 20850
Fax (301) 827-0039

Appendix J
Guidelines for Prevention of Transmission of HIV and HBV to Emergency Medical Services Personnel*: Principles of Infection Control and Their Application to EMS Personnel

This appendix addresses principles of infection control as they relate to blood-borne pathogens. This should be thought of as a subset of the more global safety measures referred to as body substance isolation. *Body substance isolation* differs from universal precautions in that it addresses a method of reducing exposure to all body substances, including blood-borne and airborne pathogens. *Universal precautions* were intended to prevent or minimize the transmission of human immunodeficiency (HIV), hepatitis B virus (HBV), and other blood-borne pathogens. This appendix is intended to expand on the issues of HIV and HBV transmission because of the significant concern often expressed by EMS personnel. It provides a historical foundation in order to better understand the concept of body substance isolation.

■ GENERAL INFECTION CONTROL

Within the health care setting, general infection control procedures have been developed to minimize the risk of patient acquisition of infection from contact with contaminated devices, objects, or surfaces or of transmission of an infectious agent from health care workers to patients. Such procedures also protect workers from the risk of becoming infected. General infection control procedures are designed to prevent transmission of a wide range of microbiologic agents and to provide a wide margin of safety in the varied situations encountered in the health care environment.

General infection control principles are applicable to other work environments where workers contact other individuals and where

---

*Adapted from Guidelines for prevention of transmission of human immunodeficiency virus and hepatitis B virus to health-care and public safety workers. MMWR 38:1–37, 1989.

transmission of infectious agents may occur. The modes of transmission noted in the hospital and medical office environment are observed in the work situations of EMS personnel as well. Therefore, the principles of infection control developed for hospital and other health care settings are also applicable to these work situations. Use of general infection control measures, as adapted to the work environments of EMS personnel, is important to protect both workers and individuals with whom they work from a variety of infectious agents, not just HIV and HBV.

Because EMS personnel work in environments that provide inherently unpredictable risks of exposures, general infection control procedures should be adapted to these work situations. Exposures are unpredictable, and protective measures may often be used in situations that do not initially appear to present risk. EMS personnel perform their duties in the community under extremely variable conditions; therefore, control measures that are simple and uniform across all situations have the greatest likelihood of worker compliance. Administrative procedures to ensure compliance also can be more readily developed than when procedures are complex and highly variable.

■ UNIVERSAL BLOOD AND BODY FLUID PRECAUTIONS TO PREVENT OCCUPATIONAL HIV AND HBV TRANSMISSION

"Universal precautions" stress that all patients should be assumed to be infectious for HIV and other blood-borne pathogens. In the hospital and other health care settings, "universal precautions" should be followed when workers are exposed to blood, certain other body fluids (amniotic fluid, pericardial fluid, peritoneal fluid, pleural fluid, synovial fluid, cerebrospinal fluid, semen, and vaginal secretions), or any body fluid visibly contaminated with blood. Since HIV and HBV transmission has not been documented from exposure to other body fluids (feces, nasal secretions, sputum, sweat, tears, urine, and vomitus), "universal precautions" do not apply to these fluids. Universal precautions also do not apply to saliva, except in the dental setting, where saliva is likely to be contaminated with blood. This point illustrates the difference between "universal precautions" and "body substance isolation" measures.

For the purpose of this appendix, human "exposure" is defined as contact with blood or other body fluids to which universal precautions apply through percutaneous inoculation or contact with an open wound, nonintact skin, or mucous membrane during the performance of normal job duties. An "exposed worker" is defined, for the purposes of this appendix, as an individual exposed, as described previously, while performing normal job duties.

The unpredictable and emergent nature of exposures encountered by EMS personnel may make differentiation between hazardous body fluids and those that are not hazardous very difficult and often impossible. For example, poor lighting may limit the EMT's ability to detect visible blood in vomitus or feces. Therefore, when EMS personnel encounter body fluids under uncontrolled, emergency circumstances in which differentiation between fluid types is difficult, if not impossible, they should treat all body fluids as potentially hazardous. This approach is more in line with the concept of body substance isolation.

The application of the principles of universal precautions to the situations encountered by these workers results in the development of guidelines for work practices, use of personal protective equipment, and other protective measures. To minimize the risks of acquiring HIV and HBV during performance of job duties, EMS personnel should be protected from exposure to blood and other body fluids as circumstances dictate. Protection can be achieved through adherence to work practices designed to minimize or eliminate exposure and through use of personal protective equipment (i.e., gloves, masks, and protective clothing), which provides a barrier between the worker and the exposure source. In some situations, redesign of selected aspects of the job through equipment modifications or environmental control can further reduce risk. These approaches to primary prevention should be used together to achieve maximal reduction of the risk of exposure.

If exposure of an individual worker occurs, medical management, consisting of collection of pertinent medical and occupational history, provision of treatment, and counseling regarding future work and personal behaviors, may reduce the risk of developing disease as a result of the exposure episode. Following episodic (or continuous) exposure, decontamination and disinfection of the work environment, devices, equipment, and clothing or other forms of personal protective equipment can reduce subsequent risk of exposures. Proper disposal of contaminated waste has similar benefits.

■ GUIDELINES FOR EMS PERSONNEL

The guidelines that appear in this section apply to all EMS personnel. This includes firefighters, first responders, paramedics, and EMTs. Job duties are often performed in uncontrolled environments that, because of a lack of time and other factors, do not allow for application of a complex decision-making process to the emergency at hand.

The general principles presented here have been developed from existing principles of occupational safety and health in conjunction with data from studies of health care workers in hospital settings. The basic premise is that workers must be protected from exposure to blood and other potentially infectious body fluids in the course of their work activities. There is a paucity of data concerning the risks these worker groups face, however, that complicates development of control principles. Therefore, the guidelines presented here are based on principles of prudent public health practice.

The following guidelines are intended to assist EMS personnel in making decisions concerning use of personal protective equipment and resuscitation equipment, as well as decontamination, disinfection, and disposal procedures.

Personal Protective Equipment

Appropriate personal protective equipment should be made available routinely by the employer to reduce the risk of exposure as defined earlier. Personal protective equipment is defined as "specialized clothing or equipment worn by an employee for protection against a hazard." General work clothes are generally not considered to be personal protective equipment. For many situations, the chance that the EMT will be exposed to blood and other body fluids to which universal precautions apply can be determined in advance. Therefore, if the chance of being exposed to blood is high (e.g., CPR, intravenous line insertion, trauma, delivering babies), the EMT should put on protective attire before beginning patient care.

Gloves

Disposable gloves (vinyl or latex) should be a standard component of emergency response equipment, and should be donned by all personnel prior to initiating any patient care tasks involving exposure to blood or other body fluids to which universal precautions apply. When the EMT anticipates that he/she may be exposed to a patient's blood or other infectious materials, gloves should be worn. Extra gloves should always be available. Considerations in the choice of disposable gloves should include dexterity, durability, fit, and the task being performed. Another basis for selection is hypersensitivity to latex. (Some health care personnel are hypersensitive to latex.) Therefore, there is no single type or thickness of glove appropriate for protection in all situations.

For situations where large amounts of blood are likely to be encountered, it is important that gloves fit tightly at the wrist to prevent blood contamination of hands around the cuff. For multiple trauma victims, gloves should be changed between patient contacts or whenever grossly contaminated, if the emergency situation allows.

- Greater personal protective equipment measures are indicated for situations where broken glass and sharp edges are likely to be encountered, such as extricating an entrapped person from an automobile. Structural fire-fighting gloves should be worn in any situation where sharp or rough surfaces are likely to be encountered.

- While wearing gloves, avoid handling personal items, such as combs and pens, that could become soiled or contaminated.

Gloves that have become contaminated with blood or other body fluids to which universal precautions apply should be removed as soon as possible, taking care to avoid skin contact with the exterior surface.

- Gloves that have become torn or punctured should be removed and replaced as soon as possible.

- Contaminated gloves should be placed and transported in bags that prevent leakage and should be disposed of or, in the case of reusable gloves, cleaned and decontaminated properly.

- Because some blood-borne pathogens may survive on surfaces for days, gloves should also be worn when decontaminating equipment or surfaces. HBV may remain viable on surfaces for 1 week or longer.

Masks, Eyewear, and Gowns

Masks, eyewear, and gowns should be present on all emergency vehicles that respond or potentially respond to medical emergencies or victim rescues. These protective barriers should be used in accordance with the level of exposure encountered. Minor lacerations or small amounts of blood do not merit the same extent of barrier use as required for exsanguinating victims or massive arterial bleeding. Management of the patient who is not bleeding, and who has no bloody body fluids present, should not routinely require use of barrier precautions.

- Masks and eyewear (e.g., safety glasses) should be worn together, or a face-shield should be used by all personnel prior to any situation where splashes of blood or other body fluids to which universal precautions apply are likely to occur (e.g., bag-valve mask ventilation when the airway or face is bloody).

- Gowns or aprons should be worn to protect clothing from splashes with blood. If large splashes or quantities of blood are present or anticipated (e.g. childbirth, major trauma patients), impervious gowns or aprons should be worn.

- The use of gowns, masks, and eyewear would be most appropriate when managing childbirth, major bleeding, or airway management techniques (intubation, suctioning) when vomiting is likely.

An extra change of work clothing should be available at all times.

Resuscitation Equipment

No transmission of HBV or HIV infection during mouth-to-mouth resuscitation has been documented. However, because of the risk of salivary transmission of other infectious diseases (e.g., herpes simplex and *Neisseria meningitidis*) and the theoretical risk of HIV and HBV transmission during artificial ventilation of trauma victims, disposable airway equipment or resuscitation bags should be used. Disposable resuscitation equipment and devices should be used once and disposed of or, if reusable, thoroughly cleaned and decontaminated after each use according to the manufacturer's recommendations.

- Mechanical respiratory assist devices (e.g., bag-valve masks, oxygen demand-valve resuscitators) should be available on all emergency vehicles and to all EMS personnel who respond or potentially respond to medical emergencies or victim rescues.

- Pocket mouth-to-mouth resuscitation masks designed to isolate EMS personnel (e.g., those with one-way valves) from contact with victims' blood and blood-contaminated saliva, respiratory secretions, and vomit should be available when mechanical devices are not readily available.

- When placing ventilation devices on emergency vehicles or in emergency equipment kits, consider placing them in a location that is quickly accessible to minimize delay in care while also providing protection to the EMT.

Infection Control Measures

As a reminder, the precautions outlined here are specifically intended for the prevention and minimization of blood-borne pathogen exposure. They do not address additional methods of infection and exposure control, nor do they address methods to reduce exposure to other potentially infectious substances. Rather, they should be considered minimum exposure control methods.

Index

Note: Page numbers in *italics* indicate figures; page numbers followed by t indicate tables.

435